CURRENT NEUROSURGICAL PRACTICE

Protection
of the
Brain from
Ischemia

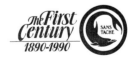

Protection of the Brain from Ischemia

Edited by

Philip R. Weinstein, M.D.

Professor and Vice Chairman
Department of Neurological Surgery
School of Medicine
University of California, San Francisco
San Francisco, California

Alan I. Faden, M.D.

Professor and Vice Chairman
Department of Neurology
School of Medicine
University of California, San Francisco
San Francisco, California

Current Neurosurgical Practice
Charles B. Wilson, M.D., Series Editor

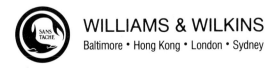

WILLIAMS & WILKINS
Baltimore • Hong Kong • London • Sydney

Editor: Carol-Lynn Brown
Associate Editor: Marjorie Kidd Keating
Copy Editor: Deborah Klenotic
Designer: Norman W. Och
Illustration Planner: Lorraine Wrzosek
Production Coordinator: Charles E. Zeller

Copyright © 1990
Williams & Wilkins
428 East Preston Street
Baltimore, Maryland 21202, USA

Accurate indications, adverse reactions, and dosage schedules for drugs are provided in this book, but it is possible that they may change. The reader is urged to review the package information data of the manufacturers of the medications mentioned.

Printed in the United States of America

Library of Congress Cataloging-in-Publication Data

Protection of the brain from ischemia / edited by Philip R. Weinstein,
    Alan I. Faden.
        p.   cm.—(Current neurosurgical practice)
    Includes index.
    ISBN 0-683-08908-0
    1. Cerebral ischemia.   I. Weinstein, Philip R.   II. Faden, Alan I.
III. Series.
    [DNLM: 1. Cerebral Ischemia—diagnosis.   2. Cerebral Ischemia—
physiopathology.   3. Cerebral Ischemia—therapy.   WL 355 P9672]
RC388.5.P74   1990
616.8'1—dc20
DNLM/DLC
for Library of Congress   89-8938
                                                                                          CIP

90 91 92 93 94
1 2 3 4 5 6 7 8 9 10

To Jill, Alex, Josh, and Josh
with appreciation for your inspiration in this search
P.R.W.

To my wife, Susan
and my children, Karine, Erik, and Julianne
A.I.F.

Foreword

It is a great honor and pleasure to introduce this volume, which has been eagerly awaited by our colleagues throughout the world. Among the developed nations, cerebral vascular disease ranks as one of the top three causes of death, and it must therefore be considered a major health hazard for humankind. Owing to elucidation of the risk factors, there has been a gradual reduction in the incidence of hemorrhagic cerebral vascular disease, but the resultant increase in longevity has been accompanied by a gradual increase in ischemic cerebral vascular disease—a trend which is likely to occur worldwide.

The effects of cerebral vascular disease, the concomitant loss of normal brain function, and the reduction or complete halt in productivity it causes have wide-ranging implications for individuals and their families, and for society at large. By the same token, the development of methods to prevent and treat this disease has importance not only for individual patients and their families but also for the nations within which they work, whether in a modest role or as a world leader affecting current and future world events. For these reasons, the development of techniques for the prevention and treatment of ischemic diseases of the brain is an issue of extreme importance for all of humanity.

The essential nature of ischemic cerebral vascular disease can be described as necrosis of brain tissue resulting from a decrease in cerebral blood flow (CBF) that is caused by stenosis or occlusion of cervical and/or intracranial arteries. Necrosis produces functional deficits in those parts of the brain and leads either to death or to survival in an impaired condition. While this pathology of cerebral vascular disease is, of course, common knowledge in medicine, it is nonetheless true that a considerable degree of uncertainty exists concerning the nature of the gradual intracerebral changes that

occur following an ischemic attack. Among several fundamental questions that remain unanswered are these: At what level of reduction in CBF and after how prolonged a duration of occlusion does damage to brain tissue begin to occur? What are the differences in these parameters between cases of focal ischemia and cases of global ischemia? With regard to recirculation following ischemia it must be said that, with the exception of morphologic findings obtained using the electron miscroscope, current research is just beginning to answer questions concerning the neurophysiology and neurochemistry of cerebral vascular disease.

In the light of these uncertainties, it is evident that an accurate evaluation of the therapeutic effects of various drugs is simply not possible. Moreover, there are significant individual differences among patients in the capacity for developing collateral pathways—a fact that makes evaluation of the prognosis following onset of cerebral vascular disease equally difficult. Considering the further problems posed by changes in various components of circulating blood and by age; blood pressure; associated disorders of the cardiac, pulmonary, and respiratory systems; diabetes; and varying degrees of arteriosclerosis, it is evident that the effect of ischemia on brain cells is an extremely complex issue.

What kinds of medical therapy are currently in use for conditions of cerebral ischemia? First of all, with regard to prevention, gradually more favorable results have been obtained by means of dietary measures to prevent arteriosclerosis and by the administration of anticoagulants, such as aspirin and warfarin, to prevent embolization and of antihypertensive drugs to prevent and/or treat hypertension. Unfortunately, with regard to therapeutic steps taken during the acute stage following the onset of ischemic cerebral vascular disease—no matter which measures have been employed—the results have been little better than those following the natural course of the disease. Logically, it is easy to imagine that by means of surgical treatment or the administration of hemolytic agents, vascular occlusions could be relieved and efforts then made to increase CBF. Such therapy, however, has been found to cause an increase in cerebral edema and cerebral hemorrhage, and for this reason attempts to induce vascular recirculation during the acute stage are now thought to be problematic. Surgical therapy, therefore, is also thought to be fruitless during the acute stage.

With regard to treatments currently in use for ischemic cerebral vascular disease, only two courses of action are open, neither of which is likely to lead to full recovery. Either the brain tissue that has been affected in the acute stage is considered beyond recovery and the patient is sent for rehabilitation with the neuronal deficits, or, alternatively, bypass surgery is performed in order to allow for some slight recovery of the brain tissue in the penumbra of the ischemic focus.

Certainly, as a matter of human compassion, serious thought should be given to the problems of prevention of ischemic cerebral vascular disease and functional recovery through rehabilitation. However, the most important questions still concern the development of therapeutic techniques that can be used effectively in the acute stage of the disease. Specifically, in order to prevent rapid deterioration of the patient's cerebral condition and to reduce the incidence of acute death, both of which are known to be a function of the interval from onset, it is essential to develop some form of therapy that can be instituted as early as possible in the acute stage. That therapy, whatever it may be, would be of extreme importance and would constitute the first positive step forward in the treatment of ischemic cerebral vascular disease. It would then be possible during that early period, while rapid deterioration of brain cells is being prevented, either to undertake vascular reconstruction or to allow for a spontaneous increase in CBF from the emergence of collateral pathways.

The most difficult and frustrating task for the neurosurgeon is to be forced simply to observe the progression of cerebral infarction following the onset of ischemia, unable to take positive action. As in managing a house on fire, the most important step would be to take protective measures at a very early stage in the event. From our own studies in animals we have found that, when cerebral flow is reduced to 40% of its normal level for a period of 3 hours, the morphology of brain cells is drastically changed and phagocytosis by leukocytes ensues 24 hours later. Needless to say, despite total occlusion of capillaries and small vessels, leukocytes manage to destroy the infarcted brain tissue. Once the brain has entered such a phase, it is already too late to take therapeutic steps.

My own interest in and study of the ischemic brain began with an attempt to prolong the permissible period of temporary vascular occlusion for radical surgery on ruptured cerebral aneurysms, and indeed this quest has become a major life's work for me. I performed my first aneurysm surgery using hypothermia on May 27, 1961, and during the following years, until 1969, I operated on many such cases. However, during that procedure complications such as cardiac arrest and skin burns were not uncommon. Throughout this period, I pondered in the back of my mind whether there might be alternative means for prolonging the permissible time for occlusion of cerebral vessels.

In contemplating results of these operations, I observed that mannitol may have been the factor which permitted prolonged occlusion of cerebral vessels without producing complications. In order to clarify the effects of drugs such as mannitol, it was first necessary to establish an experimental animal model in which infarcted foci of the same size could be produced consistently at the same site in the brain. However, it was very difficult to identify such an ideal animal model. We then found an experimental technique with which an ideal focus of infarction could be produced in virtually 100% of our animals (1). Subsequent work was then devoted to the development of related models of brain ischemia, infarction, and edema, and to a clear demonstration of the beneficial effects of agents such as mannitol and free-radical scavengers on the brain (2).

Findings concerning the protective effects produced by other drugs have led to the next step. Specifically, the anticonvulsant drug phenytoin has recently been shown to have remarkable protective effects which are brought about not by means of free-radical scavenger action, but by stabilization of the cellular membrane. As a consequence, clinically we now use a combination of three drugs, mannitol, vitamin E, and phenytoin. The combination of drugs originally used for protecting the brain from infarction was labeled the "Sendai cocktail" by young members of our department. Although significant improvements in the treatment of acute-stage cerebral infarction have been achieved, we are still but at the beginning of such research.

In addition to reviewing our own efforts, this volume describes much work done by researchers throughout the world and the most recent experimental and clinical developments concerning cerebral infarction. It contains the story of a struggle in its chapters, which describe the research being performed in various institutes in the United States and Europe, complementing the volume we of the Sendai group published with Springer Verlag in 1987 entitled, *Treatment of Cerebral Infarction*. I hope that, into the 21st century, more volumes will follow describing efforts throughout the world to address the important problems that remain to be tackled in defining new treatments to prevent cerebral infarction.

JIRO SUZUKI, M.D.
Sendai, Japan
June 1989

References

1. Sakamoto T, Tanaka S, Yoshimoto T, et al: Experimental cerebral infarction. Part 2: Electroencephalographic changes produced by experimental thalamic infarction in dogs. *Stroke* 9:214–216, 1978.
2. Suzuki J, Fujimoto S, Mizoi K, et al: The protective effect of combined administration of anti-oxidants and perfluorochemicals on cerebral ischemia. *Stroke* 15:672–679, 1984.

Note

Doctors Weinstein and Faden have created a monograph that brings together contemporary concepts of cerebral ischemia and its prevention or modification. Obvious is the care with which they chose the contributors. This volume has both depth and breadth, providing information that has never been assembled under one cover. The editors have done a truly outstanding job. When you have read these chapters, I am sure you will agree.

CHARLES B. WILSON, M.D.
June 1989

Preface

The brain's vulnerability to ischemic or hypoxic injury that may cause permanent functional loss has been the impetus for ongoing efforts to develop new and progressively more rational protective techniques. These approaches to cerebral protection and the mechanisms by which they may provide that protection are the focus of this book.

The effects of ischemia on brain tissue can be controlled, and even prevented in some instances, by a variety of physiologic, pharmacologic, and surgical techniques. Alterations in physiologic thresholds can increase the resistance of brain tissue to the effects of the insult; for example, elevation of systemic blood pressure may reverse aphasia and hemiplegia resulting from vasospasm after subarachnoid hemorrhage. In addition, maintaining perfusion that is adequate for autoregulation of cerebral blood flow, for example by carotid endarterectomy, theoretically may reduce the impact of ischemic injury to brain following hypotension caused by systemic circulatory disorders. Optimal anesthetic management may reduce the risk of ischemic stroke after temporary cerebral vascular occlusion during surgery. Certain drugs given experimentally before or after ischemia can act to prevent further deterioration of the injured tissue and secondary effects from the insult.

The authors of the chapters in this volume are among the investigators and clinicians who are actively engaged in this field. They discuss the practical and theoretical issues facing physicians who care for patients with stroke or insufficiency of cerebral vascular function and present guidelines for their treatment.

PHILIP R. WEINSTEIN
ALAN I. FADEN
June 1989

Acknowledgment

We acknowledge with respect and admiration the pioneering conceptual and experimental contributions to this field of Lindsay Symon, T.D., F.R.C.S., F.R.C.S. Ed., Professor, Gough-Cooper Department of Neurological Surgery, Institute of Neurology, British Postgraduate Medical Federation, University of London, The National Hospital, London, England.

PHILIP R. WEINSTEIN
ALAN I. FADEN
June 1989

Contributors

Harold P. Adams, Jr., M.D., Professor and Director, Division of Cerebrovascular Diseases, Department of Neurology, The University of Iowa College of Medicine, Iowa City, Iowa

Brian T. Andrews, M.D., Assistant Clinical Professor, Department of Neurological Surgery, School of Medicine, University of California, San Francisco, San Francisco, California

Jens Astrup, M.D., Professor of Neurosurgery, Department of Neurosurgery, Aarhus Municipal Hospital, Aarhus, Denmark

Gene H. Barnett, M.D., Director, Neurosurgical Intensive Care Unit, Departments of Neurosurgery and Anesthesia, The Cleveland Clinic Foundation, Cleveland, Ohio

Keith L. Black, M.D., Assistant Professor, Department of Surgery, Division of Neurosurgery, School of Medicine, University of California, Los Angeles, Los Angeles, California

Robert M. Crowell, M.D., Professor and Head, Department of Neurosurgery, University of Illinois at Chicago, Chicago, Illinois

Elizabeth A. Eelkema, M.D., Assistant Professor, Department of Radiology, Division of Neuroradiology, University Health Center of Pittsburgh, Pittsburgh, Pennsylvania

Alan I. Faden, M.D., Professor and Vice Chairman, Department of Neurology, School of Medicine, University of California, San Francisco and Chief, Neurology Service, Director, Center for Neural Injury, Veterans Administration Medical Center, San Francisco, California

J. Max Findlay, M.D., Ph.D., F.R.C.S.C., Cerebral Vascular Laboratory, Division of Neurosurgery, University of Alberta, Edmonton, Alberta, Canada

Anthony J. Furlan, M.D., Director, Cerebrovascular Program, Department of Neurology, The Cleveland Clinic Foundation, Cleveland, Ohio

Julio H. Garcia, M.D., Professor of Pathology and Director, Division of Pathology/Neuropathology, Department of Pathology and The UAB Stroke Center, The University of Alabama at Birmingham, Birmingham, Alabama

Myron D. Ginsberg, M.D., Professor of Neurology and Radiology and Director, Cerebral Vascular Disease Research Center, Department of Neurology, University of Miami School of Medicine, Miami, Florida

David A. Greenberg, M.D., Ph.D., Associate Professor, Department of Neurology, School of Medicine, University of California, San Francisco and San Francisco General Hospital Medical Center, San Francisco, California

Mark N. Hadley, M.D., Major, USAF MC, Chief of Neurological Surgery, David Grant USAF Medical Center (MAC), Travis Air Force Base, California

Van V. Halbach, M.D., Assistant Professor, Departments of Radiology and Neurological Surgery, Diagnostic and Interventional Neuroradiology Section, School of Medicine, University of California, San Francisco, San Francisco, California

Stephen T. Hecht, M.D., Assistant Professor, Departments of Radiology and Neurosurgery, Division of Neuroradiology, University Health Center of Pittsburgh, Pittsburgh, Pennsylvania

Grant B. Hieshima, M.D., Professor, Departments of Radiology and Neurological Surgery, Diagnostic and Interventional Neuroradiology Section, School of Medicine, University of California, San Francisco, San Francisco, California

Randall T. Higashida, M.D., Assistant Professor, Departments of Radiology and Neurological Surgery, Diagnostic and Interventional Neuroradiology Section, School of Medicine, University of California, San Francisco, San Francisco, California

Julian T. Hoff, M.D., Professor and Chairman, Section of Neurological Surgery, Department of Surgery, University Hospital, University of Michigan, Ann Arbor, Michigan

K.-A. Hossmann, M.D., Ph.D. Professor, Max-Planck-Institute for Neurological Research, Cologne, West Germany

Jafar J. Jafar, M.D., Associate Professor, Department of Neurosurgery, New York University, New York, New York

Jeffrey R. Kirsch, M.D., Assistant Professor, Department of Anesthesiology and Critical Care Medicine, The Johns Hopkins University, School of Medicine, Baltimore, Maryland

Niels A. Lassen, M.D., Professor of Neurosciences, Department of Clinical Physiology and Nuclear Medicine, Bispebjerg Hospital, Copenhagen, Denmark

Richard E. Latchaw, M.D., Professor of Radiology and Neurological Surgery and Interim Chairman and Chief of Neuroradiology, Department of Radiology, Division of Neuroradiology, University Health Center of Pittsburgh, School of Medicine, Pittsburgh, Pennsylvania

John R. Little, M.D., Chairman, Department of Neurosurgery and Head, Section of Cerebrovascular Surgery, The Cleveland Clinic Foundation, Cleveland, Ohio

Lawrence F. Marshall, M.D., Professor of Surgery and Neurological Surgery and Chief, Neurosurgical Services, School of Medicine, University of California Medical Center, San Diego, San Diego, California

Robert W. McPherson, M.D., Associate Professor and Chief, Neuro Anesthesia, Department of Anesthesiology and Critical Care Medicine, The Johns Hopkins University, School of Medicine, Baltimore, Maryland

Richard B. Morawetz, M.D., Professor and Chairman, Division of Neurosurgery, Department of Surgery, The University of Alabama at Birmingham, Birmingham, Alabama

Carl-Henrik Nordström, M.D., Associate Professor, Department of Neurosurgery, University Hospital, University of Lund, Laboratory for Experimental Brain Research, Lund Hospital, Lund, Sweden

Marc R. Nuwer, M.D., Ph.D., Associate Professor, Department of Neurology, University of California, Los Angeles and Reed Neurological Research Center, Los Angeles, California

L. Creed Pettigrew, M.D., Assistant Professor, Department of Neurology, University of Kentucky College of Medicine, Lexington, Kentucky

Carmela M. Picone, M.D., Assistant Professor, Department of Neurology, University of South Alabama Medical Center, Mobile, Alabama

Lawrence H. Pitts, M.D., Professor and Vice Chairman, Department of Neurological Surgery, School of Medicine, University of California, San Francisco and Chief, Neurosurgery Service, San Francisco General Hospital Medical Center, San Francisco, California

William J. Powers, M.D., Associate Professor, Departments of Neurology and Radiology, Washington University School of Medicine and Neurologist-in-Chief, Department of Neurology, The Jewish Hospital of St. Louis, St. Louis, Missouri

Jeffrey B. Randall, M.D., Chief Resident, Section of Neurosurgery, Department of Surgery, University Hospital, University of Michigan, Ann Arbor, Michigan

Peter A. Raudzens, M.D., Chief, Division of Neuroanesthesia, Barrow Neurological Institute of St. Joseph's Hospital and Medical Center, Phoenix, Arizona

Daniel M. Rosenbaum, M.D., Assistant Professor, Department of Neurology, Albert Einstein College of Medicine, Bronx, New York

Jeffrey V. Rosenfeld, M.D., F.R.A.C.S., F.R.C.S. Ed., Neurosurgeon, The Royal Melbourne Hospital, Victoria, Australia

Antonio V. Salgado, M.D., Cerebrovascular Fellow, Department of Neurology, The Cleveland Clinic Foundation, Cleveland, Ohio

Bo K. Siesjö, M.D., Professor, University of Lund, Laboratory for Experimental Brain Research, Lund Hospital, Lund, Sweden

Roger P. Simon, M.D., Professor, Department of Neurology, University of California, San Francisco and Chief, Neurology Service, San Francisco General Hospital Medical Center, San Francisco, California

Robert F. Spetzler, M.D., Director and J. N. Harber Chairman of Neurological Surgery, Barrow Neurological Institute of St. Joseph's Hospital and Medical Center, Phoenix, Arizona, and Professor and Chief, Section of Neurosurgery, University of Arizona School of Medicine, Tucson, Arizona

Thoralf M. Sundt, Jr., M.D., Professor and Chairman, Department of Neurologic Surgery, Mayo Clinic and Mayo Medical School, Rochester, Minnesota

Jiro Suzuki, M.D., Professor and Chief, Division of Neurosurgery, Tohoku University School of Medicine, Institute of Brain Disease, Sendai, Japan

Richard J. Traystman, Ph.D., Distinguished Research Professor and Director, Anesthesiology and Critical Care Medicine Research Laboratories, The Johns Hopkins University, School of Medicine, Baltimore, Maryland

Robert Vink, Ph.D., Department of Chemistry and Biochemistry, James Cook University, Townsville, Queensland, Australia

Philip R. Weinstein, M.D., Professor and Vice Chairman, Department of Neurological Surgery, School of Medicine, University of California, San Francisco and Chief, Neurosurgery Service, Veterans Administration Medical Center, San Francisco, California

Bryce Weir, M.D., C.M., M.Sc., F.R.C.S.C., F.A.C.S., Professor and Chairman, Department of Surgery, Faculty of Medicine, University of Alberta, Edmonton, Alberta, Canada

Frank M. Yatsu, M.D., Roy M. and Phyllis Gough Huffington Chair in Neurology and Professor and Chairman, Department of Neurology, Medical School, The University of Texas Health Sciences Center at Houston, Houston, Texas

Justin A. Zivin, M.D., Ph.D., Professor, Department of Neurosciences, School of Medicine, University of California, San Diego, La Jolla, California

Contents

CHAPTER ONE

Circulatory Thresholds of Brain Dysfunction and Infarction

Richard B. Morawetz, M.D.

Systemic physiologic and metabolic thresholds for failure of brain function are of practical interest to the neurologist and neurosurgeon because of their clinical applications, particularly in the intensive care unit and operating room. The events occurring during acute ischemia are initiated by a reduction or cessation of cerebral blood flow (CBF), but the biochemical processes set in motion by severe ischemia proceed in such a way that, after a critical interval, restoration of blood flow does not always reverse them (7). At that point, reversible cerebral ischemic dysfunction gives way to irreversible ischemic tissue injury. The biochemical and metabolic events occurring during acute ischemia and the processes responsible for transition from reversible to irreversible injury are not yet well understood. This chapter focuses on recognized circulatory thresholds during cerebral ischemia, emphasizing information gained from studies performed in humans and nonhuman primates.

SYSTEMIC PARAMETERS

Clinical observations indicate that impairment of brain function progressing to a reduction in or loss of consciousness or seizures can be expected to occur in conjunction with hypotension when the mean systemic blood pressure falls below 40 torr. Hypoxia resulting from reduced ventilation affects brain function, despite normal circulation, when arterial oxygen tension is reduced to below 50 torr in patients without chronic lung disease. Systemic hypoglycemia is also associated with alteration or loss of consciousness that may progress to seizures or coma.

The derangement and recovery of various metabolic processes in the brains of experimental animals subjected to ischemic and anoxic insults have been studied extensively (1, 3, 9, 10, 14, 15) and are important to our understanding of these processes. Clinicians are interested in the recovery and preservation of organized brain activity after an ischemic event and in preventing loss of neurologic function. Although specific biochemical pathways may recover completely in an experimental animal subjected to ischemia, irreversible cellular injury may have caused the loss of integrated neurologic function. Important factors related to the metabolic thresholds for failure of brain metabolism include the baseline level of brain activity, as determined by the patient's state of consciousness or activity level; the influence of intoxicants, anesthetic agents, or other drugs; and substrate availability (oxygen and glucose levels and body temperature).

The normal cerebral metabolic rate of oxygen consumption ($CMRO_2$) is 5 ml/100 g/minute. Neuronal electrical activity is abolished and infarction occurs when $CMRO_2$ in tissue falls below 1.5 to 1.7 ml/100 g/minute. Although the normal cerebral metabolic rate of glucose is also high at 2 to 6 ml/100 g/minute, deprivation of oxygen is the first ischemic metabolic parameter change to affect brain function because membrane ionic potentials are exquisitely dependent on maintenance of oxygen-dependent energy metabolism.

1

METABOLIC EFFECTS OF HYPOTHERMIA

Considerable experience has been reported regarding the protective effects of hypothermia. It is generally accepted that, when complete global cerebral ischemia occurs during cardiac arrest in the awake normothermic human, complete cessation of CBF for 5 to 6 minutes results in irreversible loss of useful brain function. However, cardiovascular surgeons routinely operate on children with complex congenital cardiac anomalies for periods of up to 60 minutes of complete cardiac standstill and circulatory arrest (8), relying on profound hypothermia for brain protection (Fig. 1.1). The multiple by which the rates of metabolic processes decrease for each 10°C decrease in body temperature is termed the Q-10 (8). Even as temperatures approach 0°C, oxygen consumption and metabolic processes continue in intact animals and in tissue slices. Profound hypothermia is used infrequently by contemporary neurosurgeons. Its useful-

ness for standard neurosurgical procedures is limited because of associated cardiac arrhythmias, which necessitate cardiopulmonary bypass for control of the rate and depth of cooling and for maintenance of perfusion.

CEREBRAL BLOOD FLOW THRESHOLDS FOR BRAIN FUNCTION

The threshold at which brain function fails because of insufficient CBF depends on the function being monitored. In the awake human or nonhuman primate, there appears to be a decline in alertness and in the speed and appropriateness of response as CBF decreases, but consciousness and neurologic function persist until CBF declines to about 20 ml/100 g/minute. At that level, focal cerebral ischemia produces failure of brain function as manifested by observable neurologic dysfunction (11, 12). Thus, occlusion of the carotid artery or middle cerebral artery (MCA) re-

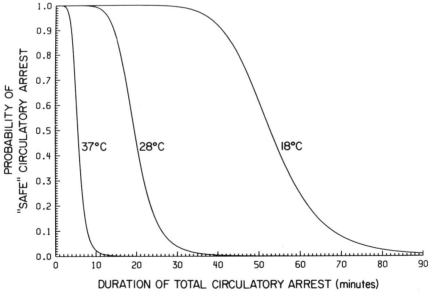

Figure 1.1. Nomogram of the estimate by Kirklin and colleagues of the probability of "safe" total circulatory arrest according to the arrest time at nasopharyngeal temperatures of 37°C, 28°C, and 18°C. Safe total circulatory arrest denotes total arrest after which no structural or functional damage has occurred. (From Kirklin JK, Kirklin JW, Pacifico AD: Deep hypothermia and total circulatory arrest. In Arciniegas E (ed): *Pediatric Cardiac Surgery.* Chicago, Year Book Medical Publishers, 1985, pp 79–85. Reproduced with permission.)

sulting in reduction of CBF to a level below 20 ml/100 g/minute produces contralateral hemiparesis or hemiplegia.

CEREBRAL FUNCTION

Brain electrical activity during acute ischemia, as monitored by electroencephalography (EEG) and measurements of somatosensory cortical evoked potentials, has been studied in anesthetized humans and in awake and anesthetized nonhuman primates. Thresholds of dysfunction vary according to state of consciousness and the anesthetic agents used but, in general, as CBF drops below a level of about 20 ml/100 g/minute in gray matter, both the EEG and the evoked response become abnormal, the EEG slowing and the evoked response showing decreased amplitude and increased latency (1–4, 17). During the early phase of acute ischemia, these abnormalities can be reversed promptly by restoration of blood flow. As CBF drops to levels of 10 to 15 ml/100 g/minute, electrical activity may be lost—although not in every case (1, 2, 16, 17). This is a reflection of cessation of synaptic activity and provides little information about either the integrity of cell membranes or ongoing metabolic processes. At lower levels of CBF, 6 ml/100 g/minute or less, there is massive release of intracellular potassium which indicates membrane failure (1). Both the cell membranes and membranes of intracellular structures, such as mitochondria, are thought to become permeable to potassium, sodium, and calcium ions (14). Membrane failure occurs rapidly in cases of normothermic cardiac arrest, and if blood flow is not restored within minutes, cell death occurs (1). Much attention has been paid to potential differences in outcome in patients and animals subjected to incomplete ischemia with low levels of residual blood flow compared to those with complete ischemia, and in hyperglycemic compared to hypoglycemic experimental animals subjected to ischemic insults, but the relevance of such findings to the functional neurologic outcome in humans experiencing an ischemic event is still unclear (14).

A most important relationship is that between the depth and the duration of cerebral ischemia. Clinically, the important events determining reversibility or irreversibility of cerebral ischemia may occur in the first few minutes or hours of an ischemic event, in most cases before a patient with acute stroke is seen by a physician. First the degree and then the duration of reduction of CBF are the critical variables during reversible cerebral ischemia; once the biochemical events mediating irreversibility have occurred, restoration of blood flow appears to be of little benefit (7).

CEREBRAL BLOOD FLOW MEASUREMENTS DURING TEMPORARY VASCULAR OCCLUSION

The clinical setting has been closely approximated in a model of cerebral ischemia in awake nonhuman primates. In a series of experiments (6, 11, 12) in monkeys *(Macaca fascicularis)*, platinum electrodes were placed in the distribution of one MCA and CBF was monitored by a hydrogen clearance technique before, during, and after a reversible ischemic event (12). After baseline CBF measurements were made, a snare ligature was placed around the origin of one MCA through a transorbital approach that obviated manipulation of the brain. When the monkey recovered from anesthesia, the MCA could be reversibly occluded for a specific interval and then the occlusion released. The neurologic status was assessed before, during, and after each cerebral ischemic event, as was focal CBF at the sites of electrode placement. In every case, the monkeys developed dense hemiparesis or hemiplegia within seconds of MCA occlusion if CBF dropped below 20 ml/100 g/minute, and reperfusion could be demonstrated following the release of MCA occlusion. Monkeys that did not die as a direct result of cerebral ischemia and infarction invariably improved neurologically or recovered to a normal neurologic state. All surviving monkeys were sacrificed 14 days after the ischemic event, and

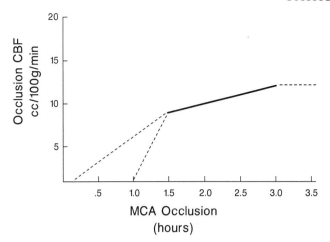

Figure 1.2. Ischemic threshold below which combinations of depth and duration of ischemia produce infarction *(solid black line).* Possible extrapolations for which firm data do not exist are also shown *(dashed lines).* CBF = cerebral blood flow; MCA = middle cerebral artery.

the areas of brain around the tips of the platinum electrodes were surveyed histologically. The presence or absence of histologic evidence of cerebral infarction was then correlated with the depth and duration of cerebral ischemia (Fig. 1.2). A well-defined threshold for development of cerebral infarction was seen: After CBF reduction to 8 ml/100 g/minute for 90 minutes of ischemia, reperfusion did not prevent infarction; the CBF threshold for infarction rose to 12 ml/100 g/minute for 180 minutes of ischemia. Periods of ischemia of less than 60 minutes' duration were well tolerated in terms of both functional recovery and histologic findings. Thus, the relationship between depth and duration of cerebral ischemia was critically important during the first 3 hours of acute ischemia in these experiments.

A clinical situation in which neurosurgeons produce well-defined reversible cerebral ischemia occurs during temporary occlusion of the carotid artery during carotid endarterectomy. The selection of methods of brain protection is a highly controversial matter (5, 13, 16). Virtually all patients undergoing carotid endarterectomy are subjected to a period of partial, reversible cerebral ischemia during the time that the carotid artery is occluded. Currently, there is no convincing evidence of any difference in outcome between patients managed with placement of a shunt

to maintain carotid blood flow bypassing the endarterectomy site and those managed without a shunt.

In an effort to better define the role of cerebral ischemia in the genesis of complications developing in patients undergoing carotid endarterectomy, 431 patients having the procedure without shunting were carefully monitored using CBF and EEG (13). CBF was monitored by injecting xenon-133 (^{133}Xe) in saline into the exposed carotid artery and following clearance of the ^{133}Xe using a single large detector placed over the Sylvian fissure ipsilateral to the side of carotid endarterectomy. Blood flow determinations were made before, during, and after the period of intraoperative carotid occlusion by monitoring clearance of ^{133}Xe from the ipsilateral hemisphere; the patients were subjected to 15 to 30 minutes of ischemia during the occlusion. EEG also was monitored before, during, and after ischemia using standard techniques. Profound cerebral ischemia with flow of less than 9 ml/100 g/minute was produced in 63 patients, and in two patients the EEG became isoelectric for many minutes. In the overall series, there was no relation between regional CBF (rCBF) during carotid occlusion and either the immediate or delayed development of complications ($\chi^2_4 = 1.02$, $p = 0.91$) or the presence of new deficits on awakening ($\chi^2_4 = 0.45$, $p = 0.98$) (Table 1.1). However, there was a signifi-

Table 1.1. Relation of Regional Cerebral Blood Flow and Development of Complications During Carotid Occlusion

Occlusion rCBF[a] (ml/100 g/min)	Number of procedures	Neurologic complications[b]	New neurologic deficit on awakening[c]
<9	63	2	2
9–13	39	1	1
13–16	77	3	2
16–20	52	1	1
>20	200	9	7
Total	431	16	13

[a] rCBF = regional cerebral blood flow.
[b] No association between rCBF and the development of complications, immediate or delayed: $\chi_4^2 = 1.02$, $p = 0.91$.
[c] No association between rCBF and the presence of new deficits on awakening: $\chi_4^2 = 0.45$, $p = 0.98$.

cant relation between rCBF and the appearance of EEG abnormalities during carotid occlusion ($\chi_4^2 = 42.04$, $p = 0.0001$) (Table 1.2). This finding emphasizes that the threshold for appearance of EEG abnormalities is substantially higher than the threshold for clinically apparent ischemic brain injury and underscores the important relationship between depth and duration of ischemia. Of additional importance is the difference in the vulnerability to ischemia of normal, healthy brain tissue and the tissue of injured brain, particularly brain that has been subjected to a previous ischemic insult. It is quite possible that injured brain is more sensitive to ischemic stress than is healthy brain, and that patients harboring ischemic lesions are therefore more vulnerable to repeated ischemic insults.

Table 1.2. Relation of Electroencephalographic Changes and Regional Cerebral Blood Flow During Carotid Occlusion[a]

Occlusion rCBF[b] (ml/100 g/min)	Number of procedures	Patients showing EEG[c] changes		70% Confidence interval (percent)
		Number	Percent	
<9	63	20	32	25–39
9–13	39	12	31	23–40
13–16	77	13	17	12–22
16–20	52	4	8	4–14
>20	200	10	5	3–7
Total	431	59	14	12–16

[a] Significant relation between rCBF during carotid occlusion and the appearance of EEG changes during occlusion: $\chi_4^2 = 42.04$, $p = 0.0001$.
[b] rCBF = regional cerebral blood flow.
[c] EEG = electroencephalography.

CBF and EEG thresholds are qualitative indicators of the tolerance of brain tissue to ischemia and give neurosurgeons guidelines for use in clinical practice. It is hoped that, in the future, specific metabolic pathways most vulnerable to ischemic injury can be identified and directly monitored.

References

1. Astrup J, Symon L, Branston NM, et al: Cortical evoked potential and extracellular K$^+$ and H$^+$ at critical levels of brain ischemia. *Stroke* 8:51–57, 1977.
2. Branston NM, Symon L, Crockard HA, et al: Relationship between the cortical evoked potential and local cortical blood flow following acute middle cerebral artery occlusion in the baboon. *Exp Neurol* 45:195–208, 1974.
3. Branston NM, Symon L, Crockard HA: Recovery of the cortical evoked response following temporary middle cerebral artery occlusion in baboons: Relation to local blood flow and pulse. *Stroke* 7:151–157, 1976.
4. Coyer PE, Simeone FA, Michele JJ: Latency of the cortical component of the somatosensory evoked potential in relation to cerebral blood flow measured in the white matter of the cat brain during focal ischemia. *Neurosurgery* 21:497–502, 1987.
5. Ferguson GG: Carotid endarterectomy: To shunt or not to shunt? *Arch Neurol* 43:615–617, 1986.
6. Garcia JH, Mitchem HC, Briggs L, et al: Transient focal ischemia in subhuman primates. *J Neuropathol Exp Neurol* 42:44–60, 1983.
7. Grotta JC: Can raising cerebral blood flow improve outcome after cerebral infarction? *Stroke* 18:264–267, 1987.
8. Kirklin JK, Kirklin JW, Pacifico AD: Deep hypothermia and total circulatory arrest. In Arciniegas E (ed): *Pediatric Cardiac Surgery.* Chicago: Year Book Medical Publishers, 1985, pp 79–85.
9. Kobayashi M, Lust WD, Passonneau JV: Concentrations of energy metabolites and cyclic nucleotides during and after bilateral ischemia in the gerbil cerebral cortex. *J Neurochem* 29:53–59, 1977.
10. Ljunggren B, Ratcheson RA, Siesjo BK: Cerebral metabolic state following complete compression ischemia. *Brain Res* 73:291–307, 1974.
11. Morawetz RB, Crowell RH, DeGirolami U, et al: Regional cerebral blood flow thresholds during cerebral ischemia. *Fed Proc* 48:49–50, 1979.
12. Morawetz RB, DeGirolami U, Ojemann RG, et al: Cerebral blood flow determined by hydrogen clearance during middle cerebral artery occlusion in unanesthetized monkeys. *Stroke* 9:143–149, 1978.
13. Morawetz RB, Zeiger HE, McDowell HA, et al: Correlation of cerebral blood flow and EEG during carotid occlusion for endarterectomy (without shunting) and neurologic outcome. *Surgery* 96:184–189, 1984.

14. Raichle ME: The pathophysiology of brain ischemia. *Ann Neurol* 13:2–10, 1983.
15. Siesjo BK: *Brain Energy Metabolism.* New York,
John Wiley & Sons, 1978.
16. Sundt TM, Sharbrough FW, Piepgras DG, et al:
Correlation of cerebral blood flow and electroencephalographic changes during carotid endarterectomy. *Mayo Clin Proc* 56:533–543, 1981.
17. Trojaborg W, Boysen G: Relation between EEG,
regional cerebral blood flow and internal carotid
artery pressure during carotid endarterectomy.
Electroencephalogr Clin Neurophysiol 34:61–69, 1973.

CHAPTER TWO

Cerebral Blood Flow: Normal Regulation and Ischemic Thresholds

Niels A. Lassen, M.D.
Jens Astrup, M.D.

REGULATION OF CEREBRAL BLOOD FLOW

Metabolic Control

The normal brain has a relatively high and rather stable global cerebral metabolic rate of oxygen during sleep, in resting wakefulness, and while performing motor and/or sensory work. Only in states of pain (21) or anxiety (24) does total cerebral oxygen uptake increase, accelerating by 20% to 30%. Cerebral blood flow (CBF), a principal determinant of the oxygen supply, is also normally higher than in other organs (approximately 50 ml/100 g/minute) and remains stable under conditions of pain and anxiety.

This picture of a fairly constant level of energy production and of energy delivery to the brain is somewhat misleading, however, because at a regional level the physiologic variations in brain activity produce corresponding changes in CBF and metabolism: More work results in a higher level of oxidative metabolism and a higher CBF. As an example, during voluntary movements of the hand both CBF and cerebral oxygen uptake increase by about 30% within a few seconds in the contralateral primary (Rolandic) sensory–motor hand area (42, 46). The technique of measurement causes a damping effect because of the presence of adjacent nonactivated cortical areas which are simultaneously recorded (20). The true amplitude of the effect of activation is therefore two to three times greater. Thus, regional increases of

CBF at 50% to 100% may occur locally during normal neuronal activity. Sensory perception also increases flow in the corresponding cortical areas. More complex tasks activate many areas simultaneously. Reading tasks activate at least 14 discrete areas—seven in each hemisphere (30). It is therefore apparent that the observed stability of the overall CBF level reflects mainly the relatively small size of the cortical areas intensely activated in the various types of brain work studied.

These findings at the regional level have firmly established, within the context of normal physiology, the general pattern of metabolic regulation of CBF (40). The term *metabolic regulation* is used to describe the linkage of variation of brain metabolism and flow. It is well known that this covariation occurs in disease states such as epileptic seizure or coma of various origins: high metabolism and flow in epileptic states; low metabolism and flow in coma (Fig. 2.1). Because the changes in metabolism are accompanied by proportional changes in flow, the internal jugular venous oxygen tension and the oxygen tension within brain tissue remain practically constant. If anything, increased activity tends to cause a slight increase in tissue partial pressure of oxygen (PtO_2). Because PtO_2 values normally are stable or even tend to increase during enhanced brain activity, it is unlikely that a local lack of oxygen triggers the mechanism that adjusts flow to match metabolism. What is it, then, that couples flow to metabolism? Although we do not have the answer to this fundamental question, at present three possibilities are being

7

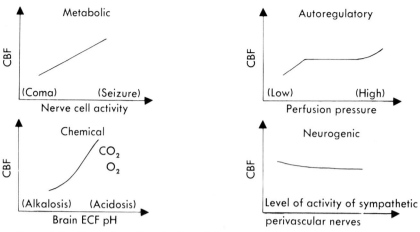

Figure 2.1.   Regulation of cerebral blood flow (CBF). ECF = extracellular fluid.

considered: The mechanism may involve increases in hydrogen (H^+), potassium (K^+), or adenosine concentrations in the extracellular fluid surrounding the brain arterioles inside the tissue. A decreasing calcium (Ca^{2+}) concentration may also play a role in relaxing the smooth muscle cells of the vessel wall.

Autoregulation

When there is a stable level of brain function, as in the resting awake state, and when normal carbon dioxide levels are maintained, CBF is remarkably stable. In particular, CBF is not influenced by variations in the cerebral perfusion pressure (CPP). The constancy of flow despite variations in the arterial pressure is called *autoregulation* (Fig. 2.1). It is an active vascular response, in that arteriolar constriction results when the distending pressure is increased and dilatation results when it is decreased.

Autoregulation of CBF occurs in many tissues other than brain, suggesting that a common mechanism is involved. The perivascular sympathetic nerves on the brain arteries are not necessary for this response (11, 47, 64), yet their stimulation modifies the autoregulation curve, shifting it toward higher pressure levels; the neurogenic control of CBF is discussed below. Because metabolic patterns differ from tissue to tissue, it appears likely that autoregulation is not caused by a metabolic mechanism

but rather results from a myogenic response of the smooth muscle cells of the arterial wall, which constrict when distending force is increased. Autoregulation of CBF is easily abolished by trauma, hypoxia, or other noxious stimuli (50). In such states the flow and apparently the pressure in the microcirculation increase with an increase in the CPP.

Autoregulation can be tested using angiotensin or trimethaphan camsylate (Arfonad, Roche Laboratories, Nutley, NJ) to vary the blood pressure over a moderate range, such as ± 20 mm Hg. These drugs do not influence the vasoconstricting muscle tone of the brain vessels, presumably because they do not readily cross the blood–brain barrier. Therefore, their effects on the cerebral resistance vessels are essentially indirect, through alterations of the blood pressure. In most patients, intracranial pressure (ICP) and cerebral venous pressure are low and are not influenced by the induced arterial pressure changes. Hence, the arterial blood pressure almost equals the CPP when the patient is in the recumbent position. But in patients with increased ICP, variations in this parameter while the drug is being infused must be taken into account.

Autoregulation of CBF explains the constancy of CBF normally found with moderate elevation of ICP. Such an elevation causes a decrease in the CPP as the cortical venous pressure increases together with the ICP: The decreased transmural pressure in the arterioles (which almost equals

CPP) causes dilatation of the arterioles (18, 55).

Autoregulation has a lower limit at a mean arterial blood pressure (MABP) of about 60 mm Hg in normotensive patients (Fig. 2.1). Below this limit, CBF decreases and the cerebral arteriovenous oxygen difference increases. At an even lower MABP (in normotensive patients, about 40 mm Hg), symptoms of cerebral ischemia in the form of mild hyperventilation, dizziness, and eventually syncope appear. Autoregulation also has an upper limit; in normotensive patients this occurs at an MABP of about 130 mm Hg (approximately 200/110 mm Hg). Above this limit the pressure breaks through the constrictor response of the arterial wall. This breakthrough is associated with a disruption of the blood–brain barrier. It has repeatedly been found that vasodilator stimuli, such as tissue acidosis, hypercapnia, or papaverine, enhance damage to the blood–brain barrier and edema formation caused by severe hypertension. Many patients with acute brain injuries have regions of brain tissue in which there is loss of autoregulation and a high flow which is known as the *luxury perfusion* syndrome (31). Such patients cannot tolerate even moderate hypertension because it causes a further rise in CBF, enhanced blood–brain barrier damage, enhanced edema formation of the vasogenic type, and rising ICP (53).

Autoregulation is modified by a shift toward the higher pressure range in chronic arterial hypertension. Apparently hypertrophied arterioles do not relax as well as normal arterioles, although they constrict better than normal arterioles do. This phenomenon characteristic of hypertrophied arterioles is of considerable clinical importance.

Chemical Control: Effects of Carbon Dioxide and Oxygen

Variations in arterial carbon dioxide tension ($PaCO_2$) exert a profound influence on CBF (Fig. 2.1). Hypercapnia causes dilation and hypocapnia causes constriction. Around the normal $PaCO_2$ of 40 mm Hg, CBF changes about 4% for each 1 mm-Hg increase or decrease in $PaCO_2$. Because it is possible to measure CBF with a random experimental error of the same order of magnitude, the effect of 1 mm-Hg variation in $PaCO_2$ can in fact be measured. Very accurate $PaCO_2$ determinations are consequently indispensable for evaluating CBF data. The effects of $PaCO_2$ changes are mediated by pH variations in the smooth muscle cells of the arteriolar wall (12, 17, 32). The pH at this site depends on the $PaCO_2$ in the blood in the arterial lumen since the gas readily diffuses across the arterial wall, and on the concentration of bicarbonate (HCO_3^-) in the cerebral spinal fluid (CSF) around the arteriole since the ions cannot freely diffuse across the wall. This dual nature of the chemical control, by $PaCO_2$ and by local CSF HCO_3^-, is of importance for understanding the vasoparalysis seen both in severe hypercapnia and in brain tissue lactic acidosis.

Chronic changes in $PaCO_2$ induce adaptive changes in CSF HCO_3^-, so that the CSF pH tends to normalize spontaneously. The cerebral vascular tone and CBF also tend to return to the normal level (8, 14, 45, 49). These adaptive changes of CSF HCO_3^- and the parallel changes of CBF occur slowly, taking 24 to 36 hours to develop or to regress. For this reason, no attempt should be made to normalize a chronically elevated $PaCO_2$ acutely in patients. If this is done, the patient may show clinical signs of acute hypocapnia, including dizziness and somnolence with subnormal CBF for several hours. This situation can be avoided by normalizing the $PaCO_2$ gradually over 1 to 2 days.

Variations in the cerebral arterial gas tension of oxygen (PaO_2) around the normal level (approximately 100 mm Hg) do not influence CBF measurably. Indeed, in moderate arterial hypoxia or hyperoxia, the unchanged CBF and oxygen uptake implies that both tissue and cerebral venous oxygen tension (PvO_2) tend to vary with PaO_2, but they vary much less than PaO_2 does. Consequently, the tissue PaO_2 cannot be considered a controlling factor in the same strict sense as tissue pH. In other words, at normal arterial gas tension levels, the pH control effect overrides PaO_2 control.

In contrast, marked arterial hypoxia

causes clear-cut cerebral vasodilatation. The threshold for a measurable flow increase is at a PaO_2 of about 50 mm Hg (26, 35). At about the same level, brain lactic acidosis caused by glycolysis develops. The importance of this acidosis for triggering the vasodilatation is not clear. If it is important, then the two strongest vasodilator stimuli known—arterial hypercapnia and arterial hypoxia—both operate by means of the pH-arteriolar wall mechanism.

Variations in the oxygen-carrying capacity of the blood, as in anemia and polycythemia, cause compensatory CBF changes, keeping cerebral PvO_2 and $PvCO_2$ normal. Therefore, no chemical stimulus for regulating flow is detectable. Because the changes in viscosity are proportional to the CBF changes, there is no reason to suspect that a change in the vascular diameter is responsible for the CBF changes.

Neurogenic Control

The arteries on the brain surface and even the larger arterioles inside the brain tissue are supplied by a network of sympathetic and parasympathetic nerve fibers that run together in the same nerve bundles (39). The sympathetic fibers originate from cells in the superior cervical ganglion, and the parasympathetic fibers originate from the facial nerve.

Studies of animals that were anesthetized and underwent only minor surgical intervention demonstrated that the pial arteries respond to norepinephrine with constriction and to acetylcholine with dilatation when the neurotransmitter agents are applied topically (28, 63). The responses were blocked by the corresponding antagonists applied in low concentrations. Yet, these antagonists do not influence the arteriolar diameter when they are applied alone and in the same low concentrations. Thus, under the conditions studied, there is no evidence of a tonic nervous control of CBF.

Electrical stimulation of the superior cervical ganglion at maximum levels results in a temporary CBF decrease in resting anesthetized animals with normal blood pressure (29). With continued stimulation

the response is small, on the order of 5% to 10% (1, 25, 36). A similar small response has been shown with continued parasympathetic stimulation (48). The small flow changes measured under these experimental conditions would appear to be of no physiologic importance. However, recent studies have revealed a physiologic role of the sympathetic nerves. When they are actively firing, the autoregulatory curve is reset so that both the upper and lower pressure thresholds are raised. Drug-induced hypotension, blocking these nerves, provides a somewhat higher CBF at the same pressure than does hemorrhagic hypotension (15). This finding is consistent with the clinical experience that drug-induced hypotension is better tolerated than is bleeding to the same pressure level. In contrast, as the upper threshold of autoregulation is also increased, hypertension induced with drugs, such as angiotensin, is less well tolerated than is hypertension induced by mechanisms involving sympathetic neural activity; for example, by baroreceptor stimulation. Because sympathetic activation is usually involved in all spontaneous acute pressure rises, as in anger, cold exposure, or isometric muscle contraction, this "resetting to the right" of the upper threshold is, physiologically speaking, the normal upper threshold. The constriction of brain arteries protects the brain against the harmful effects of hypertension, including damage to the blood–brain barrier.

Pharmacologic Control

Many drugs that have a marked effect on vascular tone in most other organs do not influence the cerebral vascular resistance because they do not cross the blood–brain barrier. For example, intracarotid injection of angiotensin or noradrenaline does not alter CBF (43).

Agents that relax the cerebral arterioles include papaverine, acetazolamide (Diamox, Lederle Laboratories, Wayne, NJ), and volatile anesthetics, and high $PaCO_2$. In particular, the cerebral vasodilation caused by high concentrations of halothane (1.5% to 2.0%) has been studied extensively. This effect is associated with an increase in cerebral blood volume which may cause ICP to rise sharply in patients with a space-occupying intracranial mass (16). This effect may be counteracted by using a lower halothane concentration and by hyperventilation. But vasodilatation cannot be completely avoided when halothane is used. For this reason, many neuroanesthesiologists recommend the use of neuroleptics and barbiturates primarily.

Agents with vasoconstrictor effects on the cerebral arterioles include theophylline, low $PaCO_2$, and most of the parenteral anesthetics, such as the barbiturates and Althesin® (Alfathesin), a mixture of two steroids—alphaxalone and alphadolone—having short-lasting anesthetic properties. Ketamine is an exception as a nonvolatile anesthetic because it causes augmentation of brain metabolism and flow. It also tends to increase ICP by the same mechanism as volatile anesthetics do, and is therefore not recommended for neuroanesthesia.

CEREBRAL BLOOD FLOW IN BRAIN TISSUE ACIDOSIS

Even a brief period of inadequate perfusion (ischemia) of the brain tissue leads to a rapid production of lactic acid. Cerebral lactic acidosis becomes very severe in patients with cardiac arrest. It develops in areas of focal ischemia, after global ischemia due to cardiac arrhythmia or arrest, and apparently also in patients with traumatic brain injury or brain tumors or other types of space-occupying lesions (41, 44). Mass effects with tissue compression and increases in ICP, which also cause episodes of ischemia, probably explain the tissue acidosis.

Brain tissue acidosis is characterized by a loss of CBF autoregulation. The luxury perfusion syndrome (31), the loss of autoregulation and high CBF, is characterized by a dissociation of flow and metabolism as the oxygen extraction ratio is reduced. Sometimes the CBF simply exceeds the normal flow rate, but more often the hyperemia is relative, that is, higher in the postischemic than in nonaffected areas. The overall level of CBF tends to be low in such clinical cases. Paradoxical flow responses tend to occur, for example, when strong vasodilator stimuli such as carbon dioxide or papaverine cause a flow decrease (intracerebral "steal") or when vasoconstrictor stimuli, such as hypocapnia or theophylline, cause a flow increase (inverse intracerebral steal). Variations in cerebral blood volume and ICP appear to underlie many of these paradoxical reactions. *False autoregulation* is a strange example of such reactions which has been described in detail by Enevoldsen and Jensen (13). Studying patients with severe traumatic head injury, they found that in areas of maximal contusion the carbon dioxide reaction was abolished or paradoxical—yet in the same areas autoregulation was maintained when the blood pressure was raised or lowered. This finding is very surprising because loss of autoregulation is the first sign of tissue injury. A rise in local tissue pressure, but not necessarily in ICP, seems to explain the paradox.

In treating ischemic brain, it is important to combat brain tissue acidosis by securing adequate oxygenation and reducing $PaCO_2$. Controlled, moderate hyperventilation and the administration of neuroleptics and barbiturates are now widely used in the intensive care of brain-injured patients, in particular in trauma cases. Another therapeutic aim is to avoid cerebral vasodilator drugs; specifically, drugs that depress respiration (e.g. morphine, meperidine) are most emphatically contraindicated in brain-injured patients with spontaneous respiration. Equally contraindicated are volatile anesthetic agents such as halothane, which can induce a most dangerous triad of hypotension, hypercapnia, and halothane-induced cerebral vasodilatation with increased ICP which is additive to the vasodilatation caused by the hypercapnia. Administration of such drugs is permissible only when ventilation and arterial blood pressure are controlled.

Recognition of these clinical principles is not based on data from CBF monitoring alone; indeed ICP monitoring has been even more useful. It is the combined pressure and flow data that constitute the conceptual basis for the intensive care of the brain-injured patient.

ISCHEMIC THRESHOLDS

Ischemia occurs when blood flow is too low to supply enough oxygen to support cellular function. With this definition, the very low CBF during severe barbiturate intoxication combined with hypothermia does not constitute ischemia because the flow suffices to sustain the very reduced metabolic level. In the normal awake state, a moderate reduction of CBF below 50 ml/100 g/minute does not elicit ischemic symptoms. This is the case as long as enough oxygen is being supplied despite the flow reduction because oxygen extraction by brain tissue can increase above its normal level of approximately 35%. Thus, because of dissociation of flow and metabolism, the moderate flow reduction remains asymptomatic. This fully compensated level of moderate CBF reduction is often termed "oligemia" in order to separate it conceptually from the more severe and symptomatic flow reduction which we call ischemia. As mentioned in the preceding section, the brain's oxygen extraction ratio is decreased in the luxury perfusion syndrome, whereas in oligemia and ischemia it is increased. For this reason, Baron et al (5) have called these low-flow states the "misery perfusion syndrome," a syndrome of impending or manifest failure of adequate oxygen supply.

During drug-induced arterial hypotension, symptoms of failing oxygen supply develop at a level of CBF of about 30 ml/100 g/minute. At this level, somnolence, dizziness, and moderate hyperventilation begin to occur. But the flow that is measured is the average flow because the measured value is dominated by the flow to the hemispheres. Therefore, this value cannot justifiably be taken to indicate the critical flow in the most sensitive structures—in the brain stem—which cause the symptoms. However, on the regional level it is possible to accurately define critical

thresholds of ischemia, thresholds below which certain aspects of the tissue's function fail. In normothermic, lightly anesthetized humans with normal hemoglobin concentration, the electroencephalogram over a hemisphere, studied during temporary carotid clamping for endarterectomy, starts to flatten when CBF falls below 20 ml/100 g/minute (54, 56). This threshold correlates very well with that of 18 to 20 ml/100 g/minute obtained by Branston et al (7) in baboons lightly anesthetized with chloralose. Using hydrogen electrodes to measure flow in the cortex, they found that below this threshold—the flow reduction being induced by clipping the middle cerebral artery (MCA) transorbitally—the evoked cortical response started to diminish. Thus, both clinical and experimental studies show that the ischemic threshold of synaptic transmission failure lies at about 20 ml/100 g/minute. In the studies in baboons (7), a lower CBF level of about 15 ml/100 g/minute was observed, below which a complete failure of evoked electrical activity was seen.

Below this ischemic threshold of electrical silence, a further (third) threshold appears to exist at a flow level of about 8 to 10 ml/100 g/minute: This is the ischemic threshold of metabolic failure. This threshold is characterized by massive efflux of cellular K^- and depletion of phosphocreatine and adenosine triphosphate (2, 4, 6). If this state of metabolic failure is sustained, ischemic tissue necrosis supervenes. But it is likely that the massive tissue acidosis developing even at somewhat higher flow levels would also kill the cells. The studies of Morawetz et al (38) showed that 2 to 3 hours of ischemia below a CBF threshold of 12 ml/100 g/minute results in infarction.

With the very important reservation that experiments of longer duration must be done, it nevertheless appears that for sustained ischemia there exists a penumbral zone of CBF between the thresholds of 20 and 15 ml/100 g/minute—perhaps even between 20 and 12 ml/100 g/minute—in which the cells do not function normally and yet may survive. It is not known how often and for how long such a half-shadow, a penumbra between life and death, prevails to be followed by reversal of paralysis of the neurons. That the state does exist, however, is suggested by the numerous cases of completely reversible focal ischemic attacks, which may last for hours. Arterial occlusion or tissue compression by a space-occupying lesion or a neurosurgeon's retractor are probably the two most frequent causes of prolonged regional brain ischemia. If neuronal paralysis is penumbral, then therapeutic measures may determine whether the brain tissue is restored or necrosis occurs. In acute vascular occlusion, elevation of the systemic blood pressure enhances collateral flow. This maneuver has recently been used to relieve focal ischemic symptoms in the postoperative period in patients operated on for arterial aneurysms (*see* Chapter 17, this volume).

It follows, from the concept of the *ischemic penumbra*, which was developed by Astrup et al (3) from the National Hospital in London, that if we could accurately measure, in the clinical setting, the reduced regional flows before and after attempted therapy—in particular in the form of vascular surgery—then the evaluation of such therapy would be vastly facilitated. Such methods are discussed at the conclusion of this chapter with precisely the idea in mind that clinical methods of measuring CBF must be evaluated in order to identify cases in which penumbral conditions exist.

We have mentioned that local ischemia may be caused by tissue compression. Because the brain is a semisolid object, the strains and stresses that occur locally may increase the tissue pressure beyond the arterial blood pressure even with a quite small increase in overall ICP. Achieving the means to compress the brain gently and lightly, and preferably only briefly, with retractors is perhaps the single most significant technical advantage attained over the past 20 to 30 years by the joint efforts of neurosurgeons and neuroanesthesiologists. Ischemia results in tissue acidosis. Hence, the relief of ischemia does not—even if the cells are not dead—immediately restore normal function. The acidotic postischemic tissue is vasoparalytic and the edema already arising during the ischemia may develop further. In the post-ischemic vasoparalytic state, the edema formation is enhanced by hypertension (22).

ISCHEMIC AND POSTISCHEMIC STROKE

In patients who have occlusion or severe spasm of a major cerebral artery, flow in the affected cortical areas is reduced depending on the efficiency of the collateral vessels. The clinical symptoms show that flow in functionally significant regions is below the ischemic threshold for normal function; that is, below 20 ml/100 g/minute. The ischemic area is typically larger on CBF studies than the hypodense area usually found on the computerized tomography (CT) scan. This observation signifies that, in ischemic stroke, edema and tissue necrosis first develop when flow is reduced to even lower levels than those abolishing neuronal activity. The border zone of the ischemic area is usually hyperemic and paradoxical vasomotor responses are observed (51).

In patients with stroke who show no arterial occlusions on angiography but on CT scans show hypodense lesions reaching the cortex, the flow is usually very high and there is luxury perfusion. Current techniques of flow measurement do not allow us to record low-flow areas in close proximity to the hyperemia (flow heterogeneity). In all likelihood, such cases represent the spontaneous lysis of the occlusion or spasm that has occurred too late to prevent tissue necrosis. Such lesions may be considered to be postischemic.

In addition to direct effects on flow and tissue function in the region supplied by the affected artery, there are important indirect effects. Distant areas may be isolated functionally when the lesion interrupts their afferent connections. In such functionally depressed but nonischemic areas, CBF is also lower than normal.

In intracerebral hemorrhage, CBF is typically reduced over large areas of the brain. Both tissue compression due to the acute hemorrhagic mass and deafferentation may play a role. In patients with transient ischemic attacks (TIAs) whose symptoms resolve within 24 hours, CBF is usually normal when the patient is studied. However, in other TIA cases, ischemic or post-ischemic (hyperemic) regions may be found in association with hypodense CT areas.

CLINICAL METHODS FOR MEASURING CEREBRAL BLOOD FLOW

Because of the complexity and three-dimensional structure of the brain, tomographic methods for CBF measurement are necessary for clinical examinations. Three such methods are being developed.

X-ray tomography enhanced by nonradioactive ("cold") xenon (Xe) (10) or by nonradioactive iodoantipyrine (9) offers the advantage of the use of an instrument routinely in widespread use. The variations in enhancement that are used for the CBF calculation are, however, small, and therefore the signal-to-noise ratio is not favorable. Hence, the actual degree of spatial resolution achieved is much less than that of the conventional CT scans. Moreover, only one level can be studied at a time (*see* Chapter 8, this volume).

Positron emission tomography (PET) permits a CBF measurement with methods based on radioactive krypton (65) or radioactive oxygen (23). In particular the latter techniques that also permit study of the brain's oxygen uptake and oxygen extraction tomographically are of importance in the context of brain ischemia (*see* Chapter 9, this volume). However, because of their cost and their logistical problems, including inconvenience for the patient, these techniques are unsuitable for routine use.

Single photon emission computerized tomography (SPECT) is based on the use of conventional gamma-emitting radioisotopes and rotating gamma camera systems. The costs and logistical problems of this technique are trivial compared to those of PET and therefore, despite being less versatile with coarser spatial resolution, SPECT is clinically more applicable. Using a highly sensitive four-camera system (52), ^{133}Xe can be used for CBF tomography. This approach has the advantage of being rapidly repeatable, completely atraumatic

to the patient, and of brief duration (4.5 minutes). It is especially useful in the study of stroke (34), TIAs (56), or vasospasm following aneurysm rupture (37). Using other isotopes such as ^{127}Xe, iodine-123-labeled amines (19, 27, 33), or technetium-99m chelates results in improvement of the spatial resolution to about 8 to 10 mm, which approaches the slice thickness of routine CT scans or magnetic resonance images.

These techniques for CBF tomography have not yet been applied routinely but this is now changing in the context of cerebral vascular surgery, where CBF studies afford a rational means of selecting patients and monitoring the hemodynamic effects of therapeutic intervention. The following case illustrates an approach that allows atraumatic evaluation of the decisive factor in collateral blood flow; namely, the arterial blood pressure distal to the arterial occlusion, the distal blood pressure.

The patient was a 68-year-old woman who had been receiving antihypertensive treatment for several years. A few months before she was admitted to the hospital,

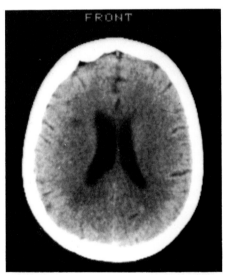

Figure 2.2. CT scan of a 68-year-old patient who had suffered a minor stroke followed by repeated orthostatic transient ischemic attacks that were relieved immediately when she sat down or fell to the lying position. CT shows a lacunar infarction deep in the left hemisphere. Note that the right side is to the right.

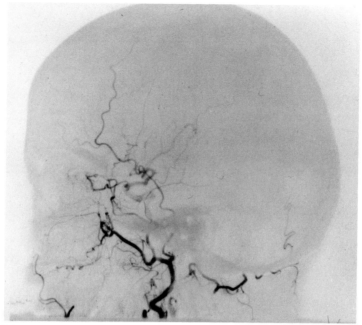

Figure 2.3. Subtraction angiography of left carotid circulation injected through the left common carotid artery in the same patient as shown in Figure 2.2. Note a left internal carotid artery occlusion and slow filling of the left anterior cerebral artery and middle cerebral artery by retrograde flow in the ophthalmic artery.

she suffered a minor stroke with motor aphasia and hemiparesis on the right side, but she made a good recovery. During her period of rehabilitation, she had repeated orthostatic TIAs consisting of weakness of the right arm and leg but had immediate relief when sitting back or falling to the lying position. This condition prompted her readmission to the hospital. Her blood pressure was moderately elevated at about 160/80 mm Hg and orthostatic hypotension was not recorded. CT showed a lacunar

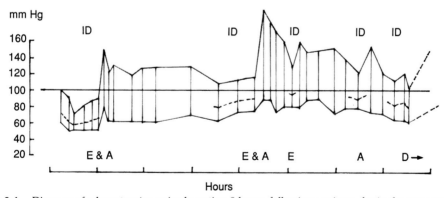

Figure 2.4. Diagram of a hypotensive episode lasting 8 hours following angiography in the same patient as shown in Figures 2.2 and 2.3. The case illustrates the crucial role of systemic blood pressure. ID denotes the presence of ischemic deficit in the form of right-sided hemiparesis and aphasia. Treatment with a β-receptor stimulating sympathomimetic amine administered orally, with angiotensin II infusion, and with dopamine infusion are denoted by E, A, and D, respectively. The dopamine drip could be gradually tapered off and stopped after some hours without blood pressure dropping below the mildly elevated baseline level. This observation, with several manifest ischemic symptoms lasting up to 1 hour (*broken lines* indicating mean arterial blood pressure) that were immediately relieved by raising the pressure, demonstrates the ischemic penumbra (3, 4) in a clinical setting.

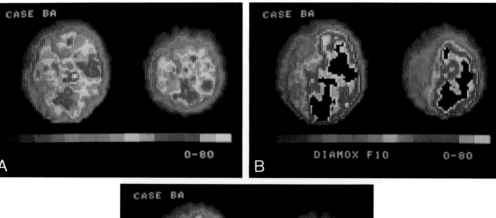

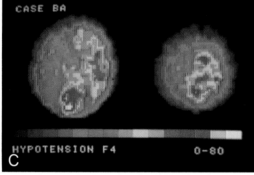

Figure 2.5. *A,* cerebral blood flow (CBF) at resting state mean arterial blood pressure (MABP) about 120 mm Hg. Color scale indicates CBF in ml/100 g/minute. Note that the patient is the same as is shown in Figures 2.2 through 2.4. *B,* the Diamox® test. CBF measurements are repeated 10 minutes after intravenous infusion of 1 g of the strong cerebral vasodilator acetazolamide (Diamox®). Note normal flow increase in nonoccluded areas and paradoxical flow decrease on the occluded side (intracerebral "steal" syndrome). Intraoperative pressure measurements with Diamox® have shown that the drug lowers distal blood pressure to even lower values. This is how the "thief," the healthy parts of the brain, manages to steal CBF from the ischemic regions, by reducing blood pressure in the collaterals by opening up side branches and thus causing the pressure to drop distally. This occurs in all cases of occlusion, even when the collaterals are adequate as evidenced by a slightly or moderately reduced distal blood pressure on the affected side. But when the collaterals are poor, then local adaptation, the autoregulatory vasodilation, is already maximal, or almost maximal, in the resting state. In this case, the drop in cerebral perfusion pressure from a low level (35 mm Hg) to an even lower level (25 mm Hg) cannot be compensated, because neither the autoregulation nor the Diamox®-induced vasodilator stimulus can further relax the local arterioles to any significant extent. Hence, flow paradoxically drops during the Diamox® test. This occurs in only a very small percentage of cases, approximately 10% in our series, of carotid occlusions. *C,* autoregulation test. CBF is repeated during controlled reduction of MABP by 20 mm Hg using Arfonad® and application of mild negative pressure to the lower body. No focal neurologic symptoms were elicited, but on the basis of the observations during the postangiographic hypotensive episode, we assume that the test was carried out very close to the ischemic threshold of synaptic (and functional) failure. Note that CBF ranges from about 35 to 40 ml/100 g/minute during this near-threshold study. These values appear to be considerably higher than the values for the ischemic threshold of approximately 20 ml/100 g/minute that must have developed during the spontaneous hypotensive episode. However, because of methodologic difficulties caused by scattered radiation (Compton scatter), the CBF method used, xenon-133 dynamic single photon emission computerized tomography, may overestimate low flows to a considerable extent.

infarction deep in the left hemisphere (Fig. 2.2). Bilateral carotid angiography indicated a left internal carotid artery occlusion and slow filling of the left anterior cerebral artery and MCA by retrograde flow in the ophthalmic artery (Fig. 2.3).

This history suggests that the orthostatic TIAs were elicited by the normal small drop in systemic blood pressure at the level of the brain caused by the upright posture, a drop in pressure reducing the distal perfusion pressure—that beyond the occlusion—to so low a level that blood flow dropped below the threshold for neuronal function. Focal ischemic neurologic deficits developed within seconds. The deficits cleared immediately when perfusion pressure and hence flow were reestablished. The crucial role of systemic blood pressure was dramatically evidenced in our patient (Fig. 2.4). Upon the accidental perivascular injection of radiopaque contrast material during carotid angiography, her blood pressure became unstable. She arrived hemiplegic and aphasic in the intensive care unit. Her MABP was about 60 to 70 mm Hg. Her ischemic deficits proved extremely sensitive to changes in MABP over the following hours, clearing completely at pressures above, and reappearing at pressures below, a critical level of about 90 to 100 mm Hg in MABP.

CBF tomography by ^{133}Xe was performed. The results of CBF tomography during the Diamox test and during the test of autoregulation are shown in Figure 2.5. As expected, resting flow (Fig. 2.5A) was lowest in the left hemisphere, where a low-flow area was seen which was much larger than the lacunar infarct on the CT scan. That this lesion was due to poor collateral flow was evidenced by the flow measurements made during a hemodynamic stress condition using 1 g of Diamox, a strong vasodilator of the cerebral microcirculation. The Diamox study (Fig. 2.5B) showed a drop in flow on the occluded left side and in increase in flow on the nonoccluded right side (the intracerebral steal of flow). A test of autoregulation (Fig. 2.5C) indicated pressure-passive flow in the left hemisphere. A reduction of MABP by about 20 mm Hg using a small dose of Arfonad and administration of mild lower body negative pressure by suction caused a drop in flow, rather than an unchanged flow, as expected in cases of unrestricted collateral supply. Both tests revealed that the local perfusion pressure to that area (distal blood pressure) was below the lowest level of autoregulation. The findings were confirmed by a very low MABP value of 33 mm Hg measured intraoperatively in the MCA branch that was subsequently used for the anastomosis during extracranial-to-intracranial bypass surgery.

This case illustrates the hemodynamic state in a patient with carotid artery occlusion whose collateral supply is so restricted that the distal arterial blood pressure is very low and collateral blood flow is dependent on systemic arterial blood pressure. The evidence points to a hemodynamic and not an embolic cause of this patient's TIAs. Moreover, her case illustrates the potential risk of acute antihypertensive treatment in occlusive cerebral vascular disease. If such a patient requires general anesthesia with surgery, caution against even a small and otherwise insignificant decrease in blood pressure is of critical importance. The recent studies by Vorstrup and colleagues (57–62) provide further details regarding the use of ^{133}Xe tomography in the context of cerebral vascular surgery.

References

1. Alm A, Bill A: The effect of stimulation of the cervical sympathetic chain on retinal oxygen tension and on uveal, retinal and cerebral blood flow in cats. *Acta Physiol Scand* 88:84–94, 1973.
2. Astrup J, Blennow G, Nilsson B: Effects of reduced cerebral blood flow upon EEG pattern, cerebral extracellular potassium, and energy metabolism in the rat cortex during bicuculline induced seizures. *Brain Res* 177:115–126, 1979.
3. Astrup J, Siesjö BK, Symon L: The state of "penumbra" in the ischemic brain: Viable and lethal thresholds in cerebral ischemia (editorial). *Stroke* 12:723–725, 1981.
4. Astrup J, Symon L, Branston NM, et al: Cortical evoked potential and extracellular K$^+$ and H$^+$ at critical levels of brain ischemia. *Stroke* 8:51–57, 1977.
5. Baron J-C, Rougemont D, Bousser MG, et al: Local CBF, oxygen extraction fraction (OEF) and CMRO$_2$: Prognostic value in recent supratentorial infarction in humans. *J Cereb Blood Flow Metab* 3 [Suppl 1]:1–2, 1983.
6. Branston NM, Strong AJ, Symon L: Extracellular potassium activity, evoked potential and tissue blood flow. *J Neurol Sci* 32:305–321, 1977.
7. Branston NM, Symon L, Crockard HA, et al: Relationship between the cortical evoked potential and local cortical blood flow following acute middle cerebral artery occlusion in the baboon. *Exp Neurol* 45:195–208, 1974.
8. Christensen MS, Brodersen P, Olesen J, et al: Cerebral apoplexy (stroke) treated with or without prolonged artificial hyperventilation. II. Cerebrospinal fluid acid–base balance and intracranial pressure. *Stroke* 4:620–631, 1974.
9. Drayer B, Coleman E, Bates M, et al: Nonradioactive iodoantipyrine-enhanced cranial computed tomography. Preliminary observations. *J Comput Assist Tomogr* 4:186–190, 1980.

10. Drayer BP, Wolfson SK Jr, Reinmuth OM, et al: Xenon-enhanced CT for analysis of cerebral integrity, perfusion, and blood flow. *Stroke* 9:123–130, 1978.

11. Eklöf B, Ingvar DH, Kågström E, et al: Persistence of cerebral blood flow autoregulation following chronic bilateral cervical sympathectomy in the monkey. *Acta Physiol Scand* 82:172–176, 1971.

12. Elliott KAC, Jasper HH: Physiological salt solutions for brain surgery: Studies of local pH and pial vessel reactions to buffered and unbuffered isotonic solutions. *J Neurosurg* 6:140–152, 1949.

13. Enevoldsen E, Jensen FT: Autoregulation and CO_2 responses of cerebral blood flow in patients with acute severe head injury. *J Neurosurg* 48:689–703, 1978.

14. Fencl V, Vale JR, Brock JA: Respiration and cerebral blood flow in metabolic acidosis and alkalosis in humans. *J Appl Physiol* 27:67–76, 1969.

15. Fitch W, MacKenzie ET, Harper AM: Effects of decreasing arterial blood pressure on cerebral flow in the baboon: influence of the sympathetic nervous system. *Circ Res* 37:550–557, 1975.

16. Fitch W, McDowall DG: Effect of halothane on intracranial pressure gradients in the presence of intracranial space-occupying lesions. *Br J Anaesth* 43:904–907, 1971.

17. Gotoh F, Tazaki Y, Meyer JS: Transport of gases through brain and their extravascular vasomotor action. *Exp Neurol* 4:48–58, 1961.

18. Häggendal E, Löfgren J, Nilsson NJ, et al: Effects of varied cerebrospinal fluid pressure on cerebral blood flow in dogs. *Acta Physiol Scand* 79:262–271, 1970.

19. Hill TC, Holman L, Lovett R, et al: Initial experience with SPECT (single-photon computerized tomography) of the brain using N-isopropyl I-123 p-iodoamphetamine: Concise communication. *J Nucl Med* 23:191–195, 1982.

20. Høedt-Rasmussen K, Sveinsdottir E, Lassen NA: Regional cerebral blood flow in man determined by intraarterial injection of radioactive inert gas. *Circ Res* 18:237–247, 1966.

21. Ingvar DH, Rosen I, Eriksson M, et al: Activation patterns induced in the dominant hemisphere by skin stimulation. In Zotterman Y (ed): *Sensory Functions of the Skin.* Elmsford, NY, Pergamon Press, 1976, pp 549–559.

22. Ito U, Ohno K, Suganuma Y, et al: Effect of steroid on ischemic brain edema. Analysis of cytotoxic and vasogenic edema occurring during ischemia and after restoration of blood flow. *Stroke* 11:166–172, 1980.

23. Jones T, Chesler DA, Ter-Pogossian MM: The continuous inhalation of oxygen-15 for assessing regional oxygen extraction in the brain of man. *Br J Radiol* 49:339–343, 1976.

24. Kety SS: Round table discussion of psychoactive drugs and anxiety, their influence on cerebral circulation and metabolism. In Ingvar DH, Lassen NA (eds): *Brain Work.* Copenhagen, Munksgaard, 1975, pp 472–474.

25. Kobayashi S, Waltz AG, Rhoton AL: Effects of stimulation of cervical sympathetic nerves on cortical blood flow and vascular reactivity. *Neurology* 21:297–320, 1971.

26. Kogure K, Scheinberg P, Reinmuth OM, et al: Mechanisms of cerebral vasodilatation in hypoxia. *J Appl Physiol* 29:223–229, 1970.

27. Kuhl DE, Barrio JR, Huang S-C, et al: Quantifying local cerebral blood flow by N-isopropyl-p-(^{123}I)iodoamphetamine (IMP) tomography. *J Nucl Med* 23:196–203, 1982.

28. Kuschinsky W, Wahl M: The functional significance of β-adrenergic and cholinergic receptors at pial arteries: A microapplication study. In Langfitt TW, McHenry, LC Jr, Reivich M, et al (eds): *Cerebral Circulation and Metabolism.* New York, Springer-Verlag, 1975, pp 470–472.

29. Lacombe P, Sercombe R, Reynier-Rebuffel AM, et al: Time course of the effects of cervical sympathetic stimulation on local CBF: Evidence for an escape phenomenon. *Acta Neurol Scand [Suppl]* 64:40–41, 1977.

30. Larsen B, Skinhøj E, Soh K, et al: The pattern of cortical activity provoked by listening and speech revealed by rCBF measurements. *Acta Neurol Scand [Suppl]* 64:268–269, 280–281, 1977.

31. Lassen NA: The luxury-perfusion syndrome and its possible relation to acute metabolic acidosis localized within the brain. *Lancet* 2:1113–1115, 1966.

32. Lassen NA, Agnoli A: The upper limit of autoregulation of cerebral blood flow—on the pathogenesis of hypertensive encephalopathy. *Scand J Clin Lab Invest* 30:113–116, 1972.

33. Lassen NA, Henriksen L, Holm S, et al: Cerebral blood-flow tomography: Xenon-133 compared with isopropyl-amphetamine-iodine-123: Concise communication. *J Nucl Med* 24:17–21, 1983.

34. Lassen NA, Henriksen L, Paulson OB: Regional cerebral blood flow in stroke by xenon-133 inhalation and emission tomography. *Stroke* 12:284–288, 1981.

35. McDowall DG: *Oxygen Measurements in Blood and Tissues.* London, Churchill Livingstone, 1966, pp 205–220.

36. Meyer NW, Klassen AC: Regional brain blood flow during sympathetic stimulation. In Langfitt TW, McHenry LC Jr, Reivich M, et al (eds): *Cerebral Circulation and Metabolism.* New York, Springer-Verlag, 1975, pp 459–461.

37. Mickey B, Vorstrup S, Voldby B, et al: Serial measurement of regional cerebral blood flow in patients with SAH using ^{133}Xe inhalation and emission computerized tomography. *J Neurosurg* 60:916–922, 1984.

38. Morawetz RB, Jones TH, Ojemann RG, et al: Regional cerebral blood flow during temporary middle cerebral artery occlusion in waking monkeys. *Acta Neurol Scand [Suppl]* 64:114–115, 1977.

39. Nielsen KC, Edvinsson I, Owman C: Cholinergic innervation and vasomotor response of brain vessels. In Langfitt TW, McHenry LC Jr, Reivich M, et al (eds): *Cerebral Circulation and Metabolism.* New York, Springer-Verlag, 1975, pp 473–475.

40. Obrist WD, Thompson H-K Jr, Wang HS, et al: Regional cerebral blood flow estimated by 133-Xenon inhalation. *Stroke* 6:245–256, 1975.

41. Olesen J: Total CO_2 lactate and pyruvate in brain biopsies taken after freezing and tissue in situ. *Acta Neurol Scand* 46:141–148, 1970.

42. Olesen J: Contralateral focal increase of cerebral

blood flow in man during arm work. *Brain* 94:635–646, 1971.

43. Olesen J: Effect of intracarotid epinephrine, norepinephrine and angiotensin on the regional cerebral blood flow in man. *Neurology* 22:978–987, 1972.

44. Palvölgyi R: Regional cerebral blood flow in patients with intracranial tumors. *J Neurosurg* 31:149–163, 1969.

45. Pannier JL, Weyne J, Demeester G, et al: Influence of changes in the acid–base composition of the ventricular system on cerebral blood flow in cats. *Pflugers Arch* 333:337–351, 1972.

46. Raichle ME, Grubb RL, Mokhtar HG, et al: Correlation between regional cerebral blood flow and oxidative metabolism. *Acta Neurol* 33:523–526, 1976.

47. Rapela CE, Green HD, Denison AB Jr: Baroreceptor reflexes and autoregulation of cerebral blood flow in the dog. *Circ Res* 21:559–568, 1967.

48. Salanga VD, Waltz AG: Regional cerebral blood flow during stimulation of tenth cranial nerve. *Stroke* 4:213–217, 1973.

49. Severinghaus JW, Chiodi H, Eger EIH, et al: Cerebral blood flow in man at high altitude: Role of cerebrospinal fluid pH in normalization of flow in chronic hypocapnia. *Circ Res* 19:274–282, 1966.

50. Shakhnovich AR, Serbinenko FA, Razumovsky AE: Functional reactivity of cerebral blood flow in patients with cerebrovascular pathology. *Acta Neurol Scand [Suppl]* 64:258–259, 1977.

51. Skyhøj Olsen T, Larsen B, Bech Skriver E, et al: Focal cerebral hyperemia measured by the intra-arterial 133-Xenon method. *Stroke* 12:736–744, 1981.

52. Stokely EM, Sveinsdottir E, Lassen NA, et al: A single photon dynamic computer-assisted tomograph (DCAT) for imaging brain function in multiple cross-sections. *J Comput Assist Tomogr* 4:230–240, 1980.

53. Strandgaard S, Olesen J, Skinhøj E, et al: Autoregulation of brain circulation in severe arterial hypertension. *Br Med J* 1:507–510, 1973.

54. Sundt TM, Sharbrough FW, Anderson RE, et al: Cerebral blood flow measurements and electroencephalograms during carotid endarterectomy. *J Neurosurg* 41:310–320, 1974.

55. Symon L, Pasztor E, Dorsch NWC, et al: Physiological responses of local areas of the cerebral circulation in experimental primates determined by the method of hydrogen clearance. *Stroke* 4:632–642, 1973.

56. Trojaborg W, Boysen G: Relation between EEG, regional cerebral blood flow and internal carotid artery pressure during carotid endarterectomy. *Electroencephalogr Clin Neurophysiol* 34:61–69, 1973.

57. Vorstrup S: Tomographic cerebral blood flow measurements i.i patients with ischemic cerebrovascular disease and evaluation of the vasodilatory capacity by the acetazolamide test (thesis, University of Copenhagen). *Acta Neurol Scand* 77 [Suppl 114]:1–48, 1988.

58. Vorstrup S, Boysen G, Brun B, et al: Evaluation of the regional cerebral vasodilatory capacity before carotid endarterectomy by the acetazolamide test. *Neurol Res* 9:10–18, 1987.

59. Vorstrup S, Brun G, Lassen NA: Evaluation of the cerebral vasodilatory capacity by the acetazolamide test before EC-IC bypass surgery in patients with occlusion of the internal carotid artery. *Stroke* 17:1291–1298, 1986.

60. Vorstrup S, Engall HC, Lindewald H, et al: Hemodynamically significant stenosis of the internal carotid artery treated with endarterectomy. Case report. *J Neurosurg* 60:1070–1075, 1984.

61. Vorstrup S, Hemmingsen R, Henriksen L, et al: Regional cerebral blood flow in patients with transient ischemic attacks studied by xenon-133 inhalation and emission tomography. *Stroke* 14:903–910, 1983.

62. Vorstrup S, Lassen NA, Henriksen L, et al: CBF before and after extracranial-intracranial bypass surgery in patients with ischemic cerebrovascular disease studied with xenon-133 inhalation tomography. *Stroke* 16:616–626, 1985.

63. Wahl M, Kuschinsky W, Bosse O, et al: Effect of 1-norepinephrine on the diameter of pial arterioles and arteries in the cat. *Circ Res* 31:248–256, 1972.

64. Waltz AG, Yamaguchi T, Regli F: Regulatory responses of cerebral vasculature after sympathetic denervation. *Am J Physiol* 221:298–302, 1971.

65. Yamamoto YL, Thompson C, Meyer E, et al: Three-dimensional topographical regional cerebral blood flow in man, measured with high efficiency mini-BGO two-ring position device using krypton-77. *Acta Neurol Scand* 60 (Suppl 72):186–187, 1979.

CHAPTER THREE

Hemodynamics of Postischemic Reperfusion of the Brain

K.-A. Hossmann, M.D., Ph.D.

Ischemia damages the brain in two different ways: directly by interfering with the blood supply of oxygen and nutrients to the brain, and indirectly by triggering a sequence of events that may cause later disturbances of the functional, biochemical, and structural integrity of the central nervous system. Among the events in the second category, hemodynamic factors are of particular importance. Gross disturbances of postischemic recirculation, nonnutritional redistribution of microcirculation, disturbances of the regulation of cerebral blood flow (CBF), and dissociation of flow and the metabolic requirements of the tissue may lead to deficiencies of supply and removal of nutrients and metabolites that may outlast the primary ischemic impact for considerable time and may become pathogenetic factors on their own.

The focus of this chapter is the pathophysiology of two major postischemic hemodynamic disturbances: the no-reflow phenomenon and the delayed postischemic hypoperfusion syndrome. Both events are multifactorial and their pathogenetic importance for postischemic cerebral revival has aroused considerable disagreement in the past. This chapter attempts to clarify some of the contradictions that may not be as controversial, however, as is frequently assumed.

NO-REFLOW PHENOMENON

The term *no-reflow* was introduced by Ames et al (4) in 1968 in order to describe the absence of vascular filling after a period of global brain ischemia (Fig. 3.1). The study was prompted by the observation

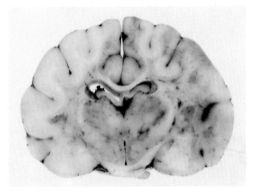

Figure 3.1. No-reflow phenomenon in a cat brain submitted to 60 minutes of global cerebral ischemia. After release of the vascular occlusion, circulating blood was marked by intravenous infusion of carbon black stain. The unstained no-reflow areas are clearly differentiated from black-stained regions with reperfusion. (From Hossmann K-A: Total ischemia of the brain. In Zülch KJ, Kaufman W, Hossmann K-A, et al (eds): *Brain and Heart Infarct*. Berlin, Springer-Verlag, 1977, pp 107–122.)

that the anoxic resistance of the central nervous tissue in vitro is not the same as it is in vivo. When the isolated retina of rabbit is completely deprived of glucose and oxygen in vitro, the evoked response to light disappears as fast as it does during circulatory arrest in vivo (3). In the in vitro situation, however, the evoked response recovers after oxygen and glucose deprivation for as long as 30 minutes (3) whereas the brain in vivo suffers irreversible injury after 8 to 10 minutes of arrested flow (46). This finding is the more surprising because the metabolic rate of the retina is as high as or higher than that of the cerebral cortex or any other part of the brain. Ames and colleagues (2, 4) therefore suspected that factors unrelated to the inherent anoxic susceptibility of the neurons are involved, which led them to investigate the patency of the vascular system after brain ischemia in vivo. Using the ingenious method of intracarotid infusion of a suspension of colloidal carbon, they found that after global ischemia exceeded a duration of 7.5 minutes circumscribed areas of the brain remained white (4). This phenomenon clearly was caused by a failure of reperfusion and, therefore, was termed the no-reflow phenomenon. Because 7.5 minutes is close to the duration of the ischemic threshold of irreversible brain damage, the suggestion was made that the vascular changes may play a crucial role in bringing the ischemic process to the point of no return and that brain parenchyma would remain viable when postischemic reperfusion was established.

Although the concept of the no-reflow phenomenon as a major pathogenetic factor in irreversible ischemic injury was new, the occurrence of postischemic hemodynamic disturbances had not escaped earlier notice. Impairment of the circulation after ischemia had been observed in a variety of tissues, including the rat adrenal gland (74), the cat heart (76), and the striated muscle of rat and dog (114). Those observations had led to the conclusion that ischemic necrosis was associated with damage to the small blood vessels (41). Hirsch et al (45) reported that the viscosity of the blood increases during ischemia and that higher than normal blood pressure is required to reperfuse the brain after circulatory arrest. Neely and Youmans (92) observed an unexpectedly high degree of recovery of the dog brain after 25 minutes of compression ischemia. They attributed the recovery to collapse of the blood vessels during ischemia which prevented the formation of microthrombi. The full significance of the no-reflow phenomenon for the pathogenesis of postischemic injury was only realized, however, when evidence was provided that prevention of this complication resulted in the return of progressing electrophysiologic and biochemical functions of the brain after normothermic cerebral-circulatory arrest of as long as 1 hour (49). Prevention of the no-reflow phenomenon thus became of central interest for the development of rational strate-

gies for prolonging the time during which the brain could be revived after ischemia.

Terminology and Localization

Although in the original terminology of Ames et al (4) the no-reflow phenomenon referred to the vascular filling defects observed after a period of global ischemia, a more detailed analysis revealed that the vascular obstruction either may resolve spontaneously or, quite the contrary, may develop after a short period of successful recirculation. Other terms like "impaired reflow" (63), "low-flow state" (121), or "primary and secondary no-reflow" (37) are therefore more appropriate. Nonetheless, the original term has become firmly established in ischemic research not only of the brain but also of other organs (29, 64, 72, 115) and, for that reason, should be maintained in order to avoid confusion with other forms of postischemic circulatory disturbances.

The localization of no-reflow is multifocal. Usually, large discrete areas are involved but multiple miliary spots have also been described. The distribution is frequently random but it may also exhibit a prevalence of either cortical or subcortical regions. Prevalence of localization may be species-dependent because cortical no-reflow is mainly observed in gerbil, dog, and monkey, whereas in rat the basal ganglia and brain stem are more severely affected (Table 3.1) (10, 14, 30, 31, 37, 62, 65, 83, 93, 129).

The appearance of no-reflow areas clearly depends on both the duration and the severity of ischemia. After complete global cerebral circulatory arrest at normal body temperature, no-reflow regions develop after 5 to 7 minutes and become prominent after 15 minutes (2, 4, 75). Following incomplete ischemia, much longer periods of ischemia are required to produce no-reflow. Several investigators reported that severe reduction of global hemispheric blood flow induced by intracranial hypertension or incomplete arterial in-flow occlusion for a duration of 15 minutes does not evoke a no-reflow phenomenon (66, 90, 118, 119), and in one study incomplete

Table 3.1.   Localization of the Region of No-Reflow After Brain Ischemia

Species	Duration of ischemia (minutes)	Type of no-reflow	Localization	Authors
Cat	30	Multifocal	Random	Ginsberg et al (30)
Dog	4–20	Large discrete	Cortex, basal ganglia, thalamus	Blinkov et al (10)
	5–15	Diffuse or multifocal	Random	Lin (83)
	6–8	Large discrete areas	Mainly cortex	Gurvitch et al (37)
	20	Miliary	Brain stem, subcortical structures	Gurvitch et al (37)
	20–30	Large discrete and miliary	Random	Norwood et al (93)
Gerbil	60	Patchy	Mainly cortex	Ito et al (62)
Monkey	10–70	Patchy	Mainly cortex	Ginsberg & Myers (31)
Rabbit	7, 5–30	Patchy	Basal ganglia, thalamus, brain stem	Cantu & Ames (14)
Rat	10–30	Patchy	Striatum, hippocampus, amygdala, thalamus, basal ganglia	Kågström et al (65)
	15	Multifocal	Brain stem, thalamus	Yamada et al (129)

global ischemia of as much as 1 to 5 hours did not result in recirculation deficits (97). Similar observations have been made after transient occlusion of the middle cerebral artery, which also results in incomplete reduction of CBF. Under these circumstances, there was no sign of the no-reflow phenomenon after periods of ischemia lasting up to 3 hours, and no-reflow usually became prominent only after 3 to 6 hours or longer (67, 87, 88). Consequently, the threshold duration of ischemia for the manifestation of no-reflow is approximately 7 minutes of complete and 3 to 6 hours of incomplete cerebral-circulatory arrest (Table 3.2) (25, 37, 62, 65–67, 75, 81, 83, 85, 88, 90, 97, 118).

The volume of no-reflow areas depends on several systemic factors and, therefore, varies in different experimental situations. At normal blood pressure and normal blood viscosity, ischemia of 7.5 minutes' duration in the rabbit causes no-reflow only in a small fraction of the total brain volume, 10 minutes of ischemia results in no-reflow in up to 35% of total brain volume, and 15 minutes results in up to 95% (2, 4). These values should be considered only as general guidelines because manipulation of systemic variables modifies the volume of no-reflow in both directions. The analysis of these factors has contributed substan-

tially to the understanding of the pathophysiology of the no-reflow phenomenon and the development of rational therapeutic procedures.

Pathophysiology

The pathophysiology of the no-reflow phenomenon is multifactorial and includes hemodynamic, vascular, and hematologic factors. In the original report of Chiang et al (17), swelling of vascular elements was considered to be the primary reason for microcirculatory occlusion, but later studies revealed that changes of blood viscosity and of the local blood perfusion pressure are of equal importance (24, 25). The role of these factors will be described separately but it should be understood that their effect is additive and that none of them is able to provoke a major degree of no-reflow on its own.

Vascular Factors

During ischemia of a duration and severity long enough to produce depolarization of cell membranes, substantial shifts of electrolytes and fluid occur between the intracellular and extracellular compartments (47, 57, 63). In the vicinity of blood

Table 3.2. Duration of Ischemia Required to Produce the No-Reflow Phenomenon

Type of ischemia	Species	Method of ischemia	Duration of ischemia	No-reflow Absent	No-reflow Present	Authors
Complete global	Dog	Cardiac arrest	5 min	+		Lin (83)
	Rabbit	Tourniquet	5 min	+		Kowada et al (75)
	Rabbit	Tourniquet	7.5 min		+	Kowada et al (75)
	Dog	Cardiac arrest	7–8 min		+	Gurvitch et al (37)
	Rat	Compression ischemia	10 min		+	Kågström et al (65)
	Rabbit	Arterial & venous occlusion	10 min		+	Fischer et al (25)
	Dog	Cardiac arrest	12 min		+	Lin & Kormano (85)
Incomplete global	Rabbit	Compression ischemia	15 min		+	Marshall et al (90)
	Rat	Four-vessel occlusion	15 min	+		Todd et al (118)
	Rat	Compression ischemia	15 min	+		Kågström et al (66)
	Hypertensive rat	Bilateral carotid artery occlusion	1–5 h	+		Ogata et al (97)
Focal	Gerbil	Carotid artery occlusion	1 h		+	Levy et al (81)
	Monkey	MCA[a] occlusion	1.5 h	+		Little et al (88)
	Monkey	MCA occlusion	3 h		+	Little et al (88)
	Cat	MCA occlusion	6 h	+		Kamijyo et al (67)
	Gerbil	Carotid artery	6 h		+	Ito et al (62)

[a]MCA = middle cerebral artery.

vessels, these shifts are particularly pronounced because the serum contained in the vessel lumen provides a reservoir of water and electrolytes that is taken up by the endothelial and perivascular glial cells (17). As a result, the capillary lumen is compressed from the outside by swollen perivascular glial processes and obstructed from the inside by endothelial blebs (17) or flaps (6). These cellular protrusions have to be distinguished from endothelial villi which are of more regular and smaller size and the formation of which correlates with the development of the delayed postischemic hypoperfusion syndrome, described in the second part of this chapter (22).

The concept of ischemic cellular swelling as the mechanism inducing microvascular occlusion conforms to the observation that no-reflow begins to develop after about 7.5 minutes of ischemia (4, 75, 82, 83). By that time, cell membranes have depolarized and the extracellular space begins to narrow, as demonstrated by electrophysiologic methods (45, 47). Therefore, it is reasonable to assume that this time also marks the beginning of the swelling of

vascular cell elements. An argument against the importance of vascular factors has been raised by Fischer et al (24), who were not able to detect major changes in the diameter of the capillary lumen. However, they performed their measurements by electron microscopy after short periods of ischemia and subsequent perfusion fixation; it cannot be excluded that the fluid shifts responsible for the morphologic alterations were reversed by the fixation process. After longer periods of ischemia which render it more difficult to reperfuse the brain vasculature with the fixative, narrowing of the capillary lumen is a prominent finding (6).

Another vascular factor that may contribute to the no-reflow phenomenon is the development of arteriolar spasm (107, 122). Three arguments have been proposed in support of such a mechanism. One is that anoxic depolarization results in an increase of extracellular potassium to more than 50 mM, which is high enough to produce pial arterial vasoconstriction in the intact animal (77). The other is that, during ischemia, vascular resistance increases by more than 100%, irrespective of the presence or absence of blood in the vascular system and this increase is only slightly reduced by dehydration with mannitol (107). Finally, microscopic observations of pial arteries revealed a decrease in the vascular diameter during ischemia (117). However, both in vivo microscopy (117) and microangiography (55) of pial arteries showed an immediate and substantial vasodilation at the moment of blood recirculation, which suggests that the reduction in vascular diameter during ischemia is due to the fall of intraluminal pressure and not to an increase of vascular tone. The vasoconstricting effect of potassium, in consequence, is counteracted by the acidosis that builds up during ischemia as a result of the accumulation of lactic acid. Because morphologic observations also failed to reveal vascular spasm (24), it is unlikely that functional alterations of vascular tone are of pathophysiologic significance for the development of the no-reflow phenomenon.

Blood Factors

According to Ames and colleagues (2, 4, 25), an increase of blood viscosity is a major component in the pathogenesis of the no-reflow phenomenon. Some authors also stress the possibility of formation of microthrombi (19, 44), but the importance of intravascular coagulation has been disputed because there is no morphologic evidence of thrombi (3, 24) and because heparin does not prevent the no-reflow phenomenon (15). The most direct evidence of viscosity changes was provided by Hirsch et al (45), who observed an increase in the screen filtration pressure of cerebral venous—but not arterial—blood shortly after the induction of global circulatory arrest. This observation would correlate with the well-known rheologic phenomenon of an increase of blood viscosity at low shear rate (27, 69), and the demonstration of sludging of erythrocytes (44) and the formation of platelet aggregates (60, 95) in cerebral vessels during ischemia. A stringent argument against the role of blood viscosity for the development of no-reflow, however, is that hypothermia reduces the development of recirculation disturbances (93) and prolongs the revival time of the brain (128), although the decreased temperature enhances blood viscosity. Therefore, it is more likely that the interaction of stagnant blood with the ischemically injured brain, and not simply blood stagnation, is responsible for the vascular obstruction. At least three pathophysiologic phenomena may contribute to this effect. One is the dehydration of intravascular blood by the ischemic brain, which can be expected to occur when the brain begins to swell and which is closely associated with the depolarization of cell membranes. This could explain why retardation of cellular depolarization by hypothermia or barbiturates also prevents the development of a no-reflow phenomenon (9, 93). The other possibility is the generation of a no-reflow promoting blood factor in the ischemic brain, as proposed by Hallenbeck and Furlow (39). This factor could be the cryoprecipitable factor VIII / von Willebrand factor protein because removal of this protein by glass wool filtration seems to improve postischemic recirculation (40). Finally, plugging of capillaries by adhering granulocytes may be involved (105), although this process is probably of greater importance for delayed postischemic hypoperfusion than for the no-reflow phenomenon.

In conclusion, analysis of the published data suggests that viscosity changes of the blood become a critical factor only after terminal depolarization of the brain has occurred. When cell membrane depolarization is prevented by either metabolic inhibition or maintenance of some blood supply, blood factors alone do not seem to provoke a no-reflow phenomenon.

Hemodynamic Factors

The severity of no-reflow depends crucially on the blood reperfusion pressure after the ischemic impact (Fig. 3.2). This has been clearly demonstrated by Fisher et al (25), who measured the volume of nonperfused brain regions after various durations of global ischemia at different reperfusion pressures. As ischemia increased from 5 to 30 minutes, the pressure

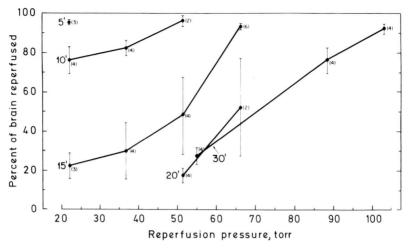

Figure 3.2. Relation between postischemic reperfusion pressure and the size of the no-reflow areas following varying durations of global brain ischemia. Note the substantial improvement of reflow with increasing perfusion pressure. (From Fischer EG, Ames A III, Lorenzo AV: Cerebral blood flow immediately following brief circulatory stasis. *Stroke* 10:423–427, 1979. Reproduced by permission of the American Heart Association, Inc.)

required to achieve reperfusion of the entire brain rose from 20 to 100 mm Hg. Similar, although less well-documented, observations have been made by numerous other authors (28, 42, 45, 54, 62). An indirect way to improve postischemic blood reperfusion is brain decompression. In the cat, restoration of CBF after prolonged global ischemia causes an increase of intracranial pressure (ICP) by as much as 70 mm Hg due to sudden postischemic brain swelling (132). Therefore, the effective blood perfusion pressure in cerebral tissue is much lower than anticipated from the systemic blood pressure level. Relief of intracranial hypertension by craniotomy substantially improves postischemic reperfusion pressure, and is presumably the reason for the observation that in animals subjected to craniotomy, postischemic metabolic recovery is faster and more homogenous than in animals with closed skull (89).

Conversely, low blood reperfusion pressure enhances no-reflow and explains the high sensitivity of the brain to cardiac arrest. Using conventional extrathoracic cardiac resuscitation procedures, the brain is exposed to a period of hypotension before spontaneous cardiac function recovers, which favors the development of no-reflow (8). When postischemic hypotension is prevented using intrathoracic car-

diac massage for the buildup of normal blood pressure levels, blood recirculation and functional recovery of the brain also improve. In fact, following 30-minute cardiac arrest in normothermic cats, the electroencephalogram and evoked potentials recovered when intracardiac massage resulted in normal blood pressure, but recovery failed when hypotension persisted during resuscitation (59).

Therapy

The multifactorial pathogenesis of no-reflow requires a multifaceted therapy that becomes more complex the longer ischemia and, in consequence, the more severe the no-reflow phenomenon (33). The most important component of this therapy is the control of postischemic blood pressure. Fischer et al (25) were able to prevent no-reflow in the rabbit after ischemia of up to 30 minutes by raising mean arterial blood pressure (MABP) to 110 mm Hg. Ito et al (62) treated no-reflow successfully in gerbils after 1-hour bilateral and 6-hour unilateral occlusion by increasing pressure above 120 mm Hg. A beneficial effect of hypertension has also been reported by various other authors (28, 54, 62). There are, however, different opinions about the effect of hypertension on survival after ischemia. Harrison et al (42) reported that hypertension prevented no-reflow after 30 minutes of bilateral occlusion in gerbils, but this did not improve postischemic mortality. On the other hand, we and others established a close relationship between prevention of no-reflow and the functional recovery process (51, 61, 89, 98). The reason for this discrepancy may be the fact that blood recirculation induces secondary disturbances that have to be treated as well. In particular, successful recirculation causes an abrupt swelling of the brain and a release of acid equivalents into the circulating blood (48, 49). The former interferes with CBF by reducing the tissue perfusion pressure, and the latter by counteracting the drug-induced blood pressure increase. For this reason, osmotic dehydration and rapid adjustment of the acid–base state of the blood are also required.

A common complication of cerebral ischemia is intravascular disseminated coagulation (52). Therefore, anticoagulation or fibrinolysis have been recommended for improving postischemic recirculation. The results of the therapy are equivocal (14, 84, 96), which is not surprising because only a minor fraction of the coagula are trapped in the cerebral circulation (60). However, prevention of coagulopathy may reduce extracerebral complications and, for this reason, may indirectly ameliorate postischemic brain damage. One of these complications is ischemia-induced pulmonary distress which has to be treated by careful control of postischemic ventilation (52).

In our laboratory, the following regimen is routinely used to minimize no-reflow after 60 minutes of complete cerebral-circulatory arrest in cats and monkeys. Five minutes before reperfusion, infusion of 20% sorbitol or mannitol (1 g/kg) and 8.4% sodium bicarbonate (3.3 mEq/kg) is started at a rate of 0.05 g/kg/minute and 0.17 mEq/kg/minute, respectively. Immediately before reperfusion, catecholamines (dopamine or norepinephrine) are infused at a rate of approximately 1 mg/minute until systolic arterial blood pressure rises to between 180 and 200 mm Hg. At this moment, recirculation is started, and infusion speed of catecholamines is reduced to maintain an MABP of about 150 mm Hg for at least 30 minutes. In addition, postischemic intravascular coagulopathy is reduced by injection of heparin (250 to 500 U), and severe ischemic or postischemic hyperglycemia by injection of insulin (1 to 2 U).

With this treatment, the initial recirculation rate after 1 hour of complete ischemia is between 20 and 40 ml/100 g/minute in 50% of experiments and above 40 ml/100 g/minute in 24% of experiments. In 26%, initial recirculation rate is less than 20 ml/100 g/minute, and it is only in these animals that functional recovery is poor (51). The development of a no-reflow phenomenon, consequently, is clearly associated with a failure of postischemic recovery. In the animals without no-reflow, on the other hand, postischemic reactive hyperemia develops after a brief interval, followed by progressive metabolic and functional recovery (49). Prevention of no-reflow thus promotes postischemic recovery even after complete cerebral-circulatory arrest of as long as 1 hour.

DELAYED POSTISCHEMIC HYPOPERFUSION

The phenomenon of delayed postischemic hypoperfusion was first described in our laboratory after a prolonged complete cerebral ischemia in cats (55), and is now widely considered to be another important pathogenetic factor of postischemic injury (Fig. 3.3). Postischemic hypoperfusion differs fundamentally from the no-reflow phenomenon, although it may be difficult to differentiate between the two processes in a particular experimental situation. In its purest form hypoperfusion develops after a transient phase of reactive hyperemia, that is, in the absence of any early postischemic recirculation disturbances. It has been observed after focal ischemia (106, 120), incomplete (118, 125) or complete (55, 73, 112) global cerebral ischemia, and cardiac arrest (82, 126). Like no-reflow, hypoperfusion appears only if ischemia exceeds a

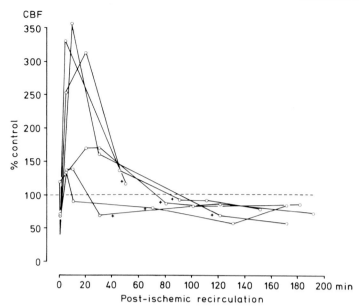

Figure 3.3. Postischemic hypoperfusion of cats submitted to 30 minutes of global cerebral ischemia. Cerebral blood flow (CBF) was measured after various recirculation times by the intraarterial xenon-133 clearance technique, and was expressed as percent of preischemic control values. After ischemia, CBF transiently increases (postischemic reactive hyperemia) but then declines below control level (postischemic hypoperfusion). Note that the beginning of spontaneous electroencephalograph activity is marked by *crosses*. (From Hossmann K-A, Lechtape-Grüter H, Hossmann V: The role of cerebral blood flow for the recovery of the brain after prolonged ischemia. *Z Neurol* 204:281–299, 1973.)

minimum duration of approximately 5 minutes (12, 82), but, in contrast, it does not increase with the duration of ischemia and does not diminish after incomplete cerebral-circulatory arrest. In fact, either 5 minutes of near-complete ischemia in gerbils (12) or 15 minutes of incomplete ischemia in rats (66) produced postischemic hypoperfusion with flow rates of less than 50% of control. In cats and monkeys, postischemic hypoperfusion seems to be slightly less severe than in rats or gerbils, particularly after ischemia of more than 30 minutes' duration (55, 58). This is surprising because after such a long duration of ischemia, the risk of no-reflow is very high.

In contrast to the severity of hypoperfusion, the temporal profile of its appearance clearly correlates with the duration of ischemia: the longer the ischemia, the later the onset of hypoperfusion. This is due to the fact that hypoperfusion is preceded by a phase of hyperemia, the duration of which increases with increasing ischemia time (55, 130). After 5 minutes of ischemia, hyper-

emia lasts only a few minutes, and postischemic hypoperfusion is present already after 10 minutes of recirculation (116). Following 30 minutes and 60 minutes of ischemia, the onset of hypoperfusion is delayed to about 45 and 90 minutes, respectively (55), and the disturbance may last as long as several days (104).

The phenomenon of delayed hypoperfusion is not restricted to ischemia alone. A similar biphasic pattern of hyperemia followed by long-lasting hypoperfusion has been described after spreading depression (79), hypoglycemia (109), and thiamine deficiency (38). Persisting hypoperfusion without preceding hyperemia occurs after subarachnoid hemorrhage (SAH) (68) and shock (18), but it is not clear whether the pathogenetic mechanism of this impairment is comparable to postischemic hypoperfusion.

Pathophysiology

In contrast to the no-reflow phenomenon that results from an obstruction of microcirculation at the capillary level, postischemic hypoperfusion is a functional process due to an increased arterial–arteriolar vascular tone. This conclusion is based on various lines of evidence. In vivo microscopy of pial arteries during and after ischemia revealed that postischemic vasodilation, which prevails during reactive hyperemia, is followed by a decrease of vascular diameter when postischemic hypoperfusion begins to develop (43, 117). The cerebral vascular system, in consequence, is not congested as during microcirculatory obstruction (44). Impairment of microcirculation by postischemic edema, as discussed in connection with the development of no-reflow, does not seem to be a pathogenetic factor either. To the contrary, postischemic edema reaches its maximum during postischemic reactive hyperemia, but it disappears when postischemic hypoperfusion becomes prominent (48). This has been demonstrated in several studies by measuring the content of brain water (131), specific gravity (119), or blood–brain barrier permeability to circulating macromolecules (116, 119), all of which are normal at the onset of postischemic hypoperfusion. Similarly, intracranial pressure, which is a function of brain edema and may reach very high levels immediately after the beginning of recirculation, normalizes before hypoperfusion develops (132). Finally, electrophysiologic function of the brain begins to recover before the onset of hypoperfusion, indicating that it begins to develop after energy state and ion homeostasis have recovered (55).

In order to determine the localization of the increased vascular tone, micropressure recordings in pial arteries have been carried out (103). This technique allows the measurement of segmental vascular resistance and, consequently, the differentiation between intracerebral (parenchymal) and extracerebral (supplying) arteries. It turned out that the resistance of intracerebral and extracerebral arteries increases to the same extent, suggesting that postischemic hypoperfusion is the result of a generalized vasospasm of the entire vascular system. This conclusion is confirmed by angiography (55) which revealed not only narrowing of intracerebral vessels,

but also a substantial constriction of the extracerebral supplying arteries, such as the carotid and vertebral arteries.

The increased vascular tone of the intracerebral and extracerebral vascular bed is associated with a peculiar disturbance of the regulation of blood flow which may also explain the transition of reactive hyperemia to hypoperfusion. During reactive hyperemia the cerebral vascular bed is paralyzed, and vascular tone does not respond to either changes in blood pressure or arterial carbon dioxide (CO_2) (78). Autoregulation and CO_2 reactivity are therefore completely abolished. This type of regulation disturbance changes when reactive hyperemia ceases and postischemic hypoperfusion begins to develop. At this time autoregulation but not CO_2 reactivity begins to recover (55, 111) and CBF stabilizes at a subnormal level (Fig. 3.4). A similar disturbance of vascular reactivity has also been observed during delayed hypoperfusion induced by other pathologic processes, such as spreading depression (123) or SAH (68, 91), indicating that these processes may share a common pathogenetic mechanism.

The reason for the dissociation between autoregulation and CO_2 reactivity is still unclear. Some of the therapeutic studies discussed below suggest that either an imbalance of the equilibrium between thromboxane A_2 (TXA_2) and prostacyclin (PGI_2) (99) or the calcium-mediated processes (127) may be involved, but these conclusions are disputed. It has also been considered that postischemic activation of the central sympathetic system may cause the release of excessive amounts of norepinephrine, but this hypothesis was refuted by demonstrating that neither preischemic lesions of the locus ceruleus (11) nor the application of sympatholytic agents (55, 117) are able to relieve the vascular spasms.

Recently, adhesions to the vascular wall of formed blood cell elements, in particular platelets and neutrophilic granulocytes, have been discussed as a contributing factor to flow impairment (5, 36, 105). Such adhesions may be induced by conformational changes of the luminal side of endothelial cells that result in the formation of regular arrays of microvilli (22). A major

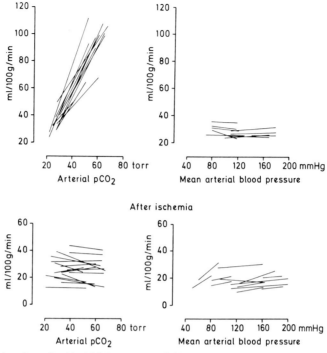

Figure 3.4. Arterial carbon dioxide (CO_2) reactivity *(left)* and autoregulation *(right)* of cerebral blood flow before and after 60 minutes of global cerebral ischemia in cats. CO_2 reactivity was tested by increasing arterial PCO_2 with CO_2 added to the inspired air, and autoregulation was tested by increasing blood pressure with intravenous infusion of catecholamines. After ischemia, CO_2 reactivity is completely abolished but autoregulation is preserved over a range from 80 to 200 mm Hg. (From Hossmann K-A, Lechtape-Grüter H, Hossmann V: The role of cerebral blood flow for the recovery of the brain after prolonged ischemia. *Z Neurol* 204:281–299, 1973.)

pathogenetic role of platelet adhesion, however, can be dismissed. By pre-ischemic labeling of platelets, intravascular accumulation could be demonstrated during the early recirculation period, but platelets disappeared from the cerebral vasculature before postischemic hypoperfusion became manifest (60). It has not been established whether granulocytes behave in a similar way, but even reversible adhesions to the vascular wall may produce long-lasting effects because granulocytes are known to trigger the generation of hydroxyl radicals that may interfere directly or indirectly with the reactivity of the vascular system (21). An argument in favor of this hypothesis is the slight but significant improvement of hypoperfusion after preischemic depletion of neutrophilic granulocytes with antineutrophilic serum (5, 36) On the other hand, neither the

production of oxygen radicals with the xanthine–xanthine oxidase system nor production of hydroxyl radicals with hydrogen peroxide and ferrous sulfate is able to produce prolonged vasospasm (124). The role of free radicals, therefore, remains to be clarified.

The pathophysiologic significance of postischemic hypoperfusion for the supply of nutrients to the brain is also unclear and has been controversial in the past. In some situations, the decrease of CBF is apparently coupled to a parallel decrease of glucose and oxygen consumption which suggests that the reduction in flow accompanies a primarily metabolic lesion of the brain (7, 101). In other experimental conditions, CBF and metabolic rate of the brain are dissociated, and secondary tissue hypoxia may ensue (Fig. 3.5) (50, 80). Therefore, it is impossible to decide at the pres-

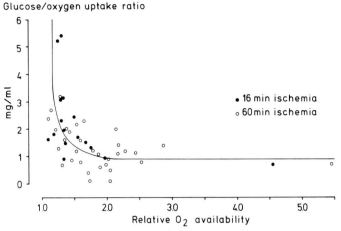

Figure 3.5. Dependency of the cerebral glucose/oxygen uptake ratio from relative tissue oxygen availability during postischemic hypoperfusion following 16 minutes *(closed circles)* or 60 minutes *(open circles)* of global cerebral ischemia. The glucose/oxygen uptake ratio was determined from arterial cerebral venous differences, and the relative oxygen availability by relating absolute oxygen availability to oxygen consumption. Note the sharp increase of the glucose/oxygen uptake ratio with declining relative oxygen availability, indicating that anaerobic glucose utilization is stimulated when postischemic oxygen availability does not match the oxygen requirements of the brain. Relative oxygen availability decreases as a function of postischemic hypoperfusion and is independent of the duration of ischemia. (From Hossmann K-A: Cerebral dysfunction related to local and global ischemia of the brain. In Hoffmeister F, Müller C (eds): *Brain Function in Old Age. Evaluation of Changes and Disorders.* Berlin, Springer-Verlag, 1979, pp 385–393.)

ent time if postischemic hypoperfusion is an epiphenomenon or a pathogenetic factor on its own. However, it is very unlikely that without adequate control of CBF any other therapeutic approach for improving postischemic recovery will be successful. Adequate treatment of postischemic hypoperfusion, in consequence, is of greatest importance regardless of the causal relationship between ischemic injury and flow impairment.

Therapy

In principle, postischemic hypoperfusion and the resulting metabolic disturbances can be ameliorated by reducing vascular tone, improving the rheologic properties of the blood, and reducing the oxygen and glucose requirements of the tissue. All these approaches have been explored, although with remarkably little success. The following is a brief account of the more important investigations in this field.

Reduction of vascular tone has been at-tempted pharmacologically and by interfering with the molecular processes resulting in vascular spasm. For the former purpose, so-called vasoactive drugs have been tested such as papaverine, aminophylline, Hydergine (ergoloid mesylates, Sandoz Pharmaceuticals, East Hanover, NJ), or PGI_2 (55, 70). In addition, antiserotoninergic and various α-adrenergic blocking and β-adrenergic stimulating agents were used (55, 117). It appears that vascular tone can, in fact, be slightly reduced with these drugs, but even with intracarotid infusion this effect is only achieved at a dose that causes peripheral vasodilation and thus a drop in blood pressure. The relief of vascular tone is counteracted by the reduction in cerebral perfusion pressure, and the net effect on CBF is almost nil.

Relief of increased vascular tone has also been attempted by interfering with the equilibrium between TXA_2 and PGI_2. TXA_2 is synthesized by platelets and is a potent vasoconstrictor, whereas PGI_2, which is synthesized in the vascular wall, has a vasodilating effect. CBF can therefore be expected to improve when TXA_2 synthesis is inhibited or PGI_2 is increased. However, neither PGI_2 infusion (70), nor the specific inhibition of TXA_2 synthesis (100) was able to improve postischemic hypoperfusion. Inhibiting TXA_2 synthesis with a less specific agent, ibuprofen, reversed postischemic hypoperfusion, suggesting that other eicosanoid metabolites may be involved (35). The identity of these metabolites, however, has not been determined and it is not known whether the increase of flow is associated with an improvement of function.

Another interesting approach for treating postischemic hypoperfusion is the application of calcium antagonists because increased calcium fluxes are thought to contribute to ischemic brain injury (23, 108). The results are equivocal. Following global ischemia in dogs for a duration of 10 to 20 minutes, the calcium antagonists nimodipine and lidoflazine were able to improve postischemic hypoperfusion (102, 127), but in cats submitted to 1 hour of global ischemia, flunarizine did not have any beneficial effect (56). Moreover, different opinions also exist about the functional significance of this approach. Steen et al (113) reported an improvement of neurologic function, but Sakabe et al (102) and Smith et al (110) did not observe such an effect, even though mean CBF increased. The latter authors also noted that after therapy, CBF was extremely inhomogeneous with areas of hyperemia and hypoemia in close vicinity suggesting that the increase of flow is not nutritive (110).

The only way to increase CBF despite persistently high vascular tone is to decrease blood viscosity. Several authors have used isovolemic hemodilution for this purpose (16, 34, 53, 84), but the metabolic rate of oxygen or the functional recovery does not substantially improve because the oxygen-carrying capacity of the blood decreases as much as flow improves (71). A more promising approach may be hemodilution with fluorocarbons (129).

In view of these unsatisfactory results, attempts have been made to ameliorate the effects of reduced oxygen supply by either reducing the oxygen consumption of the tissue or preventing mitochondrial damage (86). Oxygen consumption was lowered by hypothermia (71) or by a high dose of barbiturates (9, 32, 71), and the mitochondrial respiratory efficiency by the use of calcium antagonists (94). The latter approach was attempted under the assumption that postischemic flooding of the cytosol with calcium may direct the mitochondrial respiratory capacity to the sequestration of calcium rather than the synthesis of adenosine triphosphate (26).

The reported data are equivocal and require further analysis. Barbiturates at first seemed to ameliorate postischemic brain damage (9), but when tested again, they failed to reduce the misrelationship between oxygen delivery and oxygen consumption (71) and did not improve functional recovery (32). Hypothermia is protective when initiated before (128) or during ischemia (13) but fails to improve the misrelationship between oxygen supply and oxygen consumption during postischemic recirculation (71). Calcium antagonists may improve ischemic injury in the selectively vulnerable regions (1, 20), but they seem to be without effect in other parts of the brain in which postischemic hypoperfusion develops as well. The therapeutic problem of treating postischemic hypoperfusion, in consequence, remains unsolved and requires further investigation.

PERSPECTIVE

The analysis of the hemodynamics of resuscitation has led to the differentiation between two forms of postischemic flow disturbances: the no-reflow phenomenon and the postischemic hypoperfusion syndrome. The no-reflow phenomenon is clearly a limiting factor for postischemic resuscitation, and its successful prevention results in the restitution of complex biochemical and electrophysiologic functions after complete cerebral-circulatory arrest of as long as 1 hour.

The pathophysiologic role of postischemic hypoperfusion, in contrast, is less clear. Despite extensive experimentation, it has not been established if postischemic hypoperfusion is an epiphenomenon of postischemic brain injury or a pathogenetic factor on its own. At present, no reliable therapeutic procedure is available to prevent the development of postischemic hypoperfusion. Therefore, it is not known if postischemic recovery will improve in the absence of hypoperfusion. However, in awaiting clarification of this question, postischemic hypoperfusion should be considered as a potentially harmful complication that is likely to aggravate all other postischemic disturbances that may interfere with tissue oxygenation, such as postischemic respiratory distress, postischemic coagulopathy or postischemic brain edema. Similarly, the analysis of molecular events leading to ischemic brain damage should always consider the possibility of additional hemodynamic disturbances that may interfere with the pathologic process and therefore may further impair the ultimate postischemic outcome.

References

1. Alps BJ, Hass WK: The potential beneficial effect of nicardipine in a rat model of transient forebrain ischemia. *Neurology* 37:809–814, 1987.

2. Ames A III: Incidence and significance of vascular occlusion in focal and diffuse ischemia. In Langfitt TW, McHenry LC Jr, Reivich M, et al (eds): *Cerebral Circulation and Metabolism.* New York, Springer-Verlag, 1975, pp 551–554.

3. Ames A III, Gurian BS: Effects of glucose and oxygen deprivation on function of isolated mammalian retina. *J Neurophysiol* 26:617–634, 1963.

4. Ames A III, Wright RL, Kowada M, et al: Cerebral ischemia. II. The no-reflow phenomenon. *Am J Pathol* 52:437–453, 1968.

5. Arfors K, Grögaard B, Gerdin B: Neutrophils and delayed hypoperfusion in cerebral cortex after cerebral ischemia in the rat (abstract). *Fed Proc* 45:1156, 1986.

6. Arsenio-Nunes ML, Hossmann K-A, Farkas-Bargeton E: Ultrastructural and histochemical investigation of the cerebral cortex of cat during and after complete ischemia. *Acta Neuropathol (Berl)* 26:329–344, 1973.

7. Beckstead JE, Tweed WA, Lee J, et al: Cerebral blood flow and metabolism in man following cardiac arrest. *Stroke* 9:569–573, 1978.

8. Bircher N, Safar P, Stewart R: A comparison of standard "mast"-augmented and open-chest CPR in dogs. *Crit Care Med* 8:147–152, 1980.

9. Bleyaert Al, Nemoto EM, Safar P, et al: Thiopental amelioration of brain damage after global ischemia in monkeys. *Anesthesiology* 49:390–398, 1978.

10. Blinkov SM, Larina VN, Putsillo MV: Experimental study of cerebral microcirculatory bed. Communication I. Perfusion of the cerebral vasculo-

11. Blomqvist P, Lindvall O, Wieloch T: Delayed postischemic hypoperfusion: Evidence against involvement of the noradrenergic locus ceruleus system. *J Cereb Blood Flow Metab* 4:425–429, 1984.

12. Blomqvist P, Wieloch T: Ischemic brain damage in rats following cardiac arrest using a long-term recovery model. *J Cereb Blood Flow Metab* 5:420–431, 1985.

13. Busto R, Dietrich WD, Globus MYT, et al: Small differences in intraischemic brain temperature critically determine the extent of ischemic neuronal injury. *J Cereb Blood Flow Metab* 7:729–738, 1987.

14. Cantu RC, Ames A III: Distribution of vascular lesions caused by cerebral ischemia. Relation to survival. *Neurology* 19:128–132, 1969.

15. Cantu RC, Snyder M: Effect of anticoagulants, vasodilators, and dipyridamole on postischemic cerebral vascular obstruction. *J Surg Res* 2:70–71, 1972.

16. Chan R, Leniger-Follert E: Effect of isovolemic hemodilution on oxygen supply and electrocorticogram in cat brain during focal ischemia and in normal tissue. *Int J Microcirc Clin Exp* 2:297–313, 1983.

17. Chiang J, Kowada M, Ames A III, et al: Cerebral ischemia. III. Vascular changes. *Am J Pathol* 52:455–476, 1968.

18. Christenson JT, Kuikka JT, Owunwanne A, et al: Cerebral circulation during endotoxic shock with special emphasis on the regional cerebral blood flow in vivo. *Nucl Med Commun* 7:531–540, 1986.

19. Crowell JW, Smith EE: Effect of fibrinolytic activation on survival and cerebral damage following periods of circulatory arrest. *Am J Physiol* 186:283–285, 1956.

20. Desphande JK, Wieloch T: Flunarizine, a calcium entry blocker, ameliorates ischemic brain damage in the rat. *Anesthesiology* 64:215–224, 1986.

21. Diener AM, Beatty PG, Ochs HD, et al: The role of neutrophil membrane glycoprotein 150 (GP-150) in neutrophil-mediated endothelial cell injury in vitro. *J Immunol* 135:537–543, 1985.

22. Dietrich WD, Busto R, Ginsberg MD: Cerebral endothelial microvilli: Formation following global forebrain ischemia. *J Neuropathol Exp Neurol* 43:72–83, 1984.

23. Farber JI: The role of calcium in cell death. *Life Sci* 29:1289–1295, 1981.

24. Fischer EG, Ames A III, Hedley-Whyte ET, et al: Reassessment of cerebral capillary changes in acute global ischemia and their relationship to the "no-reflow phenomenon." *Stroke* 8:36–39, 1977.

25. Fischer EG, Ames A III, Lorenzo AV: Cerebral blood flow immediately following brief circulatory stasis. *Stroke* 10:423–427, 1979.

26. Fiskum G: Involvement of mitochondria in ischemic cell injury and in regulation of intracellular calcium. *Am J Emerg Med* 2:147–153, 1983.

27. Gaehtgens P, Marx P: Hemorheological aspects of the pathophysiology of cerebral ischemia. *J Cereb Blood Flow Metab* 7:259–265, 1987.

28. Gänshirt H, Zylka W: Überlebenszeit, Erholungslatenz und Elektrocorticogram des Warmblü-

capillary network after circulatory arrest. *Zh Vopr Neirokhir* 1:38–42, 1981.

tergehirns in ihrer Abhängigkeit vom Blutdruck. *Pflügers Arch* 256:181–194, 1952.

29. Gavin JB, Humphrey SM, Herdson PB: The no-reflow phenomenon in ischemic myocardium. *Int Rev Exp Pathol* 25:361–383, 1983.

30. Ginsberg MD, Budd WW, Welsh FA: Diffuse cerebral ischemia in the cat: I. Local blood flow during severe ischemia and recirculation. *Ann Neurol* 3:482–492, 1978.

31. Ginsberg MD, Myers RE: The topography of impaired microvascular perfusion in the primate brain following total circulatory arrest. *Neurology* 22:998–1011, 1972.

32. Gisvold SE, Safar P, Hendrickx HH, et al: Thiopental treatment after global brain ischemia in pigtailed monkeys. *Anesthesiology* 60:88–96, 1984.

33. Gisvold SE, Safar P, Rao G, et al: Multifaceted therapy after global brain ischemia in monkeys. *Stroke* 5:803–812, 1984.

34. Gottstein U: Evaluation of isovolemic hemodilution. *Clin Hemorheol* 4:133–149, 1984.

35. Grice SC, Chappel ET, Prough DS, et al: Ibuprofen improves cerebral blood flow after global cerebral ischemia in dogs. *Stroke* 18:787–791, 1987.

36. Grögaard B, Schürer L, Gerdin B, et al: The role of polymorphonuclear leukocytes in postischemic delayed hypoperfusion. In Novelli GP, Ursini F (eds): *Oxygen Free Radicals in Shock*. Basel, Karger, 1986, pp 74–78.

37. Gurvitch AM, Blinkov SM, Valanchute AL, et al: Types of no-reflow phenomenon observed during arrest of cerebral circulation and postischemic period. *Crit Care Med* 4:132–135, 1976.

38. Hakim AM: Effect of thiamine deficiency and its reversal on cerebral blood flow in the rat. Observations on the phenomena of hyperperfusion, "no reflow," and delayed hypoperfusion. *J Cereb Blood Flow Metabol* 6:79–85, 1986.

39. Hallenbeck JM, Furlow TW Jr: Influence of several plasma fractions on post-ischemic microvascular reperfusion in the central nervous system. *Stroke* 9:375–382, 1978.

40. Hallenbeck JM, Furlow TW Jr: Influence of factor VIII/von Willebrand factor protein (F VIII/vWF) and F VIII/vWF-poor cryoprecipitate on post-ischemic microvascular reperfusion in the central nervous system. *Stroke* 12:93–97, 1981.

41. Harman JW: The significance of local vascular phenomena in the production of ischemic necrosis in skeletal muscle. *Am J Pathol* 24:625–641, 1948.

42. Harrison MJG, Sedal L, Arnold J, et al: No-reflow phenomenon in the cerebral circulation of the gerbil. *J Neurol Neurosurg Psychiatry* 38:1190–1193, 1975.

43. Hart MN, Sokoll MD, Davies LR, et al: Vascular spasm in cat cerebral cortex following ischemia. *Stroke* 9:52–57, 1978.

44. Hekmatpanah J: Cerebral blood flow dynamics in hypotension and cardiac arrest. *Neurology* 23:174–180, 1973.

45. Hirsch H, Breuer M, Künzel HP, et al: Über die Bildung von Thrombocytenaggregaten und die Änderung des Hämatokrits durch komplette Gehirnischämie. *Dtsch Z Nervenheil* 186:58–66, 1964.

46. Hirsch H, Schneider M: Überlebens-, Erholungs- und Wiederbelebungszeit des Gehirns bei Normo-

und Hypothermie. In Olivecrona H, Tönnis W (eds): *Handbuch der Neurochirurgie*. Berlin, Springer-Verlag, 1968, pp 509–552.

47. Hossmann K-A: Cortical steady potential, impedance and excitability changes during and after total ischemia of cat brain. *Exp Neurol* 32:163–175, 1971.

48. Hossmann K-A: Development and resolution of ischemic brain swelling. In Pappius HM, Feindel W (eds): *Dynamics of Brain Edema*. Berlin, Springer-Verlag, 1976, pp 219–227.

49. Hossmann K-A: Total ischemia of the brain. In Zülch KJ, Kaufman W, Hossmann K-A, et al (eds): *Brain and Heart Infarct*. Berlin, Springer-Verlag, 1977, pp 1–124.

50. Hossmann K-A: Cerebral dysfunction related to local and global ischemia of the brain. In Hoffmeister F, Müller C (eds): *Brain Function in Old Age. Evaluation of Changes and Disorders*. Berlin, Springer-Verlag, 1979, pp 385–393.

51. Hossmann K-A: Resuscitation potentials after prolonged cerebral ischemia in cats. *Crit Care Med* 16:964–971, 1988.

52. Hossmann K-A, Hossmann V: Coagulopathy following experimental cerebral ischemia. *Stroke* 8:249–254, 1977.

53. Hossmann K-A, Kerckhoff W van den, Matsuoka Y: Treatment of cerebral ischemia by hemodilution. *Bibl Haematol* 47:77–85, 1981.

54. Hossmann K-A, Kleihues P: Reversibility of ischemic brain damage. *Arch Neurol* 29:375–384, 1973.

55. Hossmann K-A, Lechtape-Grüter H, Hossmann V: The role of cerebral blood flow for the recovery of the brain after prolonged ischemia. *Z Neurol* 204:281–299, 1973.

56. Hossmann K-A, Paschen W, Csiba L: Relationship between calcium accumulation and recovery of cat brain after prolonged cerebral ischemia. *J Cereb Blood Flow Metab* 3:346–353, 1983.

57. Hossmann K-A, Sakaki S, Zimmerman V: Cation activities in reversible ischemia of the cat brain. *Stroke* 8:77–81, 1977.

58. Hossmann K-A, Zimmerman V: Resuscitation of the monkey brain after 1 hour complete ischemia. I. Physiological and morphological observations. *Brain Res* 81:59–74, 1974.

59. Hossmann V, Hossmann K-A: Return of neuronal function after prolonged cardiac arrest. *Brain Res* 60:423–438, 1973.

60. Hossmann V, Hossmann K-A, Takagi S: Effect of intravascular platelet aggregation on blood recirculation following prolonged ischemia of the cat brain. *J Neurol* 222:159–170, 1980.

61. Ianotti F, Hoff J: Ischemic brain edema with and without reperfusion: An experimental study in gerbils. *Stroke* 14:562–567, 1983.

62. Ito U, Ohno K, Yamaguchi T, et al: Transient appearance of "no-reflow" phenomenon in Mongolian gerbils. *Stroke* 11:517–521, 1980.

63. Jamison RL: The role of cellular swelling in the pathogenesis of organ ischemia. *West J Med* 120:205–218, 1974.

64. Jennings RB, Sommers HM, Kaltenbach JP, et al: Electrolyte alterations in acute myocardial ischemic injury. *Circ Res* 14:260–269, 1964.

65. Kågström E, Smith M-L, Siesjö BK: Local cerebral

blood flow in the recovery period following complete cerebral ischemia in the rat. *J Cereb Blood Flow Metab* 3:170–182, 1983.

66. Kågström E, Smith M-L, Siesjö BK: Recirculation in the rat brain following incomplete ischemia. *J Cereb Blood flow Metab* 3:183–192, 1983.

67. Kamijyo Y, Garcia JH, Cooper J: Temporary regional cerebral ischemia in the cat. A model of hemorrhagic and subcortical infarction. *J Neuropathol Exp Neurol* 36:338–350, 1977.

68. Kamiya K, Kuyama H, Symon L: An experimental study of the acute stage of subarachnoid hemorrhage. *J Neurosurg* 59:917–924, 1983.

69. Kee DB Jr, Wood JH: Rheology of the cerebral circulation. *Neurosurgery* 15:125–131, 1984.

70. Kerckhoff W van den, Hossmann K-A, Hossmann V: No effect of prostacyclin on blood flow, regulation of blood flow and blood coagulation following global cerebral ischemia. *Stroke* 14:724–730, 1983.

71. Kerckhoff W van den, Matsuoka Y, Paschen W, et al: Influence of barbiturates, hypothermia and hemodilution on post-ischemic metabolism and functional recovery following cerebrocirculatory arrest in cats. In Spatz M, Mrsulja BB, Rakic LJ, et al (eds): *Circulatory and Developmental Aspects of Brain Metabolism.* New York, Plenum, 1980, pp 103–122.

72. Kloner RA, Ganote CE, Jennings RB: The "no-reflow" phenomenon after temporary coronary occlusion in the dog. *J Clin Invest* 54:1496–1508, 1974.

73. Koch KA, Jackson DL, Schmiedl M, et al: Total cerebral ischemia: Effect of alterations in arterial PCO_2 on cerebral microcirculation. *J Cereb Blood Flow Metab* 4:343–349, 1984.

74. Kovács K, Carroll R, Tapp E: Temporary ischemia of the adrenal gland. *J Pathol Bacteriol* 91:235–240, 1966.

75. Kowada M, Ames A III, Majno G, et al: Cerebral ischemia. I. An improved experimental method for study: Cardiovascular effects and demonstration of an early lesion in the rabbit. *J Neurosurg* 28:150–157, 1968.

76. Krug A, de Rochemont W, Korb G: Blood supply of the myocardium after temporary coronary occlusion. *Circ Res* 19:57–62, 1966.

77. Kuschinsky W, Wahl M, Bosse O, et al: Perivascular potassium and pH as determinants of local pial arterial diameter in cats. A microapplication study. *Circ Res* 31:240–247, 1972.

78. Lassen NA: The luxury-perfusion syndrome and its possible relation to acute metabolic acidosis localized within the brain. *Lancet* 2:1113–1115, 1966.

79. Lauritzen M, Jorgensen MB, Diemer NH, et al: Persistent oligemia of rat cerebral cortex in the wake of spreading depression. *Ann Neurol* 12:469–474, 1982.

80. Levy DE, Pike CL, Uitert RL van: Delayed dissociation of cerebral blood flow and metabolism following stroke in gerbils. *Neurology* 28:378–379, 1978.

81. Levy DE, Uitert RL van, Pike CL: Delayed postischemic hypoperfusion: A potentially damaging consequence of stroke. *Neurology* 29:1245–1252, 1979.

82. Lin S-R: Angiographic studies of cerebral circulation following various periods of cardiac arrest. A preliminary study in the dog. *Invest Radiol* 9:374–385, 1974.

83. Lin, S-R: Cerebral circulation after cardiac arrest. Angiographic and carbon black perfusion studies. *Radiology* 117:627–632, 1975.

84. Lin S-R: The effect of dextran and streptokinase on cerebral function and blood flow after cardiac arrest. An experimental study on the dog. *Neuroradiology* 16:340–342, 1978.

85. Lin S-R, Kormano M: Cerebral circulation after cardiac arrest. Microangiographic and protein tracer studies. *Stroke* 8:182–188, 1977.

86. Linn F, Paschen W, Grosse-Ophoff B, et al: Mitochondrial respiration during recirculation after prolonged ischemia in cat brain. *Exp Neurol* 96:321–333, 1987.

87. Little JR, Kerr FWL, Sundt TM: Microcirculatory obstruction in focal cerebral ischemia. Relationship to neuronal alterations. *Mayo Clinic Proc* 50:264–270, 1975.

88. Little JR, Kerr FWL, Sundt TM: Microcirculatory obstruction in focal cerebral ischemia: An electron microscopic investigation in monkeys. *Stroke* 7:25–30, 1976.

89. Marcy VR, Welsh FA: Correlation between cerebral blood flow and ATP content following tourniquet-induced ischemia in cat brain. *J Cereb Blood Flow Metab* 4:362–367, 1984.

90. Marshall LF, Durity F, Lounsbury R, et al: Experimental cerebral oligemia and ischemia produced by intracranial hypertension. Part 1: Pathophysiology, electroencephalography, cerebral blood flow, blood–brain barrier, and neurological function. *J Neurosurg* 43:308–317, 1975.

91. Mendelow AD, McCalden TA, Hattingh J, et al: Cerebrovascular reactivity and metabolism after subarachnoid hemorrhage in baboons. *Stroke* 12:58–65, 1981.

92. Neely WA, Youmans JR: Anoxia of canine brain without damage. *JAMA* 183:1085–1087, 1963.

93. Norwood WI, Norwood CR, Castaneda AR: Cerebral anoxia: Effect of deep hypothermia and pH. *Surgery* 86:203–209, 1979.

94. Nowicki JP, MacKenzie ET, Young AR: Brain ischemia, calcium and calcium antagonists. *Pathol Biol* 30:282–288, 1982.

95. Obrenovitch TP, Hallenbeck JM: Platelet accumulation in regions of low blood flow during the postischemic period. *Stroke* 16:224–234, 1985.

96. O'Connor M, Lin S-R, King A, et al: Evaluation of therapeutic mechanisms of plasma expander and fibrinolytic agent following cardiac arrest. Experimental study on the dog (abstract). *Microvasc Res* 17:S166, 1979.

97. Ogata J, Fujishima M, Tamaki K, et al: An ultrastructural study of developing cerebral infarction following bilateral carotid artery occlusion in spontaneously hypertensive rats. *Acta Neuropathol (Berl)* 40:171–177, 1977.

98. Osburne RC, Halsey JH Jr: Cerebral blood flow. A predictor of recovery from ischemia in the gerbil. *Arch Neurol* 32:457–461, 1975.

99. Pickard J, Tamura A, Stewart M, et al: Prostacyclin, indomethacin and the cerebral circulation. *Brain Res* 197:425–431, 1980.

100. Prough DS, Kong D, Watkins WD, et al: Inhibition of thromboxane A_2 production does not improve post-ischemic brain hypoperfusion in the dog. *Stroke* 17:1272–1276, 1986.

101. Pulsinelli WA, Levy DE, Duffy TE: Regional blood flow and metabolism in postischemic brain (abstract). *Stroke* 11:126, 1980.

102. Sakabe T, Nagai I, Ishikawa T, et al: Nicardipine increases cerebral blood flow but does not improve neurologic recovery in a canine model of complete cerebral ischemia. *J Cereb Blood Flow Metab* 6:684–690, 1986.

103. Schmidt-Kastner R, Hossmann K-A, Grosse-Ophoff B: Pial artery pressure after one hour of global ischemia. *J Cereb Blood Flow Metab* 7:109–117, 1987.

104. Schmidt-Kastner R, Grosse-Ophoff B, Hossmann K-A: Delayed recovery of CO_2 reactivity after one hour's complete ischaemia of cat brain. *J Neurol* 233:367–369, 1986.

105. Schmidt-Schönbein GW: Capillary plugging by granulocytes and the no-reflow phenomenon in the microcirculation. *Fed Proc* 46:2397–2401, 1987.

106. Shigeno T, Teasdale GM, McCulloch J, et al: Recirculation model following MCA occlusion in rats. Cerebral blood flow, cerebrovascular permeability, and brain edema. *J Neurosurg* 63:272–277, 1985.

107. Siemkowicz E: Cerebrovascular resistance in ischemia. *Pflügers Arch* 388:243–247, 1980.

108. Siesjö BK: Calcium and ischemic brain damage. *Eur Neurol* 25:45–56, 1986.

109. Siesjö BK, Abdul-Rahman A: Delayed hypoperfusion in the cerebral cortex of the rat in the recovery period following severe hypoglycemia. *Acta Physiol Scand* 106:375–376, 1979.

110. Smith M-L, Kågström E, Rosén I, et al: Effect of the calcium antagonist nimodipine on the delayed hypoperfusion following incomplete ischemia in the rat. *J Cereb Blood Flow Metab* 3:543–546, 1983.

111. Snyder JV, Nemoto EM, Carroll RG, et al: Intracranial pressure, brain blood flow regulation and glucose and oxygen metabolism after 15 minutes of circulatory arrest in dogs (abstract). *Stroke* 4:342, 1973.

112. Snyder JV, Nemoto EM, Carroll RG, et al: Global ischemia in dogs: Intracranial pressures, brain blood flow and metabolism. *Stroke* 6:21–27, 1975.

113. Steen PA, Newberg LA, Milde JH, et al: Nimodipine improves cerebral blood flow and neurologic recovery after complete cerebral ischemia in the dog. *J Cereb Blood Flow Metab* 3:38–43, 1983.

114. Strock PE, Majno G, Diethelm G: Protection of the vascular patency of ischemic dog limbs by various perfusate solutions. In Norman J (ed): *Organ Perfusion and Preservation.* New York, Appleton-Century-Crofts, 1967, p 27.

115. Summers WK, Jamison RL: The no-reflow phenomenon in renal ischemia. *Lab Invest* 25:635–643, 1971.

116. Suzuki R, Yamaguchi T, Kirino T, et al: The effects of 5-minute ischemia in Mongolian gerbils. I. Blood-brain barrier, cerebral blood flow, and local cerebral glucose utilization changes. *Acta Neuropathol (Berl)* 60:207–216, 1983.

117. Takagi S, Cocito L, Hossmann K-A: Blood recirculation and pharmacological responsiveness of the cerebral vasculature following prolonged ischemia of cat brain. *Stroke* 8:707–712, 1977.

118. Todd NV, Picozzi P, Crockard HA: Quantitative measurement of cerebral blood flow and cerebral blood volume after cerebral ischaemia. *J Cereb Blood Flow Metab* 6:338–341, 1986.

119. Todd NV, Picozzi P, Crockard HA: Recirculation after cerebral ischemia. Simultaneous measurement of cerebral blood flow, brain edema, cerebrovascular permeability and cortical EEG in the rat. *Acta Neurol Scand* 74:269–278, 1986.

120. Traupe H, Kruse E, Heiss W-D: Reperfusion of focal ischemia of varying duration: Postischemic hyper- and hypoperfusion. *Stroke* 13:615–622, 1982.

121. Tweed WA, Wade JG, Davidson WJ: Mechanisms of the "low-flow" state during resuscitation of the totally ischemic brain. *J Canad Sci Neurol* 4:19–23, 1977.

122. Wade JG, Amtorp O, Sörensen SC: No-flow state following cerebral ischemia. Role of increase in potassium concentration in brain interstitial fluid. *Arch Neurol* 32:381–384, 1975.

123. Wahl M, Lauritzen M, Schilling L: Change of cerebrovascular reactivity after cortical spreading depression in cats and rats. *Brain Res* 411:72–80, 1987.

124. Wei E, Christman CW, Kontos HA, et al: Effects of oxygen radicals on cerebral arterioles. *Am J Physiol* 248:H157–H162, 1985.

125. Welsh FA, O'Connor MJ: Secondary decline of blood flow during postischemic recirculation of cat brain (abstract). *Stroke* 11:126, 1980.

126. White BC, Winegar CD, Jackson RE, et al: Cerebral cortical perfusion during and following resuscitation from cardiac arrest in dogs. *Am J Emerg Med* 2:128–138, 1983.

127. White BC, Winegar CD, Wilson RF, et al: Calcium blockers in cerebral resuscitation. *J Trauma* 23:788–794, 1983.

128. White RJ: Cerebral hypothermia and circulatory arrest. Review and commentary. *Mayo Clin Proc* 53:450–458, 1978.

129. Yamada H, Chujo T, Kashiki Y, et al: Studies on isolated rat brain perfusion with emulsion of fluorocarbon. Proceedings of the Xth International Congress for Nutrition: Symposium on Perfluorochemical Artificial Blood. Kyoto/Osaka, Igakushobo Medical Publisher, 1975, pp 121–134.

130. Zimmer R, Lang R, Oberdörster G: Post-ischemic reactive hyperemia of the isolated perfused brain of the dog. *Pflügers Arch* 328:332–343, 1971.

131. Zimmerman V, Hossmann K-A: Resuscitation of the monkey brain after one hour's complete ischemia. II. Brain water and electrolytes. *Brain Res* 85:1–11, 1975.

132. Zimmerman V, Hossmann V, Hossmann K-A: Intracranial pressure after prolonged cerebral ischemia. In Lundberg N, Pontén U, Brock M (eds): *Intracranial Pressure II.* Berlin, Springer-Verlag, 1975, pp 177–182.

CHAPTER FOUR

Glycolytic Metabolism in Brain Ischemia

Myron D. Ginsberg, M.D.

The characteristics of glycolytic and oxidative metabolism in the normal and abnormal brain have been comprehensively examined in a recent monograph (51), and metabolic events in ischemia have been extensively reviewed (52, 53). In this chapter, several aspects of glycolytic metabolism of particular current interest will be emphasized: (a) regional assessment of altered glycolysis in ischemia; (b) influence of elevated plasma glucose on ischemic brain injury; and (c) recent observations concerning hydrogen ion dyshomeostasis in ischemia.

LOCAL CEREBRAL GLUCOSE UTILIZATION IN ISCHEMIA

Introduction of the powerful 2-deoxyglucose autoradiographic method for measuring local cerebral glucose utilization (54) has permitted the analysis of altered glycolytic metabolism at the regional level during cerebral ischemia. However, there are methodologic considerations that raise questions about the application of this method in ischemia. They result from possible variations in values for the rate constants and the so-called *lumped constant* of the mathematical model. These considerations have been evaluated by several workers (15, 23, 38). Recently, it has become possible to determine the lumped constant regionally by an autoradiographic strategy using methylglucose (19, 38). If circumstances that clearly violate the model assumptions are avoided (e.g. cerebral blood flow [CBF] so reduced as to impede 2-deoxyglucose delivery to tissue), the

method may be judiciously used to gain insights into the pathophysiology of brain ischemia (56).

We (17) were the first to report abnormalities of local brain glucose utilization occurring in cats following 90 minutes of unilateral middle cerebral artery (MCA) and common carotid artery occlusions. A core of greatly suppressed glucose utilization was found in the caudate nucleus, surrounded by a variable rim of apparently increased glucose consumption, possibly attributable to anaerobic glycolysis. (The 2-deoxyglucose method cannot distinguish between aerobic and anaerobic glucose metabolism.) An association between locally increased 2-deoxyglucose uptake and mild to moderate anaerobic perturbations of brain high-energy phosphate metabolite levels was established by Welsh et al (61) by direct assay of regional tissue samples. A double-radiotracer analysis of both local glucose utilization (^{14}C-2-deoxyglucose) and local blood flow (^{3}H-antipyrine) showed that increased glucose utilization tends to occur only in brain regions having a CBF reduction below 39% of control levels (16) (Fig. 4.1). Postischemic studies in this model have revealed foci of enhanced cortical glucose utilization following short recirculation periods. These studies suggest that metabolic recovery appears to progress more rapidly in the caudate nucleus than in the cerebral cortex (16).

Blood flow–metabolism relationships in MCA occlusion were investigated extensively by Tanaka et al (56) in the cat. Using the radiolabeled microsphere technique, they assessed blood flow both at the end of the ischemic period and after 4 hours of recirculation. They correlated these measurements with local glucose utiliza-

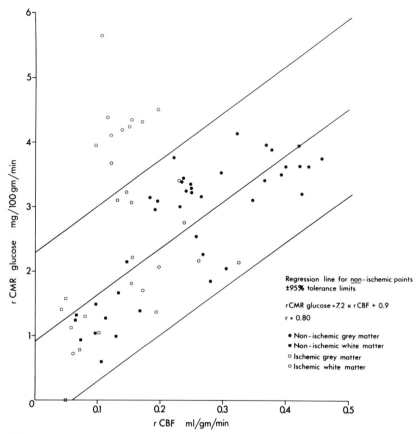

Figure 4.1. Regional cerebral blood flow (rCBF) plotted versus regional cerebral metabolic rate for glucose (rCMR glucose) as assessed in multiple regional samples taken from the ischemic and nonischemic forebrain of cats anesthetized with pentobarbital and subjected to 90 minutes of unilateral middle cerebral artery and common carotid artery occlusions. The majority of ischemic samples lie within the 95% tolerance limits of the regression line established on the basis of points from the nonischemic hemisphere. A minority of samples, all representing ischemic gray matter tissue, lie outside the tolerance limits; these represent zones of relative glucose hypermetabolism, occurring at CBF levels below 40% of control. (Figure courtesy of MD Ginsberg and M Reivich.)

tion at 4 hours of recirculation and with light-microscopic histology in adjacent brain blocks of the same cat. In the central MCA territory, intraischemic blood flow values below 30% of control were associated with a broad range of glucose metabolic rates (0% to 270% of control values) during the postischemic period, and with widely varying degrees of histologic injury. However, when intraischemic CBF had been reduced below 5% of control, glucose utilization showed a consistent and severe depression during recirculation and was accompanied by severe histologic damage (56). Local blood flow of below 40% of control during *recirculation* also correlated

with marked depression of local postischemic glucose utilization and with severe histologic damage. In contrast, when recirculatory blood flow was 40% to 115% of control, the glycolytic rate was found to be increased to an average of 154% of control; histologic damage in those regions was generally mild. Similar results were obtained in the peripheral MCA territory. These findings suggest a persistent anaerobic glycolysis during the recirculation period, despite recovery of CBF to levels greater than those normally associated with anaerobiosis. This pattern may thus be an accompaniment of early tissue injury.

Evidence in support of the role of relative glycolytic hypermetabolism in the genesis of ischemic neuronal injury was provided by studies in a rat model of graded focal ischemia produced by unilateral carotid artery occlusion and elevated intracranial pressure—a model giving rise to a gradient of hemodynamic and metabolic perturbations, with the most profound energy metabolite depletion and blood flow reduction occurring in the lateral striatum and lateral neocortex (2). Surprisingly, light microscopy revealed the striatum to be the predominant locus of ischemic neuronal damage, whereas the neocortex was much less prominently affected (12). Postischemic glucose metabolism and blood flow were assessed by a double-label radioisotopic strategy. At 2 hours of recirculation following a 30-minute ischemic insult, the striatum proved to be unique in exhibiting a disproportionately elevated glucose metabolism to blood flow ratio (Fig. 4.2). In contrast, the less affected lateral neocortex exhibited a normal metabolism to blood flow ratio (12). These results suggest that the resumption of a high level of glucose metabolism, disproportionate to blood flow, in the early postischemic state might play a contributory role in the process of neuronal injury.

A subsequent study, carried out in the rat four-vessel occlusion model, implicated striatal dopamine in this process. In that study, unilateral striatal dopamine depletion, produced by a previous lesion of the substantia nigra, was found both to diminish the magnitude of postischemic metabolism/blood flow uncoupling (21) and to confer a marked protection against ischemic neuronal death in that structure, as assessed both histologically and by uptake of the radiotracer calcium-45 (20). These results suggest that the maintenance of a normal metabolism/blood flow interrelationship following ischemia may be a necessary, if not sufficient, factor in ensuring ultimate tissue viability.

An apparent glucose hypermetabolism has been observed within the marginal zone of a developing thrombotic cortical infarct produced in the rat by a photochemical method (8), both at 4 hours and at 5 days after injury. At the 4-hour time point, this zone proved on histologic examination to correspond to a region of normal-sized but moderately hyperchromatic neurons interspersed among occasional dark, shrunken neurons with preserved neuropil. In contrast, the hypermetabolic zone 5 days after infarct coincided with a field of intense macrophage infiltration. The findings in this study suggest that the capacity to mount a hypermetabolic response early after ischemia presupposes at least an intermediate degree of tissue viability.

Other studies support the view that increased local glucose utilization in the postischemic brain is not ipso facto evidence of severe injury. For example, a recent study combining autoradiography with direct measurement of tissue metabolite levels has shown areas of increased postischemic local glucose utilization to be confined to zones of relatively minor alteration of energy metabolites (57). As noted earlier, after ischemia, increased 2-deoxyglucose uptake may be observed in the zones where CBF is sufficiently recovered to make persistent ischemia unlikely to be serving as ongoing stimulus to anaerobic metabolism (56).

Whereas marked postischemic depression of local glucose utilization has been shown to coincide with major local changes in lactate and high-energy phosphates (57) and would appear to signal an inhibition of glycolytic metabolism, intermediate degrees of depressed glucose utilization have been observed in brain regions with normal high-energy metabolite levels (57). Similar findings have been observed in global transient forebrain ischemia, in which a postischemic depression of glucose utilization (45) appears to coexist with recovery of high-energy metabolites (43). The responsible mechanism in this case may be a diminution of neural function. It has been shown, for example, that following transient forebrain ischemia in the rat, resting glucose utilization is suppressed and, simultaneously, the previously ischemic somatosensory cortex is refractory to physiologic stimulation; the latter impairment resolves only slowly, over a period of several days (7).

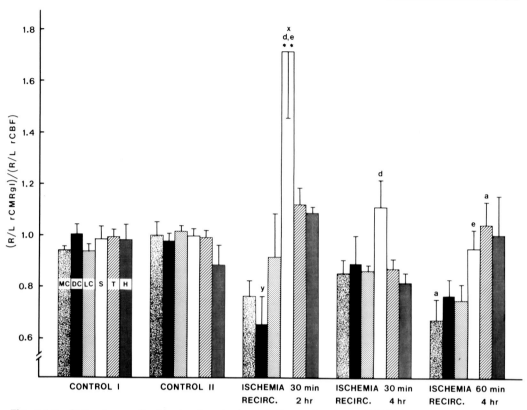

Figure 4.2. Ratio of normalized regional cerebral metabolic rate for glucose (rCMRgl) to normalized regional cerebral blood flow (rCBF) in the control period and following transient unilateral forebrain ischemia in the rat. The normalized regional metabolic and hemodynamic data were derived by dividing regional values from the ischemic hemisphere of individual rats by the corresponding values from the homologous (contra-lateral) nonischemic region, and subsequently obtaining group averages (± standard error of the mean). The postischemic striatum (S), following 30 minutes of ischemia and 2 hours of recirulation, shows a significant elevation of its metabolism/blood flow ratio ($p < 0.01$), whereas this ratio is normal in the previously ischemic lateral cortex (LC), which had received an equivalent degree of ischemia. R/L = right/left; MC = medial cortex; DC = dorsolateral cortex; T = thalamus; H = hippocampus; Recirc = recirculation. (From Ginsberg MD, Graham DI, Busto R: Regional glucose utilization and blood flow following graded forebrain ischemia in the rat: Correlation with neuropathology. *Ann Neurol* 18:470–481, 1985.)

INFLUENCE OF ELEVATED PLASMA GLUCOSE ON ISCHEMIC BRAIN INJURY

Global Ischemia

A seminal advance in our understanding of the pathophysiology of ischemic brain injury occurred with the recognition that whether an animal was fed or fasted bore a direct relation to the degree of injury sustained during transient circulatory arrest. Although in retrospect the obser-

vations of earlier investigators were explicable on this basis (3, 4, 10, 29), the definitive observation was made serendipitously by Myers and Yamaguchi (35). These workers were examining the behavioral and neuropathologic sequelae of cardiac arrest in juvenile rhesus monkeys which had previously been trained in pattern discrimination and color discrimination tasks. The monkeys were typically deprived of food for 12 to 24 hours preceding circulatory arrest, and they were hydrated with physiologic saline solution. Cardiac arrest was induced by intravenously administered potassium chloride. However, two monkeys were hydrated instead with 100 to 200 ml of 5% dextrose solution administered within 10 to 15 minutes of circulatory arrest. Despite a similar duration of arrest, dramatically different outcomes ensued. The saline-infused monkeys typically recovered respiratory activity and pupillary responsiveness quickly following resuscitation, regained consciousness at 2 to 11 hours, eventually exhibited full neurologic recovery, and performed visual discrimination tasks with the same accuracy as before the cardiac arrest. Pathologic examination showed either intact brains or a pattern of injury restricted to nuclear structures of the brain stem, cerebellar Purkinje cells, and hippocampus. In marked contrast, the two monkeys receiving glucose infusions just before cardiac arrest remained comatose, developed repetitive generalized myoclonic discharges, became decerebrate and opisthotonic, and exhibited dilated fixed pupils and vasomotor instability. Their brains showed mild edema and widespread necrosis of cortex and basal ganglia (35).

Siemkowicz and Hansen (50) confirmed this observation in rats that were subjected to 10 minutes of complete ischemia by inflation of a pneumatic neck cuff to 600 to 700 mm Hg. Normoglycemic animals (mean blood glucose level, 7.8 mmol/liter) sustained only minor neurologic deficits and were capable of 3-week survival. In contrast, hyperglycemic rats (mean blood glucose level, 24 mmol/liter) remained comatose, failed to regain spontaneous respiration, exhibited myoclonic and tonic seizure activity, and died within 12 hours (50).

We (18, 60) have examined the implications of glucose pretreatment from a metabolic and hemodynamic perspective, making use of a previously validated model of global cerebral ischemia produced by basilar and bilateral common carotid artery occlusions plus hypotension in the pentobarbital-anesthetized cat (11, 13, 59). During ischemia, blood flow assessed by the autoradiographic method was virtually absent throughout the cerebral hemispheres, with persistence of minimal flow (0.01 to 0.11 ml/g/minute) in scattered per-

isulcal and subpial areas. Following 15 minutes of ischemia and 90 minutes of normotensive recirculation in cats not receiving glucose, local blood flow was reduced uniformly to about 31% of control levels throughout gray and white matter structures—exemplifying the phenomenon of postischemic hypoperfusion described in a variety of animal ischemia models (28, 45). In contrast, animals receiving 1.5 g/kg of 50% dextrose solution immediately before ischemia exhibited a heterogeneous postischemic blood flow pattern, with severe hypoperfusion of large portions of the cortical mantle yet normal to increased blood flow in adjacent areas. With a longer ischemic insult (30 minutes), dextrose pretreatment caused widespread, profound postischemic hypoperfusion throughout the forebrain. A close correlation was observed between local brain blood flow and regional energy metabolite patterns: Zones of higher postischemic blood flow showed significant recovery of adenosine triphosphate (ATP) and phosphocreatine and only moderately elevated lactate levels, whereas zones of lower flow corresponded to areas with persistently depleted energy metabolites and associated lactate elevation (18).

Regional metabolism was studied more extensively in this model using transcalvarial freezing for preservation of cerebral metabolites (41) followed by NADH* fluorescence photography and regional enzymatic–fluorometric metabolite assays. Although generally equal degrees of metabolite depletion were observed in dextrose-pretreated and nonpretreated cats at the end of the period of ischemia, the former group exhibited more severely impaired *post*ischemic restitution of brain ATP, phosphocreatine, and lactate levels; dextrose pretreatment also increased the number of brain regions which failed to resynthesize ATP and phosphocreatine during recirculation.

In the studies noted earlier (18, 60), dextrose infusion before ischemia elevated plasma glucose levels to approximately 35 to 67 mmol/liter and brain glucose levels

---

*NADH = reduced form of nicotinamide—adenine dinucleotide.

by approximately 2.5 times. In addition, it is probable that residual blood flow during the ischemic insult itself permitted ongoing delivery of glucose to tissue. This was the source of the somewhat higher tissue lactate levels observed at the end of the ischemic insult and the source of marked lactate elevations which persisted regionally in the postischemic brain at levels as high as 40 to 60 mmol/kg. In their earlier studies, Ljunggren et al (30) produced a wide range of both plasma and brain glucose levels by administering either insulin or glucose to rats. They were able to demonstrate, at the conclusion of 5 minutes of complete cerebral ischemia, that brain glucose was virtually depleted and a corresponding spectrum of cerebral lactate elevations was observed, varying over a fourfold range from the hypoglycemic to the hyperglycemic group.

Pulsinelli et al (47) demonstrated in the rat that a mild to moderate (twofold to threefold) elevation of blood glucose is sufficient to exacerbate the sequelae of transient high-grade forebrain ischemia. Fasted, saline-treated control rats, following 20 minutes of ischemia, showed no evidence of neurologic dysfunction 24 hours later, whereas glucose-pretreated rats developed seizures during the first 24 postischemic hours, and many died. The neuropathologic score following 24-hour survival indicated much more extensive ischemic cell change in neocortex, striatum, hippocampus, and cerebellum in glucose-pretreated rats than in the controls. It is interesting that administration of equivalent amounts of glucose *during* or following ischemia did not significantly affect the neuropathologic outcome except in the cerebellum. The effect of postischemic glucose administration was studied by Welsh et al (60), and though a suggestive metabolic impairment was observed, the overall effect was not as great as with glucose pretreatment. Mannitol, administered in an effort to duplicate the osmotic effects of glucose pretreatment, did not accentuate ischemic neuropathology in the rat (47) and was associated in cats with less extensive pathology than was glucose (60). These results are consistent with the conclusion that the effect of glucose pretreatment is largely unrelated to an osmotic action.

Focal Vascular Occlusion

As noted above, the initial studies of hyperglycemia complicating ischemia were carried out in models of transient reversible global ischemia. Until recently, there were few comparable studies of this issue in the setting of focal thrombotic vascular occlusion. Brint et al (1), in an abstract report, noted increased infarct volume in a hyperglycemic rat model of MCA and common carotid artery occlusion. Myers et al (34) and de Courten-Myers et al (5), using the cat model of MCA occlusion, showed that hyperglycemia exacerbated brain edema and increased mortality.

More recent studies have suggested that the effect of hyperglycemia in cerebral infarction is more complex than was previously recognized. We (14) studied the problem in a model of unilateral cortical infarction induced photochemically in Wistar rats (by the interaction of intravenously administered dye with light-irradiation of the brain (58)). Infarct areas were assessed planimetrically following 7-day survival. Hyperglycemia was produced by intraperitoneal dextrose administration 15 minutes before the induction of infarction. Surprisingly, infarct volumes in rats with plasma glucose levels in the range of 15 to 34 mmol/liter were significantly smaller (approximately 25%) than infarct volumes in rats with plasma glucose levels in the range of 10 mmol/liter or lower. Comparable amounts of intraperitoneal mannitol, by contrast, produced somewhat larger infarct volumes. It was hypothesized that the small but definite beneficial effect of hyperglycemia in this model of end-arteriolar thrombotic infarction might possibly be attributable to improvement of local energy metabolism at the periphery of the lesion during its early period of expansion. Studies to be described later in this chapter have served further to clarify this phenomenon.

To study focal ischemia in greater detail, Prado et al (42) studied two different rat models of focal vascular occlusion, taking care to quantitate infarct volume separately in the neocortex (a collaterally perfused structure) and the striatum (a structure having end-arterial perfusion). In Wistar rats with MCA thrombosis coupled with temporary bilateral common carotid artery occlusions, higher preischemic plasma glucose levels were strongly correlated with larger cortical infarct volumes, the volume approximately doubling as plasma glucose increased from 6 to 31 mmol/liter. In contrast, the size of the striatal infarct was not correlated with plasma glucose level. The latter finding was confirmed in the Sprague-Dawley rat— a strain in which MCA occlusion gives rise to a much larger striatal infarct. In these studies, also, despite glucose levels ranging from 5.4 to 44 mmol/liter, striatal infarct volume was unrelated to the plasma glucose level. In both the model of photochemically induced microvascular occlusion (9, 58) and striatal infarction (22), the occluded vessels are nonanastomosing (end-arterial) vascular channels, so that no possibility exists of "rescue" from collateral arterial beds. When flow is severely and permanently reduced to a zone without collateral supply, the extent of tissue injury appears to be determined primarily by the topography of blood flow reduction and is not exacerbated by increasing plasma glucose. A contrasting situation occurs in the neocortex, wherein collateral circulation persists during ischemia produced by MCA occlusion. In this case, the degree of tissue acidosis in the incompletely ischemic marginal zones may be modulated by the ongoing transport of glucose from blood to brain and its anaerobic conversion to lactic acid. The latter is influenced by the plasma glucose level.

Myers et al (34) have contributed the interesting observation that, when MCA occlusion is temporary, hyperglycemia strongly increases the likelihood of death from cerebral edema upon release of vascular occlusion. Furthermore de Courten-Myers et al (5) have shown that, if MCA occlusion is permanent, increased plasma glucose at the time of MCA occlusion increases infarct size, whereas hyperglycemia instituted after occlusion appears to accentuate mortality secondary to cerebral edema.

Nedergaard and Astrup (36), studying MCA occlusion in normoglycemic Wistar rats, showed that spontaneous transient deflections of the direct current (DC) potential arise from the cortical infarct rim and are associated with local elevations of the rate of glucose utilization as reflected by phosphorylation of radiolabeled 2-deoxyglucose. In hyperglycemic rats, however, these DC potential deflections are greatly diminished and 2-deoxyglucose phosphorylation remains normal. The investigators inferred from these findings that spontaneous recurrent transient increases of extracellular potassium occurring at the infarct rim may serve to stimulate glucose metabolism in normoglycemic rats, but that this response is suppressed in rats with hyperglycemia. This group demonstrated a sharp transitional zone between infarcted and normal tissue in hyperglycemic rats, whereas in normoglycemic rats with MCA occlusion there is a larger zone of incomplete infarction—that is, neuronal necrosis with intact neuropil (37). An autoradiographic study from this laboratory (38) has corroborated the finding that there is enhanced glucose utilization in border zones surrounding an ischemic focus in normoglycemic animals, whereas this phenomenon is diminished in hyperglycemia. Thus, hyperglycemia enlarges zones of cortical infarction but may protect against selective neuronal necrosis at the periphery of the infarct. This protective mechanism may be relevant to our finding of hyperglycemia-associated reduction of infarct size in the model of photochemically induced cortical microvascular thrombosis (14).

HYPERGLYCEMIA IN HUMAN ISCHEMIC STROKE SYNDROMES

Despite a wealth of data from experiments in animals, attempts to show a significant influence of hyperglycemia on human cerebral infarction have proved difficult, possibly because of the considerable variability in clinical ischemic stroke as well as the problem of patient randomization. Melamed (32) showed that, regardless of whether or not patients were diabetic, hyperglycemia present at the time of ischemic cerebral infarction was associated with a greater short-term mortality. This finding was interpreted as an indication of a greater "stress response" in patients with larger infarcts, but may possibly reflect an exacerbating effect of hyperglycemia on stroke. Pulsinelli et al (46) reported both retrospective and prospective observations in this area. The retrospective analysis compared diabetic with nondiabetic patients admitted to a single hospital with the diagnosis of ischemic stroke; mean blood glucose levels at the time of admission were 5.9 mmol/liter for the diabetic patients and 14.4 mmol/liter for those without diabetes. The groups were well matched both demographically and with respect to their histories of vascular illness. Diabetic patients had a significantly greater proportion of poor neurologic outcomes (46%) than the nondiabetic group (24%) and a greater number of both stroke-related and total in-hospital deaths. In the prospective component of this study, a separate nondiabetic population with ischemic stroke was analyzed with respect to blood glucose levels above or below 6.7 mmol/liter, as measured at the time of hospital admission. Relative to the group with elevated blood glucose levels on admission, a greater proportion of patients with levels below 6.7 mmol/liter were able to return to work after recovering from their stroke, although this difference was of only marginal statistical significance.

Mohr et al (33) also assessed this relationship through the National Institute of Neurological and Communicative Disorders and Stroke Data Bank. Analyzing data from 412 patients with well-documented admission glucose levels, they found that increased mortality rates correlated with higher admission glucose values but found no evidence of an effect of blood glucose levels either on the acute course of stroke during the first 24 hours or on outcome in subgroups of patients with large atherothrombotic infarctions, intraparenchymal hemorrhage, or lacunar infarction. When patients were analyzed by subgroups, assigned according to admission blood glucose level in 1.1 mmol/liter (20 mg/dl) increments, patients with admission glucose levels below 5.5 mmol/liter (100 mg/dl) had lower mortality rates, but above this value no relationship to blood glucose levels was apparent.

RELATIVE SEVERITY OF INJURY OF COMPLETE VERSUS INCOMPLETE CEREBRAL ISCHEMIA

The deleterious influence of severe tissue lactic acidosis is closely related to the issue of relative severity of injury in complete versus incomplete cerebral ischemia. The experiments of Hossmann et al (24, 25) suggested that greater injury to the brain resulted from prolonged periods of *in*complete ischemia than from complete ischemia; this conclusion has been reached by other investigators as well (39, 40). Siesjö (52) has suggested that the degree of tissue acidosis is a crucial determinant of outcome in ischemia, whether complete or incomplete. Rehncrona et al (49) showed that excessive lactate accumulation in the ischemic brain precludes recovery, irrespective of the degree of residual CBF during ischemia. These investigators also showed a progressive deterioration of mitochondrial function after incomplete, but not after complete, ischemia (48). In contrast, other workers (31, 55) have reported a better outcome in patients with incomplete as opposed to complete ischemia when the duration of ischemia is relatively brief and brain lactate levels are less than 17 mmol/kg.

Experiments designed to yield a more definitive outcome were performed by Yoshida et al (62) and Dietrich et al (6), who used rat models of either incomplete or complete ischemia for 1 hour. Both degrees of ischemia were produced by a similar procedure—a combination of bilateral common carotid artery occlusion, systemic hypotension, and elevation of cerebral spinal fluid pressure. The degree of intracranial hypertension was adjusted to produce the required grade of ischemia. Brain lactate levels were 16 to 19 mmol/kg in the rats with incomplete ischemia and 11 to 13 mmol/kg in those with complete ischemia. In the cerebral cortex, the degree of metabolic recovery was similar after complete and incomplete ischemia whereas in subcortical regions, less recovery was seen following complete ischemia (62). Perfusion defects were evident in both the cortical and subcortical regions following 25 minutes of complete ischemia, but not following the same period of incomplete ischemia (6). Whereas incomplete ischemia gave rise only to ischemic neuronal alterations in selectively vulnerable regions, complete ischemia was associated in addition with focal parenchymal necrosis, vascular stasis, and ultrastructural evidence of perivascular astrocytic swelling with luminal compression (6). Thus, in the absence of profound tissue lactic acidosis, the presence of residual blood flow during prolonged ischemia appears to improve postischemic reperfusion, promote recovery of brain energy metabolism in subcortical regions, and prevent frank tissue necrosis. The failure of incomplete ischemia without profound tissue lactic acidosis to exacerbate tissue injury would argue against a possible role of peroxidative degradative processes in contributing to injury in the setting of residual circulation during ischemia.

HYDROGEN ION DYSHOMEOSTASIS IN BRAIN ISCHEMIA

Kraig et al (26) examined the relationship between interstitial hydrogen ion content and tissue lactate during complete ischemia produced by cardiac arrest in rats. Plasma glucose levels ranged from normoglycemic to profoundly hyperglycemic. In rats with blood glucose levels of 3 to 7 mmol/liter, brain lactate levels rose 8 to 13 mmol/kg and pH declined by 0.44 units. In contrast, in rats with blood glucose levels of 17 to 80 mmol/liter, the brain lactate

values were 16 to 31 mmol/kg during ischemia and brain interstitial pH fell by 1.07 units. Graphic analysis of all points (Fig. 4.3) showed a relatively constant interstitial pH of 6.81 until tissue lactate levels reached 13 mmol/kg, at which point interstitial pH declined abruptly to approximately 6.18, where it remained as tissue lactate levels increased. That this curve does not resemble the curve produced by in vitro titration of a cortical homogenate suggests that, during complete ischemia, the interstitial hydrogen ion is not in equilibrium with hydrogen ion in other brain compartments. Kraig et al (26) emphasize that a variety of physiochemical buffering and ion-transport mechanisms exist to deal with excess intracellular hydrogen ion. They hypothesize that the abrupt interstitial pH transition during complete ischemia may coincide with brain *infarction* and may reflect failure of the brain cells' plasma membranes to regulate intracellular hydrogen ions by transport mechanisms. These workers have implicated glial cells as a final site of continued acid production in ischemia (27).

PERSPECTIVE

Hyperglycemia present before ischemia or during incomplete ischemia serves to elevate glucose transport into brain tissue and, thereby, to promote profound tissue acidosis through anaerobic glycolysis during the ischemic period. In an effort to explain the mechanism governing the transition from isolated ischemic neuronal necrosis to frank tissue infarction it has been pointed out (44) that cerebral acidosis enhances the release of ferrous iron, which may in turn catalyze the formation of active oxygen radical species, initiating lipid peroxidation. This has been proposed as a possible mechanism of ischemic brain infarction.

Acknowledgments—Dr. Ginsberg is the recipient of a Jacob Javits Neuroscience Investigator Award. His research is supported by U.S. Public Health Service Grants NS 05820, NS 22603 and NS 21720, and by a Grant-in-Aid from the American Heart Association.

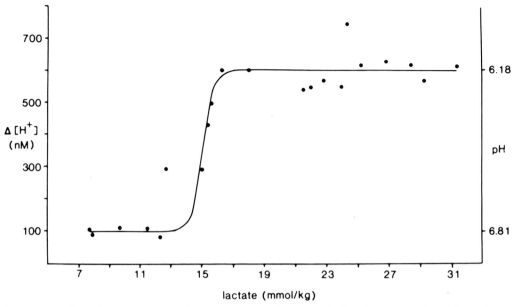

Figure 4.3. Peak changes in brain interstitial hydrogen ion concentration (as measured with ion-selective micropipettes) plotted with respect to lactate levels assessed by enzymatic–fluorometric techniques in tissue frozen in liquid nitrogen at the time of peak hydrogen ion change, during complete cerebral ischemia in the rat. (From Kraig RP, Pulsinelli WA, Plum F: Hydrogen ion buffering during complete brain ischemia. *Brain Res* 342:281–290, 1985.)

References

1. Brint S, Kraig R, Kiessling M, et al: Hyperglycemia augments infarct size in focal experimental brain ischemia (abstract). *Ann Neurol* 18:127, 1985.
2. Busto R, Ginsberg MD: Graded focal cerebral ischemia in the rat by unilateral carotid artery occlusion and elevated intracranial pressure: Hemodynamic and biochemical characterization. *Stroke* 16:466–476, 1985.
3. Campbell JA: Increase of resistance to oxygen want in animals on certain diets. *Q J Exp Physiol* 28:231–241, 1938.
4. Craven C, Chinn H, MacVicar R: Effect of carrot diet and restricted feeding on the resistance of the rat to hypoxia. *J Aviat Med* 21:256–258, 1950.
5. de Courten-Myers GM, Myers RE, Schoolfield L: Effects of serum glucose concentration at and following middle cerebral artery occlusion on infarct size in cats (abstract). *Neurology* 37 (Suppl 1):130, 1987.
6. Dietrich WD, Busto R, Yoshida S, et al: Histological and hemodynamic consequences of complete versus incomplete ischemia in the rat. *J Cereb Blood Flow Metab* 7:300–308, 1987.
7. Dietrich WD, Ginsberg MD, Busto R: Effect of transient cerebral ischemia on metabolic activation of a somatosensory circuit. *J Cereb Blood Flow Metab* 6:405–413, 1986.
8. Dietrich WD, Ginsberg MD, Busto R, et al: Photochemically-induced cortical infarction in the rat.

2. Acute and subacute alterations in local glucose utilization. *J Cereb Blood Flow Metab* 6:195–202, 1986.
9. Dietrich WD, Watson BD, Busto R, et al: Photochemically-induced cerebral infarction. I. Early microvascular alterations. *Acta Neuropathol (Berl)* 72:315–325, 1987.
10. Friede R, van Houten W: Relations between postmortem alterations and glycolytic metabolism in the brain. *Exp Neurol* 4:197–204, 1961.
11. Ginsberg MD, Budd WW, Welsh FA: Diffuse cerebral ischemia in the cat. I. Local blood flow during severe ischemia and recirculation. *Ann Neurol* 3:482–492, 1978.
12. Ginsberg MD, Graham DI, Busto R: Regional glucose utilization and blood flow following graded forebrain ischemia in the rat: Correlation with neuropathology. *Ann Neurol* 18:470–481, 1985.
13. Ginsberg MD, Graham DI, Welsh FA, et al: Diffuse cerebral ischemia in the cat. III. Neuropathological sequelae of severe ischemia. *Ann Neurol* 5:350–358, 1979.
14. Ginsberg MD, Prado R, Dietrich WD, et al: Hyperglycemia reduces the extent of cerebral infarction in rats. *Stroke* 18:570–574, 1987.
15. Ginsberg MD, Reivich M: Use of the 2-deoxyglucose method of local cerebral glucose utilization in the abnormal brain: Evaluation of the lumped constant during ischemia. *Acta Neurol Scand [Suppl 72]* 60:226–227, 1979.
16. Ginsberg MD, Reivich M, Giandomenico A: Re-

gional brain glucose metabolism during recovery from transient cerebral ischemia. *Acta Neurol Scand [Suppl 64]* 56:128–129, 1977.

17. Ginsberg MD, Reivich M, Giandomenico A, et al: Local glucose utilization in acute focal cerebral ischemia: Local dysmetabolism and diaschisis. *Neurology* 27:1042–1048, 1977.

18. Ginsberg MD, Welsh FA, Budd WW: Deleterious effect of glucose pretreatment on recovery from diffuse cerebral ischemia in the cat. *Stroke* 11:347–354, 1980.

19. Gjedde A, Diemer NH: Autoradiographic determination of regional brain glucose content. *J Cereb Blood Flow Metab* 3:303–310, 1983.

20. Globus MY-T, Ginsberg MD, Dietrich WD, et al: Substantia nigra lesion protects against ischemic damage in the striatum. *Neurosci Lett* 80:251–256, 1987.

21. Globus MY-T, Ginsberg MD, Harik SI, et al: Role of dopamine in ischemic striatal injury: Metabolic evidence. *Neurology* 37:1712–1719, 1987.

22. Grand W: Microsurgical anatomy of the proximal middle cerebral artery and the internal carotid artery bifurcation. *Neurosurgery* 7:151, 1980.

23. Hawkins RA, Phelps ME, Huang S-C, et al: Effect of ischemia on quantification of local cerebral glucose metabolic rate in man. *J Cereb Blood Flow Metab* 1:37–51, 1981.

24. Hossmann K-A, Kleihues P: Reversibility of ischemic brain damage. *Arch Neurol* 29:375–384, 1973.

25. Hossmann K-A, Zimmerman V: Resuscitation of the monkey brain after 1 h complete ischemia. I. Physiological and morphological observations. *Brain Res* 81:59–74, 1974.

26. Kraig RP, Pulsinelli WA, Plum F: Hydrogen ion buffering during complete brain ischemia. *Brain Res* 342:281–290, 1985.

27. Kraig RP, Pulsinelli WA, Plum F: Carbonic acid buffer changes during complete brain ischemia. *Am J Physiol* 250:R348–R357, 1986.

28. Levy DE, Van Uitert RL, Pike CL: Delayed postischemic hypoperfusion: A potentially damaging consequence of a stroke. *Neurology* 29:1245–1252, 1979.

29. Lindenberg R: Patterns of CNS vulnerability in acute hypoxaemia, including anaesthesia accidents. In Schade J, McMenemy WH (eds): *Selective Vulnerability of the Brain in Hypoxemia.* Philadelphia, FA Davis, 1963, pp 189–210.

30. Ljunggren B, Norberg K, Siesjö BK: Influence of tissue acidosis upon restitution of brain energy metabolism following total ischemia. *Brain Res* 77:173–186, 1974.

31. Marshall LF, Graham DI, Durity F, et al: Experimental cerebral oligemia and ischemia produced by intracranial hypertension. Part 2: Brain morphology. *J Neurosurg* 43:318–322, 1975.

32. Melamed E: Reactive hyperglycaemia in patients with acute stroke. *J Neurol Sci* 29:267–275, 1976.

33. Mohr JP, Rubenstein L, Edelstein SZ, et al: Approaches to pathophysiology of stroke through the NINCDS data bank. In Plum F, Pulsinelli WA (eds): *Cerebrovascular Diseases* (Transactions of the Fourteenth Research [Princeton-Williamsburg] Conference). New York, Raven Press, 1985, pp 63–68.

34. Myers R, de Courten-Myers G, Schoolfield L: Increased mortality from hemispheral edema from release of MCA occlusion (abstract). *Stroke* 18:279, 1987.

35. Myers RE, Yamaguchi S: Nervous system effects of cardiac arrest in monkeys. Preservation of vision. *Arch Neurol* 34:65–74, 1977.

36. Nedergaard M, Astrup J: Infarct rim: Effect of hyperglycemia on direct current potential and (^{14}C)2-deoxyglucose phosphorylation. *J Cereb Blood Flow Metab* 6:607–615, 1986.

37. Nedergaard M, Diemer NH: Focal ischemia of the rat brain, with special reference to the influence of plasma glucose concentration. *Acta Neuropathol (Berl)* 73:131–137, 1987.

38. Nedergaard M, Jakobsen J, Diemer NH: Autoradiographic determination of cerebral glucose content, blood flow, and glucose utilization in focal ischemia of the rat brain: Influence of the plasma glucose concentration. *J Cereb Blood Flow Metab* 8:100–108, 1988.

39. Nordström C-H, Rehncrona S, Siesjö BK: Restitution of cerebral energy state, as well as of glycolytic metabolites, citric acid cycle intermediates and associated amino acids after 30 minutes of complete ischemia in rats anaesthetized with nitrous oxide or phenobarbital. *J Neurochem* 30:479–486, 1978.

40. Nordström C-H, Rehncrona S, Siesjö BK: Effects of phenobarbital in cerebral ischemia. Part II. Restitution of cerebral energy state, as well as of glycolytic metabolites, citric acid cycle intermediates and associated amino acids after pronounced incomplete ischemia. *Stroke* 9:335–343, 1978.

41. Pontén U, Ratcheson RA, Salford LG: Optimal freezing conditions for cerebral metabolites in rats. *J Neurochem* 21:1127–1138, 1973.

42. Prado R, Ginsberg MD, Dietrich WD, et al: Hyperglycemia increases infarct size in collaterally perfused but not end-arterial vascular territories. *J Cereb Blood Flow Metab* 8:186–192, 1988.

43. Pulsinelli WA, Duffy TE: Regional energy balance in rat brain after transient forebrain ischemia. *J Neurochem* 40:1500–1503, 1983.

44. Pulsinelli WA, Kraig RP, Plum F: Hyperglycemia, cerebral acidosis, and ischemic brain damage. In Plum F, Pulsinelli WA (eds): *Cerebrovascular Diseases* (Transactions of the Fourteenth Research [Princeton-Williamsburg] Conference). New York, Raven Press, 1985, pp 201–210.

45. Pulsinelli WA, Levy DE, Duffy TE: Regional cerebral blood flow and glucose metabolism following transient forebrain ischemia. *Ann Neurol* 11:499–509, 1982.

46. Pulsinelli WA, Levy DE, Sigsbee B, et al: Increased damage after ischemic stroke in patients with hyperglycemia with or without established diabetes mellitus. *Am J Med* 74:540–544, 1983.

47. Pulsinelli WA, Waldman S, Rawlinson D, et al: Moderate hyperglycemia augments ischemic brain damage: A neuropathologic study in the rat. *Neurology* 32:1239–1246, 1982.

48. Rehncrona S, Mela L, Siesjö BK: Recovery of brain mitochondrial function in the rat after complete and incomplete cerebral ischemia. *Stroke* 10:437–446, 1979.

49. Rehncrona S, Rosen I, Siesjö BK: Brain lactic acidosis and ischemic cell damage. 1. Biochemistry and neurophysiology. *J Cereb Blood Flow Metab* 1:297–311, 1981.

50. Siemkowicz E, Hansen AJ: Clinical restitution following cerebral ischemia in hypo-, normo- and hyperglycemic rats. *Acta Neurol Scand* 58:1–8, 1978.

51. Siesjö BK: *Brain Energy Metabolism.* Chichester, John Wiley & Sons, 1978.

52. Siesjö BK: Review. Cell damage in the brain: A speculative synthesis. *J Cereb Blood Flow Metab* 1:155–185, 1981.

53. Siesjö BK: Review article. Cerebral circulation and metabolism. *J Neurosurg* 60:883–908, 1984.

54. Sokoloff L, Reivich M, Kennedy C, et al: The (^{14}C) deoxyglucose method for measurement of local cerebral glucose utilization: Theory, procedure, and normal values in the conscious and anesthetized albino rat. *J Neurochem* 28:897–916, 1977.

55. Steen PA, Michenfelder JD, Milde JH: Incomplete versus complete cerebral ischemia: Improved outcome with a minimal blood flow. *Ann Neurol* 6:389–398, 1979.

56. Tanaka K, Greenberg JH, Gonatas NK, et al: Regional flow–metabolism couple following middle cerebral artery occlusion in cats. *J Cereb Blood Flow Metab* 5:241–252, 1985.

57. Tanaka K, Welsh FA, Greenberg JH, et al: Regional alterations in glucose consumption and metabolite levels during postischemic recovery in cat brain. *J Cereb Blood Flow Metab* 5:502–511, 1985.

58. Watson BD, Dietrich WD, Busto R, et al: Induction of reproducible brain infarction by photochemically initiated thrombosis. *Ann Neurol* 17:497–504, 1985.

59. Welsh FA, Ginsberg MD, Rieder W, et al: Diffuse cerebral ischemia in the cat. II. Regional metabolites during severe ischemia and recirculation. *Ann Neurol* 3:493–501, 1978.

60. Welsh FA, Ginsberg MD, Rieder W, et al: Deleterious effect of glucose pretreatment on recovery from diffuse cerebral ischemia in the cat. II. Regional metabolite levels. *Stroke* 11:355–363, 1980.

61. Welsh FA, Greenberg JH, Jones SC, et al: Correlation between glucose utilization and metabolite levels during focal ischemia in cat brain. *Stroke* 11:79–84, 1980.

62. Yoshida S, Busto R, Martinez E, et al: Regional brain energy metabolism after complete versus incomplete ischemia in the rat in the absence of severe lactic acidosis. *J Cereb Blood Flow Metab* 5:490–501, 1985.

CHAPTER FIVE

Neurochemical Determinants of Ischemic Cell Damage

Carl-Henrik Nordström, M.D.
Bo K. Siesjö, M.D.

The dysfunction and cell damage that occur following cerebral ischemia are primarily caused by interference with cellular energy production. Because of lack of oxygen, oxidative phosphorylation is arrested and synthesis of adenosine triphosphate (ATP), active transport, and biosynthesis cease within a very short period (76). As a result of cellular energy failure, transmembrane ionic gradients are dissipated and degradation of structural components begins.

For many years, it was thought that irreversible cellular damage unavoidably occurs after only a few minutes of complete cerebral ischemia. This opinion has been modified during the past decade (105). Provided that the conditions for recovery are optimal, short-term restoration of brain functions may be achieved after periods of ischemia lasting as long as 60 minutes (44–46). Reasonably good long-term recovery of brain functions has been achieved in experimental trials after arrest of the cerebral circulation for 10 to 12 minutes in dogs (96, 97, 120) and 14 to 17 minutes in monkeys (34, 67, 74, 118). Furthermore, different brain cells vary substantially in their sensitivity to ischemia. Essentially, cerebral ischemia can give rise to two types of cellular damage. First, if the ischemia is of brief or moderate duration, only neurons are killed and there is no destruction of glial and vascular cells. Neuronal necrosis is then usually restricted to the selectively vulnerable regions: to pyramidal cells in the hippocampus and neocortex; to neurons in the caudate putamen and thalamus; and to other subcortical nuclei (10, 85, 113). Second, following a more severe and protracted ischemic insult, there is a pattern of dense laminar necrosis or infarction (30, 31, 82). The duration of ischemia, however, is only one of the factors determining whether the damage will affect only neurons or will progress to infarction (85, 113). In hyperglycemic subjects, for example, destruction of glial cells, swelling of tissue, and infarction are more prominent features of ischemia, suggesting that the degree of cellular lactic acidosis is also important (71, 83, 104). At present, it seems probable that different mechanisms are responsible for producing selective neuronal vulnerability as compared to cerebral infarction.

Therapeutic measures aimed at the protection of the brain from ischemia should be based on a knowledge of the pathophysiologic and biochemical processes involved. As a basis for the subsequent discussion of mechanisms promoting ischemic brain damage, we first review briefly certain aspects of metabolic changes occurring during ischemia and recirculation.

CEREBRAL METABOLIC CHANGES DURING ISCHEMIA

Energy Metabolism

Following a sudden interruption of cerebral circulation, the energy reserves of the brain are rapidly depleted. The oxygen stores of brain tissue are negligible and can sustain normal energy demands for only a few seconds (103). Apart from available phosphocreatine (PCr) and ATP, only the ATP that is formed during anaerobic glycolysis can subsequently be used during ischemia. The changes occurring during ischemia may be summarized in four equations (Eq.):

$$ATP + HOH \rightarrow ADP + P_i + H^+, \qquad (5.1)$$
$$PCr + ADP + H^+ \rightarrow Cr + ATP, \qquad (5.2)$$
$$ADP + ADP \rightarrow ATP + AMP, \qquad (5.3)$$
$$Glucose + 2\ ADP + P_i \rightarrow 2$$
$$lactate^- + 2H^+ + 2\ ATP, \qquad (5.4)$$

in which HOH = water, ADP is adenosine diphosphate, P_i is inorganic phosphate, Cr is creatine, and AMP is adenosine monophosphate. During ischemia, much of the available ATP is used by the membrane-bound ATPases for maintaining ionic gradients (Fig. 5.1). ATP is then hydrolyzed to yield ADP and inorganic phosphate (P_i; Eq. 5.1). Equations 2 and 3 illustrate reactions catalyzed respectively by creatine kinase and adenylate kinase, both of which retard the depletion of ATP. During anaerobic glycolysis two molecules of ATP are formed for each glucose molecule (Eq. 5.4). PCr is depleted within the first minute of complete cortical ischemia in the rat and ATP approaches its minimal value within 2 minutes (Fig. 5.2). As lactate accumulation continues for a somewhat longer period, some additional ATP must be produced. This glycolytically produced ATP is probably used for ion transportation. If the ischemia is severe but not complete (i.e. if oxygen delivery is insufficient for aerobic metabolism) additional glucose will be supplied for anaerobic metabolism and lactate formation. The consequence of this exaggerated lactic acidosis will be discussed shortly.

In the absence of oxygen, mitochondrial production of ATP ceases. Even if some oxygen is delivered to the tissue, mitochondrial ATP production is probably negligible. In vitro studies show a marked reduction in the respiration rates of mitochondria (25, 89); poor mitochondrial function has also been shown in vivo, especially if tissue pH decreases substantially (41).

If the restoration of circulation to the

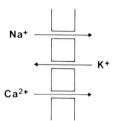

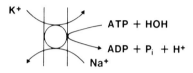

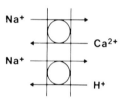

Figure 5.1. Passive ion leakage causes potassium (K^+) to leave cells and sodium (Na^+) and calcium (Ca^{2+}) to enter, as well as the energy-requiring processes which achieve repumping of the ions. Adenosine triphosphate (ATP) is used directly by the Na^+/K^+-ATPase, which exchanges three Na^+ for two K^+. The Na^+ gradient thus created can be used to extrude Ca^{2+} or hydrogen (H^+). ADP = adenosine diphosphate; P_i = inorganic phosphate; HOH = water.

brain is prompt and efficient, there can be a surprisingly rapid normalization of the cerebral energy stores, even after periods of complete ischemia lasting up to 60 minutes (27, 44–46, 61, 74, 86). A correspondingly rapid normalization of mitochondrial respiratory capacity in vitro has also been documented (41, 89).

Although the processes leading to the breakdown of cellular structure are precipitated by energy failure, ATP depletion may not be the only cause, or the direct cause, of these events. ATP depletion triggers a cascade of reactions, such as loss of ionic homeostasis and enhanced anaerobic glycolysis with secondary effects on lipid and protein metabolism. It is also sus-

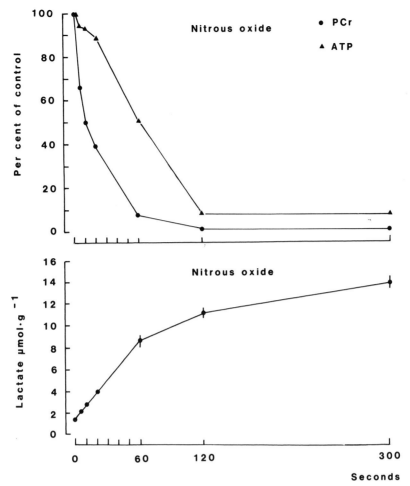

Figure 5.2.   Rate of changes in cerebral cortical concentrations of phosphocreatine (PCr), adenosine triphosphate (ATP), and lactate during total ischemia in rats. (Adapted from Nilsson B, Norberg K, Nordström C-H, et al: Rate of energy utilization in the cerebral cortex of rats. *Acta Physiol Scand* 93:569–571, 1975.)

pected that some of the most harmful reactions are produced during recirculation/reoxygenation.

Ion Homeostasis

Changes in the cortical extracellular concentrations of potassium (K$^+$), calcium Ca^{2+}), sodium (Na$^+$), and chloride (Cl$^-$), and concomitant changes in the volume of the extracellular fluid (ECF), occur during complete ischemia (39, 75) (Fig. 5.3). During the first phase (1.5 to 2 minutes after ischemia), extracellular K$^+$ rises slowly toward a value of 10 to 15 mM and extra-

cellular Ca^{2+}, Na$^+$, and Cl$^-$ remain essentially unaltered. The gradual reduction in ECF space (to about 80% of normal), however, may indicate a slow leakage of Na$^+$ and Cl$^-$ into the cells (42). In the second phase, a sudden increase in extracellular K$^+$ takes place, the extracellular concentrations of Ca^{2+}, Na$^+$, and Cl$^-$ fall, and simultaneous reduction of ECF volume to about 50% of control is observed (39, 44). This rapid breakdown of ion homeostasis occurs when PCr and ATP concentrations approach zero (Fig. 5.2); that is, the point at which energy-dependent ion transport can no longer match passive ionic fluxes caused by the electrochemical gradients.

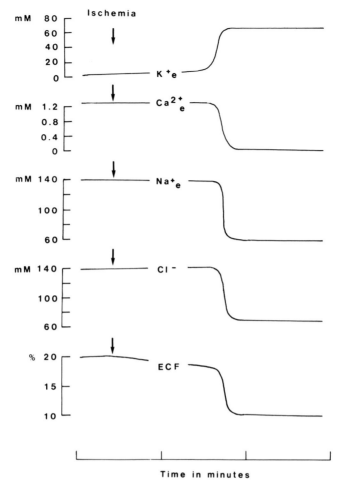

Figure 5.3. Changes occurring in cerebral cortical concentrations of volume of extracellular potassium (K^+_e), calcium (Ca^{2+}_e), sodium (Na^+_e), chloride (Cl^-), and extracellular fluid (ECF) during complete ischemia. Although K^+ shows an early, slow rise in concentration, the major ion fluxes occur about 90 seconds after interruption of circulation.

The very rapid ionic fluxes during this second phase probably indicate a sudden increase in membrane permeability to all participating ions (39, 75, 107).

The duration of the first, slow phase of ionic changes can be influenced by two factors. Because the ATP present during ischemia is used primarily for transmembrane ion transport, the duration of this phase depends on the amounts of glycolytically produced ATP during ischemia: Preischemic hyperglycemia prolongs and preischemic hypoglycemia shortens this phase (38, 102).

The duration of the slow phase also depends on the preischemic leak of ions, the functional state of the tissue, and the preischemic metabolic rate (3). The time to terminal depolarization can be maximized by lowering the metabolic rate or increasing the glucose stores. Whereas the time from the start of ischemia to terminal depolarization is 40 seconds in rats having generalized seizure activity, it is more than 4 minutes in barbiturate-anesthetized rats maintained at a body temperature of 27°C. The protective effect of hypothermia in brain ischemia is of clinical importance. The protective effect of hyperglycemia is overshadowed by the subsequent, additional, and usually detrimental lowering of pH.

Changes in Acid–Base Balance

During the first 5 minutes of complete cerebral ischemia in the rat, lactate levels increase (Fig. 5.2). The ischemic brain does not exchange electrolytes, fluids, or gases with the surrounding tissues. The metabolic acids produced cause the liberation of carbon dioxide (CO_2) from bicarbonate, which is retained within the tissue (57, 60). Under these conditions, there is a close relation between the amount of lactate accumulated and the reduction in intracellular pH.

Normal preischemic stores of glucose and glycogen suffice to increase lactate content during complete ischemia to 12 to 14 μmol g^{-1} (Fig. 5.2), causing a reduction in intracellular pH from approximately 7.0 to 6.4. The lactate values obtained depend on the preischemic nutritional state. Un-

der experimental conditions in which preischemic blood glucose levels were maintained at 2.4 μmol ml^{-1} (hypoglycemia), 7.8 μmol ml^{-1} (normoglycemia), and 28 μmol ml^{-1} (hyperglycemia), the ischemic lactate concentrations were 4.8, 12.1, and 20.7 μmol g^{-1}, respectively, and the estimated intracellular pH values were 6.83, 6.42, and 6.05, respectively (60). In severe, incomplete ischemia, the degree of lactic acidosis depends on the plasma glucose concentration as well as residual blood flow. Under these circumstances, the accumulation of lactate may considerably exceed 20 μmol g^{-1} (71, 79, 91, 114).

Provided that the ischemia is of moderate duration and reperfusion is adequate, restoration of cellular metabolism causes rapid normalization of intracellular pH (62, 114). Figure 5.4 illustrates recovery of tissue lactate content and intracellular pH in

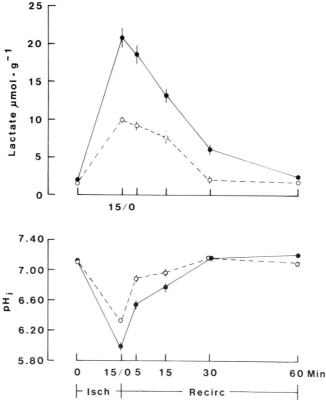

Figure 5.4. Changes in tissue lactate content and in average intracellular pH (pH$_i$) during and after ischemia of 15 minutes' duration. Isch = ischemia, Recirc = recirculation. (From Smith M-L, Hanwehr R von, Siesjö BK: Changes in extracellular and intracellular pH in the brain during and after ischemia in hyperglycemic and in moderately hypoglycemic rats. *J Cereb Blood Flow Metab* 6:574–583, 1986.)

moderate hypoglycemia and hyperglycemia after 15 minutes of experimental ischemia. The normalization of intracellular
pH is caused by extrusion of H^+ by the
transmembrane Na^+/H^+ exchange (Fig.
5.1), washout of accumulated CO_2 by the
circulation, and oxidation of accumulated
lactate. Because the Na^+/H^+ antiporter
is stimulated at low intracellular pH values
(35, 63, 84, 93), a rapid extrusion of H^+
would be anticipated when the extracel-
lular/intracellular Na^+ gradient is restored.
However, at a low extracellular pH level,
extracellular H^+ competes with Na^+. A
prompt reduction of carbon dioxide tension (PCO_2) and intravenous infusion of a
base encourages rapid normalization of intracellular pH. Of course, if ischemia is of
longer duration or if recirculation is inadequate, normal mitochondrial function is
not resumed and the acidosis is not reversed.

Lipid and Protein Metabolism

Pathways of phospholipid metabolism
are shown in Figure 5.5. The turnover of
inosine phosphoglyceride (GPI) involves
the breakdown of GPI to diphosphoglyceride (DG), and the cycle of reactions is
completed by energy-dependent reformation of GPI from DG. This cycle is connected to the metabolism of other phospholipids by a reversible pathway for base
exchange. In the general turnover of phospholipids, lysophospholipids are formed
which may be reacylated at the expense of
ATP.

As originally described by Bazan (5, 6),
ischemia is accompanied by a rapid accumulation of free fatty acids (FFAs). The
magnitude of the increase in FFA concentration observed during complete ischemia
and during severe incomplete ischemia is
similar (92) (Fig. 5.6), indicating that the
severity of intracellular acidosis does not
influence the release of FFA.

Several factors promote the degradation
of phospholipids during ischemia. First,
the liberation of transmitter substances and
the ensuing influx of Ca^{2+} into the cells
activate phospholipase A_2 (Fig. 5.5). Second, there is evidence that a substantial

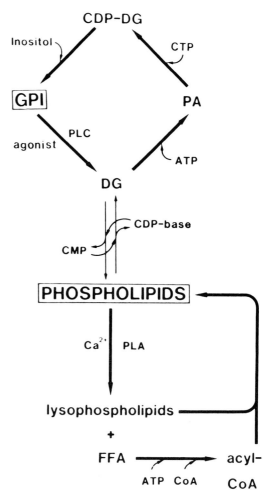

Figure 5.5. Turnover of inosine phosphoglyceride
(GPI) and resynthesis of phospholipids from their
degradation products. CDP = cytidine diphosphate;
DG = diphosphoglyceride; CTP = cytidine triphosphate; PLC = phospholipase C; PA = phosphatidic
acid; ATP = adenosine triphosphate; CMP = cytidine monophosphate; Ca^{2+} = calcium; PLA = phospholipase A; FFA = free fatty acid; CoA = coenzyme
A.

proportion of the FFAs formed during the
initial ischemic period results from activation of phospholipase C (1, 131). This enzyme is stimulated when several transmitters interact with synaptic membranes. As
the formation of inositol triphosphate trig-
gered by phospholipase C liberates Ca^{2+}
from intracellular stores (8), phospholipases C and A_2 may act in concert to raise
cytosolic Ca^{2+}, Third, the energy depletion during ischemia precludes resynthesis
of membrane phospholipids.

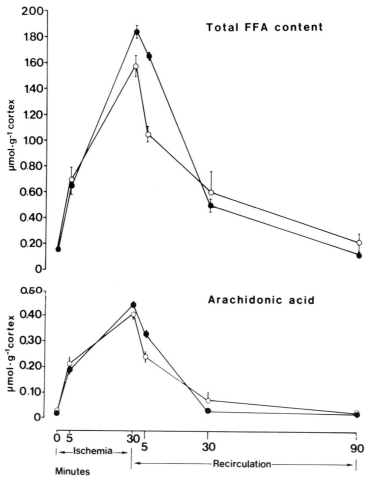

Figure 5.6. Total free fatty acid (FFA) concentrations *(upper panel)* and arachidonic acid concentration in rat cerebral cortex subjected to transient complete *(filled symbols)* and severe incomplete ischemia *(open symbols)*. (From Rehncrona S, Westerberg E, Åkesson B, et al: Brain cortical fatty acids and phospholipids during and following complete and severe incomplete ischemia. *J Neurochem* 38:84–93, 1982.)

One FFA showing a pronounced increase during ischemia is arachidonic acid (Fig. 5.6). Following recirculation of the tissue, there is a gradual decrease in FFA concentration (92, 131). During the initial phase of recirculation there is clearly sufficient oxygen and arachidonic acid to trigger a cascade of reactions along the cyclooxygenase and lipoxygenase pathways. Increased production of prostaglandins, thromboxanes, and leukotrienes will subsequently occur (68, 104, 129).

Cessation of the oxygen supply arrests all anabolic reactions but allows most catabolic reactions to proceed. Consequently, during ischemia, protein synthesis is completely blocked (9, 17, 21). Disaggregation of the polyribosomes, however, does not occur until oxygen is resupplied (17, 21).

MECHANISMS OF ISCHEMIC BRAIN DAMAGE

The neurochemical determinants of ischemic cell damage are based on the depletion of cellular energy stores and the ensuing derangement of ion homeostasis, acid–base homeostasis, and phospholipid and protein metabolism.

Acidosis and Ischemic Brain Damage

The first studies correlating the outcome following transient ischemia with level of cerebral glucose supply were published in 1976 (69, 72, 77). In that year, our group reported that rats showed better cerebral metabolic recovery after 30 minutes of complete ischemia than following a similar period of severe, incomplete ischemia (77). The remaining trickle of blood flow in the rats subjected to incomplete ischemia may impair outcome as a consequence of either continued supply of oxygen or glucose, the latter aggravating tissue lactic acidosis. In a series of experiments, Myers (69, 72) and Yamaguchi (72) showed that recovery from ischemia or hypoxia was impaired in monkeys who ingested food or had a preischemic glucose infusion (69, 72). These initial observations were confirmed in experimental studies examining clinical restitution, short-term metabolic recovery, postischemic blood recirculation, and histopathologic outcome (33, 51, 70, 71, 73, 78, 87, 90, 91, 101, 125). Thus, the exacerbation of ischemic brain damage by acidosis includes postischemic failure of mitochondrial metabolism, seizures, edema, and widespread neuronal damage. Either postischemic seizures or edema could aggravate this damage because seizures increase metabolic rate and edema may impede adequate recirculation.

If a normal perfusion pressure is obtained promptly upon recirculation, then transient ischemia is followed by a period of reactive hyperemia which, in turn, is followed by a secondary reduction of flow, usually called delayed hypoperfusion (50). Although some studies indicate that hyperglycemia may further compromise blood flow during ischemia and give rise to perfusion defects during recirculation (22, 33, 130), a similar degree of deterioration of cortical energy state during ischemia and a similar rate of restoration of high-energy phosphate compounds were reported in moderately hypoglycemic and markedly hyperglycemic animals (43, 114). In these experiments, isolated mitochondria from both groups of animals recovered their respiratory functions at similar rates (43).

These data indicate that the final deterioration of function and metabolism occurring in the hyperglycemic animals after 18 to 24 hours is preceded by a period of apparent normalization of energy metabolism. However, this interval is inversely proportional to the duration of the ischemia, and after ischemia of long duration the perfusion defects may appear in the immediate recirculation period (51). It is then difficult to differentiate between a true no-reflow phenomenon (2) and a rapidly developing, secondary deterioration of flow.

The difference in lactate concentration between hypoglycemic and hyperglycemic groups persists for a period of time during recirculation (Fig. 5.4). Ischemia is accompanied by accumulation of endogenously formed osmoles that lead to edema upon recirculation (47). A large part of these osmoles is due to lactate. Thus, one might expect an exaggeration of postischemic edema in hyperglycemic animals. In a comparison of normoglycemic and hyperglycemic rats (122), the specific gravity of tissue from cortex and caudate putamen obtained after 10 minutes of forebrain ischemia (Fig. 5.7) showed a transient increase in tissue water content during the first 3 to 6 hours after ischemia. Both groups also developed a secondary increase in tissue water content after 24 hours. This late edema was transient in the normoglycemic rats and more pronounced in hyperglycemic animals. Hyperglycemic rats did not recover; they developed seizures resulting in a further increase in tissue water and a secondary perturbation of ion homeostasis. These findings indicate that severe acidosis during ischemia may lead to delayed brain injury.

In normoglycemic animals, transient ischemia is known to cause neuronal damage in certain selectively vulnerable regions (10). In contrast, in glucose-infused animals, neuronal damage is widespread, tissue edema is pronounced ("status spongiosus"), and the lesions are characterized by marked clumping of nuclear chromatin (51, 70, 71, 87). In a recent series of studies, the effects of hyperglycemia on postischemic histopathology have been further characterized, with three principal find-

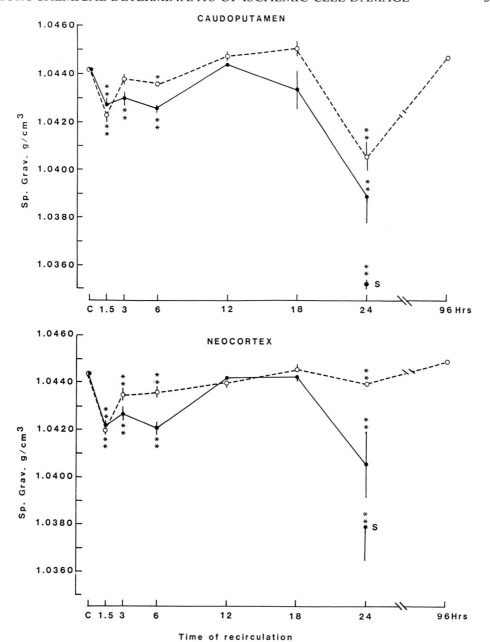

Figure 5.7. Specific gravity (Sp. Grav.) measured in caudoputamen *(top)* and neocortex *(bottom)* at different times after recirculation in normoglycemic *(open symbols)* and hyperglycemic *(filled symbols)* animals. The filled symbol marked with "S" denotes the group with seizures. The graph illustrates the biphasic edema after ischemia. (From Smith M-L, Siesjö BK: Acidosis-related brain damage: Immediate and delayed events. In Somjen G (ed): *Mechanisms of Cerebral Hypoxia and Stroke*. New York, Plenum, 1988, pp 57–71.

ings (115, 116): *(a)* hyperglycemia shortens the maturation period, that is, it reduces the time lag before histopathologic alterations are observed; *(b)* hyperglycemia increases the severity of the lesions; and *(c)*

a specific type of lesion encompassing unilateral or bilateral necrosis of the substantia nigra, pars reticulata (SNPR) is observed.

The pathogenesis of postischemic sei-

zures is far from clear. It has been speculated, however, that neurons involved in
the normal inhibitory control of seizure
activity are injured during ischemia (112).
It is widely accepted that, apart from a
local inhibitory control, there is also a γ-
aminobutyric acid (GABA)-ergic system
which exerts a more general influence on
neuronal excitability. This system is con-
stituted by the neurons in SNPR, which
may be central to preventing generaliza-
tion of local seizure activity (28, 29, 48, 66).
In all probability, the relationship between
the occurrence of postischemic seizures and
the observed histopathologic lesions in
SNPR is complex. The observation that
spongiotic lesions in SNPR appear very
soon after an ischemic event, however,
has led to the suggestion that this damage
represents a combined excitotoxic and acidosis-related effect (117); excitotoxic damage is discussed later in this chapter.

The molecular mechanisms explaining
the deleterious effects of extreme acidosis
during ischemia are only incompletely
known. A low intracellular pH inhibits
mitochondrial phosphorylation (41). It has
also been proposed that glial cells may
choose to regulate intracellular pH during
acidosis, thereby sacrificing their volume
regulation (53, 54, 106, 107). Thus, severe
acidosis may exacerbate early damage with
failure of energy metabolism, progressive
edema, and secondary compromise of microcirculation. However, in the experiments just discussed (Fig. 5.7), glucose-
infused animals did not show much accen-
tuation of the initial edema. The ultimate
deterioration occurred after a delay during
which normal tissue water content is found.

The mechanisms contributing to the delayed alteration of membrane function that
leads to cellular edema and generalized
seizure activity remain speculative. Possibly the insult gives rise to an injury that
prevents long-term recovery, although
short-term restitution seems to be adequate. For example, if the primary lesion
causes permanent damage to deoxyribo-
nucleic acid (DNA) or protein synthesis
(9), it would first become manifest when
the cell's preischemic stores of essential
proteins were depleted. It has been suggested previously that severe acidosis
may cause denaturation of proteins and nu-

cleic acids (51). Such denaturation may
be a result of low pH as such, but may
also reflect damage resulting from interaction of free radicals with membrane
components.

Free Radicals and Reperfusion Damage

For several years, it has been speculated
that free-radical reactions contribute to cell
damage during ischemia (11, 19, 26, 37,
104, 109). Free radicals such as the superoxide anion ($\cdot O_2^-$) normally participate in
a variety of cellular reactions: they are generated in the respiratory chain; they take
part in reactions catalyzed by cyclooxygenase and lipoxygenase; they are formed in
the xanthine oxidase reaction; and they
arise during autooxidation of many substances, including catecholamines. During
recirculation, an increase in the formation
of free radicals can be anticipated (104).
These reactions include the release, reuptake, and oxidation of catecholamines, the
oxidation of polyenoic FFAs, and the oxidation of hypoxanthine accumulated during ischemia. They reflect the restoration
of homeostasis after the metabolic cascade
which occurred during the ischemia. We
recognize that many of them represent
Ca^{2+}-triggered cascades; for example, Ca^{2+}
influx and release is, at least in part, responsible for lipolysis and accumulation of
arachidonic acid, as discussed earlier. Furthermore, McCord (65) has suggested that
oxidation of hypoxanthine and xanthine to
$\cdot O_2^-$ occurs because the normally predominant xanthine dehydrogenase (which does
not produce $\cdot O_2^-$) is converted to xanthine
oxidase by a protease, activated by Ca^{2+}.

Although free-radical mechanisms provide a logical and probable explanation for
the development of brain damage after
ischemia, there is actually little experimental evidence that such reactions are important. At present, there is experimental
support for the view that free-radical reactions may contribute to cerebral vasospasm and vascular damage caused by
trauma (56, 98, 124), but it is less well
established that such reactions are responsible for the damage affecting neurons or
glial cells. From a theoretical point of view,

it is also difficult to explain why the most likely product in most free-radical reactions, the relatively untoxic $\cdot O_2^-$ ion, should cause damage to cells that have an abundance of enzymatic and nonenzymatic scavenger systems. This may relate to the deleterious effect of extreme acidosis.

Acidosis enhances free-radical reactions in vitro (108). This effect may be explained by noting that a low pH $\cdot O_2^-$ is converted to its hydrated form (HO_2) which is more lipid soluble and prooxidant (32). Alternatively, as suggested by Barber and Bernheim (4), acidosis may promote free-radical reactions by releasing prooxidant iron from proteins such as ferritin and transferrin. It is likely that a more injurious free-radical species (OH·) is formed when iron catalyzes the reaction between $\cdot O_2^-$ and H_2O_2 (36, 37). Normally, iron in the form of Fe^{3+} is tightly bound to ferritin and transferrin. The $\cdot O_2^-$ formed during recirculation may reduce this Fe^{3+}, which is then released and possibly chelated to compounds of lower molecular weight where it may act as a prooxidant. We suggest that acidosis acts similarly by causing the release of iron from ferritin and transferrin. In support of this notion it has been reported that such low-molecular-weight iron chelates increase during postischemic recirculation (55).

Recently, it has been suggested that iron-catalyzed free-radical damage to DNA may be partly responsible for ischemic cell injury (55, 58). Certainly there may be several connections among the derangement of intracellular pH regulation during ischemia, iron metabolism, and free-radical reactions during recirculation. Because free-radical reactions are known to propagate slowly in the plane of membranes, such mechanisms may also explain why some ischemic damage first appears after a seemingly injury-free interval.

Intracellular Calcium and Cell Death

Under physiologic conditions, intracellular Ca^{2+} serves as a key regulator of a multitude of cellular functions. During excitation of neurons, the opening of voltage-sensitive calcium channels (VSCCs) and agonist-operated calcium channels (AOCCs) allows intracellular Ca^{2+} to rise. This event results in two types of metabolic effects: (a) Ca^{2+}, either directly or after binding to regulator proteins like calmodulin, modulates the functional state of cellular enzymes and the functional state of membrane channels; and (b) a rise in intracellular Ca^{2+} influences the rate-limiting steps in the citric acid cycle and thus augments metabolic rate and ATP formation. This effect is exerted on rate-limiting intramitochondrial dehydrogenases (20, 40).

A breakdown of Ca^{2+} homeostasis may be a mechanism responsible for ischemic cell damage (88, 104, 107, 109, 110) (Fig. 5.8). During ischemia, an influx of Ca^{2+} occurs through VSCCs and AOCCs. Simultaneously, lack of ATP and of oxygen prevents Ca^{2+} extrusion and sequestration of Ca^{2+} by mitochondria and endoplasmic reticulum. On the basis of the ability of Ca^{2+} to activate lipases and proteases in micromolar concentrations (52, 99), Ca^{2+}-related damage may occur if cytosolic Ca^{2+} concentrations increase substantially. Proteolysis and Ca^{2+}-induced disaggregation of microtubuli might then disrupt the cytoskeleton and its anchorage to plasma membranes. Moreover, toxic products of phospholipid hydrolysis, such as lyso-phospholipids, FFAs, and leukotrienes, may adversely affect membrane structure and function (11, 109, 110).

With respect to noncerebral tissues, the Ca^{2+} hypothesis has recently been questioned (12). It is not known whether Ca^{2+} accumulation precedes cell damage or occurs as a result of it. In vitro, cells that ultimately die in response to anoxia or poisons often fail to show an increase in intracellular Ca^{2+}. It has also been emphasized that a shortage of ATP may produce effects similar to those attributed to an elevated Ca^{2+} concentration, such as actions on proteolysis and lipolysis (59). Because there is normally a rapid turnover of certain phospholipids, energy depletion would result in the accumulation of FFAs and other degradation products simply by preventing resynthesis. The turnover of proteins may cause a corresponding dissolution of the cytoskeleton, resulting in plasma membrane dysfunction and blebbing (59, 119).

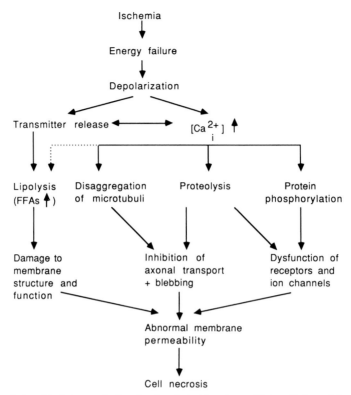

Figure 5.8. The relationship between ischemia, depolarization, loss of intracellular calcium (Ca^{2+}_i) homeostasis, and presumed Ca^{2+}_i-related, pathologic events. Because lipolysis occurs mainly by phospholipase C activity, a rise in Ca^{2+}_i may not be an important cause of the accumulation of free fatty acids (FFAs).

These alternative mechanisms do not, however, exclude the possibility that Ca^{2+} influx is an important mediator of ischemic cell damage. When the Ca^{2+} hypothesis was advanced to explain neuronal damage, it was assumed that Ca^{2+} influx through VSCCs could explain cell damage in states of ischemia, hypoglycemia, and status epilepticus, as well as the phenomenon of selective vulnerability (104). Recent results in vitro support the concept of such Ca^{2+}-related damage but suggest a different route of Ca^{2+} influx (13, 14, 95). These and other studies indicate that the adverse effect of Ca^{2+} is exerted at neuronal sites with a high density of AOCCs gated by excitatory amino acids.

Excitotoxic Damage

Excitotoxins have been implicated in the pathogenesis of a variety of neurologic diseases, and during the past few years this field of research has produced an explosion of information. Originally, the involvement of excitatory amino acids was proposed to account for neuronal necrosis in chronic degenerative neurologic disorders and epilepsy (18, 80, 100). Similar pathophysiologic mechanisms have also been suggested to cause brain damage in states of ischemia and hypoglycemia (7, 49, 93, 111, 126, 127), two conditions which may show dendrosomatic, axon-sparing features consistent with excitotoxic lesions. In each of those conditions, the extracellular concentrations of glutamate and aspartate increase markedly, probably because release is enhanced and reuptake is inhibited.

Glutamate and aspartate are ubiquitous excitatory transmitters within the central nervous system (16, 24, 123). Three major postsynaptic receptor types, which are mainly localized to the dendritic regions, have been identified. These receptors are selectively stimulated by the neurotoxins kainate, quisqualate, and N-methyl-D-aspartate (NMDA), respectively (Fig. 5.9). Their relative distributions within the central nervous system differ, they mediate different functional responses, and they are blocked by different antagonists. The NMDA-receptor complex is now believed to be a member of a superfamily of proteins, including receptors and ion channels for the neurotransmitters acetylcholine, glycine, and GABA. Recent information indicates that the NMDA receptors are linked to phenomena such as long-term potentiation, regulation of synaptic differentiation during brain development, learning, and memorizing.

There is now ample evidence that excitatory amino acid receptors are, at least in part, responsible for neuronal damage during ischemia as well as hypoglycemia: (a) glutamate induces excessive swelling and neuronal death in vitro in neuronal cultures subjected to hypoxic conditions (13, 15, 94); (b) glutamate and aspartate are found in high concentrations in the ECF during ischemia and during postischemic recirculation (7); (c) transection of major

putative glutamatergic excitatory input to the hippocampus ameliorates ischemic damage (128); (d) local injections of a glutamate-receptor antagonist appear to protect the hippocampus against ischemic damage in experimental forebrain ischemia (111); and (e) noncompetitive NMDA antagonists reduce the size of the ischemic lesion following experimental occlusion of the middle cerebral artery (81).

The molecular mechanisms underlying excitotoxic lesions are still obscure but may tentatively be discussed according to Figure 5.9, which illustrates schematically two types of ionic channels gated by glutamate. The involvement of Ca^{2+} in the activation of this receptor has only recently been clarified (16, 64). When glutamate acts on kainate and quisqualate receptors, the conductance for Na^+ probably increases, allowing an influx of Na^+ because of its steep electrochemical gradient. This influx of Na^+ forces Cl^- to enter through normal or activated anion channels, and, for osmotic reasons, water passes into the cell and dendritic edema may develop (95, 121). When glutamate interacts with the

Agonist-operated channels

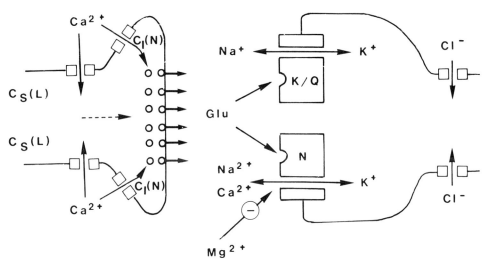

Figure 5.9. Presynaptic voltage-sensitive calcium channels as well as two types of postsynaptic channels gated by glutamate receptors. The presynaptic channels are assumed to be of the L and N types, the L type being sensitive (C_s) and the N type insensitive (C_i) to calcium antagonists of the dihydropyridine class. Agonist-operated channels, which are activated by glutamate, have been assumed to be gated by kainate/quisqualate (K/Q) or by NMDA (N) receptors. Normally, only the latter is supposed to open a conductance for calcium. Ca^{2+} = calcium; Na^+ = sodium; K^+ = potassium; Mg^{2+} = magnesium; Glu = glucose; Cl^- = chloride. (From Siesjö BK: Historical overview: Calcium, ischemia and death of brain cells. *Ann NY Acad Sci* 522:638–661, 1988.)

NMDA receptor, Ca^{2+} enters the cell. The increase in Ca^{2+} conductance is strongly antagonized by magnesium, which normally blocks the channel. This block is relieved during membrane depolarization. Thus, two events are required to provoke Ca^{2+} influx: depolarization of the cell membrane and activation of the NMDA receptor.

The sudden changes of extracellular concentrations of Na^+, Cl^-, and Ca^{2+} occurring after 60 to 90 seconds of complete cerebral ischemia (Fig. 5.3) are caused by neuronal depolarization and sudden release of excitatory amino acids (EEAs). Consequently, at this point massive influxes of Na^+, Ca^{2+} and Cl^- and an influx of water occur. Since the channel gated by the kainate–quisqualate receptor is probably equally permeable to all monovalent cations, a sudden influx of H^+ through that channel might be anticipated. A localized intracellular acidosis may then occur among the cascade of reactions elicited by excitatory amino acids. Furthermore, it has recently been observed that toxicity of kainate to cerebellar neurons in vitro may be prevented by inhibition of the enzyme xanthine oxidase (23). This observation suggests that excitotoxin-induced neuronal damage may also be mediated by superoxide radicals.

Excitotoxic postsynaptic damage occurring after ischemia may be due to several cooperating mechanisms: local increase in intracellular Ca^{2+}; osmolytic damage of dendrites; local acidosis; and free-radical reactions. In a recent series of in vitro experiments (14, 15), some aspects of glutamate neurotoxicity were clarified. Glutamate was found to produce morphologic changes in mature, but not in immature, cortical neurons. Furthermore, the results indicate that the neurotoxicity of glutamate has two components. During the first phase, a marked neuronal swelling occurs which is dependent on extracellular Na^+ and Cl^- and which can be mimicked by high K^+. The second component occurs later and is characterized by gradual neuronal disintegration. This damage is dependent on extracellular Ca^{2+} and is probably mediated by transmembrane influx of Ca^{2+}. Finally, the results indicate that the lethal Ca^{2+} entry takes place via AOCCs and that NMDA receptors may play a dominant role in mediating glutamate neurotoxicity.

PERSPECTIVE

Experimental data at present indicate that several mechanisms are involved in the development of ischemic brain damage. It seems very probable that the mechanisms responsible for selective neuronal vulnerability are different from those causing glial swelling and extensive brain edema. Moreover, during the period of recirculation, functional aberrations such as epileptic seizure activity contribute to the ultimate damage.

Several studies indicate that selective neuronal vulnerability is, at least in part, an excitotoxic lesion. Although the molecular mechanisms are not accurately known, it seems probable that Ca^{2+} influx through NMDA-activated channels is of considerable importance and that osmolytic damage to dendrites and dendritic spines may contribute to neuronal damage.

The molecular mechanisms promoting glial destruction, laminar necrosis, and ultimately infarction are less well delineated. In these lesions, tissue edema is a dominating feature and one may speculate that the inability of the cells to regulate their volume may be a primary defect. This might occur if the cells regulate their intracellular pH at the expense of their volume regulation. When ischemia is accompanied by delayed acidosis-related damage, a pH-related damage to protein structure and function seems likely to occur. Such a lesion could gradually increase and ultimately cause gross membrane dysfunction. Although the experimental evidence is weak at present, the primary damage to membrane components could be due to iron-catalyzed free-radical reactions enhanced by the drastic lowering of pH.

References

1. Abe K, Kogure K, Yamamoto H, et al: Mechanisms of arachidonic acid liberation during ischemia in gerbil cerebral cortex. *J Neurochem* 48: 503–509, 1987.

2. Ames A III, Wright RL, Kowada M, et al: Cerebral ischemia. II. The no-reflow phenomenon. *Am J Pathol* 52:437–453, 1968.

3. Astrup J, Rehncrona S, Siesjö BK: The increase in extracellular potassium concentration in the ischemic brain in relation to the preischemic functional activity and cerebral metabolic rate. *Brain Res* 199:161–174, 1980.

4. Barber AA, Bernheim F: Lipid peroxidation: Its measurement, occurrence, and significance in animal tissues. *Adv Gerontol Res* 2:355–403, 1967.

5. Bazan NG: Effects of ischemia and electroconvulsive shock on free fatty acid pool in the brain. *Biochim Biophys Acta* 218:1–10, 1970.

6. Bazan NG: Free arachidonic acid and other lipids in the nervous system during ischemia and after electroshock. In Porcellati G, Amaducci L, Galli C (eds): *Function and Metabolism of Phospholipids in the Central and Peripheral Nervous Systems*. New York, Plenum, 1976, pp 317–335.

7. Benveniste H, Drejer J, Schousboe A, et al: Elevation of the extracellular concentrations of glutamate and aspartate in rat hippocampus during transient cerebral ischemia monitored by intracerebral microdialysis. *J Neurochem* 43:1369–1374, 1984.

8. Berridge MJ: Inositol triphosphate and diacylglycerol as second messengers. *Biochem J* 220:345–360, 1984.

9. Bodsch W, Takahashi K, Barbier A, et al: Cerebral protein synthesis and ischemia. *Prog Brain Res* 63:197–210, 1985.

10. Brierley JB, Graham DI: Hypoxia and vascular disorders of the central nervous system. In Adams JH, Corsellis JAN, Duchen LW (eds): *Greenfield's Neuropathology*, ed 4. London, Edward Arnold, 1984, pp 125–207.

11. Chan PH, Fishman RA: Free fatty acids, oxygen free radicals, and membrane alterations in brain ischemia and injury. In Plum F, Pulsinelli W (eds): *Cerebrovascular Diseases* (Transactions of the Thirteenth Research [Princeton] Conference). New York, Raven Press, 1985, pp 161–171.

12. Cheung JY, Bonventre JV, Malis CD, et al: Calcium and ischemic injury. *N Engl J Med* 314:1670–1676, 1986.

13. Choi DW: Glutamate neurotoxicity in cortical cell culture is calcium dependent. *Neurosci Lett* 58:293–297, 1985.

14. Choi DW: Ionic dependence of glutamate neurotoxicity. *J Neurosci* 7:369–379, 1987.

15. Choi DW, Maulucci-Gedde M, Kriegstein AR: Glutamate neurotoxicity in cortical cell culture. *J Neurosci* 7:357–368, 1987.

16. Collingridge GL: Long-term potentiation in the hippocampus: Mechanisms of initiation and modulation by neurotransmitters. *TIPS* 6:407–411, 1985.

17. Cooper HK, Zalewska, T, Kawamaki S, et al: The effect of ischemia and recirculation on protein synthesis in the rat brain. *J Neurochem* 28:929–934, 1977.

18. Coyle JT, Bird SJ, Evans RH, et al: Excitatory amino acid neurotoxins: Selectivity, specificity, and mechanisms of action. *Neurosci Res Program Bull* 19:330–337, 1982.

19. Demopoulos H, Flamm E, Seligman M, et al: Molecular pathology of lipids in CNS membranes. In Jöbsis FF (ed): *Oxygen and Physiological Function*. Dallas, Professional Information Library, 1977, pp 491–508.

20. Denton RM, McCormack JG: Ca^{2+} transport by mammalian mitochondria and its role in hormone action. *Am J Physiol* 249:E543–E554, 1985.

21. Dienel GA, Pulsinelli WA, Duffy T: Regional protein synthesis in rat brain following acute hemispheric ischemia, *J Neurochem* 35:1216–1226, 1980.

22. Dietrich WD, Busto R, Yoshida S, et al: Histopathological and hemodynamic consequences of complete versus incomplete ischemia in the rat. *J Cereb Blood Flow Metab* 7:300–308, 1987.

23. Dykens JA, Stern A, Trenkner E: Mechanism of kainate toxicity to cerebellar neurons in vitro is analogous to reperfusion tissue injury. *J Neurochem* 49:1222–1228, 1987.

24. Fagg GE: L-glutamate, excitatory amino acid receptors and brain function. *TINS* 8:207–210, 1985.

25. Fiskum G: Involvement of mitochondria in ischemic cell injury and in regulation of intracellular calcium. *Am J Emerg Med* 1:147–153, 1983.

26. Flamm E, Demopoulos HB, Seligman ML, et al: Free radicals in cerebral ischemia. *Stroke* 9:445–447, 1978.

27. Folbergrová, J, Ljunggren B, Norberg K, et al: Influence of complete ischemia on glycolytic metabolites, citric acid cycle intermediates, and associated amino acids in the rat cerebral cortex. *Brain Res* 80:265–279, 1974.

28. Gale K: Mechanisms of seizure control mediated by gamma-aminobutyric acid: Role of the substantia nigra. *Fed Proc* 44:2414–2424, 1985.

29. Gale K: Role of the substantia nigra in GABA-mediated anticonvulsant action. *Adv Neurol* 44:343–364, 1986.

30. Garcia JH: Experimental ischemic stroke: A review. *Stroke* 15:5–14, 1984.

31. Garcia JH, Kalimo H, Kamijyo Y, et al: Cellular events during partial cerebral ischemia. I. Electron microscopy of feline cerebral cortex after middle-cerebral-artery occlusion. *Virchows Arch [B]* 25:191–206, 1977.

32. Gebicki JA, Bielsky BHJ: Comparison of the capacities of the perhydroxyl and the superoxide radicals to initiate chain oxidation of linoleic acid. *J Am Chem Soc* 103:7020–7022, 1981.

33. Ginsberg MD, Frank AW, Budd WW: Deleterious effect of glucose pretreatment on recovery from diffuse cerebral ischemia in the cat. *Stroke* 11:347–354, 1980.

34. Gisvold SE, Safar P, Rao G, et al: Multifaceted therapy after global brain ischemia in monkeys. *Stroke* 15:803–812, 1984.

35. Grinstein S, Rothstein A: Mechanisms of the regulation of the Na^+/H^+ exchanger: Topical review. *J Membr Biol* 90:1–12, 1986.

36. Halliwell B, Gutteridge JMC: The importance of free radicals and catalytic metal ions in human diseases. *Mol Aspects Med* 8:89–193, 1985.

37. Halliwell B, Gutteridge JMC: Oxygen radicals and the nervous system. *TINS* 8:22–26, 1985.

38. Hansen AJ: The extracellular potassium concentration in brain cortex following ischemia in hypo- and hyperglycemic rats. *Acta Physiol Scand* 102:324–329, 1978.

39. Hansen AJ: Effects of anoxia on ion distribution in the brain. *Physiol Rev* 65:101–148, 1985.

40. Hansford RG: Relation between mitochondrial calcium transport and control of energy metabolism. *Rev Physiol Biochem Pharmacol* 102:1–72, 1985.

41. Hillered L, Ernster L, Siesjö BK: Influence of in vitro lactic acidosis and hypercapnia on respiratory activity of isolated rat brain mitochondria. *J Cereb Blood Flow Metab* 4:430–437, 1984.

42. Hillered L, Siesjö BK, Arfors KE: Mitochondrial response to transient forebrain ischemia in the rat. *J Cereb Blood Flow Metab* 4:438–446, 1984.

43. Hillered L, Smith M-L, Siesjö BK: Lactic acidosis and recovery of mitochondrial function following forebrain ischemia in the rat. *J Cereb Blood Flow Metab* 5:259–266, 1985.

44. Hossmann K-A: Treatment of experimental cerebral ischemia. *J Cereb Blood Flow Metab* 2:275–297, 1982.

45. Hossmann K-A: Post-ischemic resuscitation of the brain: Selective vulnerability versus global resistance. *Prog Brain Res* 63:3–17, 1985.

46. Hossmann K-A, Kleihues P: Reversibility of ischemic brain damage. *Arch Neurol* 29:375–384, 1973.

47. Hossmann K-A, Zimmerman V: Resuscitation of the monkey brain after 1 hour's complete ischemia. I. Physiological and morphological observations. *Brain Res* 81:59–74, 1974.

48. Iadarola MJ, Gale K: Substantia nigra: Site of anticonvulsant activity mediated by gamma-aminobutyric acid. *Science* 218:1237–1240, 1982.

49. Jørgensen MB, Diemer NH: Selective neuron loss after cerebral ischemia in the rat. Possible role of transmitter glutamate. *Acta Neurol Scand* 66:536–546, 1982.

50. Kågström E, Smith M-L, Siesjö BK: Recirculation in the rat brain following incomplete ischemia. *J Cereb Blood Flow Metab* 3:183–192, 1983.

51. Kalimo H, Rehncrona S, Söderfeldt B, et al: Brain lactic acidosis and ischemic cell damage: 2. Histopathology. *J Cereb Blood Flow Metab* 1:313–327, 1981.

52. Katz AM, Messineo FC: Lipid membrane interactions and the pathogenesis of ischemic damage in the myocardium. *Circ Res* 48:1–16, 1981.

53. Kempski O, Staub F, von Rosen F, et al: Molecular mechanisms of glial swelling in vitro. *Neurochem Pathol* 9:109–114, 1988.

54. Kimelberg KH, Rose JW, Barron KD, et al: Astrocytic swelling in head injury: Beneficial effects of an inhibitor of anion exchange transport and glutamate uptake in glial cells. *Neurochem Pathol,* in press.

55. Komara JS, Nayini NR, Bialick HA, et al: Brain ion delocalization and lipid peroxidation following cardiac arrest. *Ann Emerg Med* 15:384–389, 1986.

56. Kontos HA: Oxygen radicals in cerebral vascular injury. *Circ Res* 57:508–516, 1985.

57. Kraig RP, Pulsinelli WA, Plum F: Carbonic acid buffer changes during complete brain ischemia. *Am J Physiol* 250:R348–R357, 1986.

58. Krause GS, Joyce KM, Nayini NR, et al: Cardiac arrest and resuscitation: Brain iron delocalization during reperfusion. *Ann Emerg Med* 14:1037–1043, 1985.

59. Lemasters JJ, Diguiseppi J, Nieminen AL, et al: Blebbing, free Ca^{2+} and mitochondrial membrane potential preceding cell death in hepatocytes. *Nature* 325:78–81, 1987.

60. Ljunggren B, Norberg K, Siesjö BK: Influence of tissue acidosis upon restitution of brain energy metabolism following total ischemia. *Brain Res* 77:173–186, 1974.

61. Ljunggren B, Ratcheson RA, Siesjö BK: Cerebral metabolic state following complete compression ischemia. *Brain Res* 73:291–307, 1974.

62. Mabe H, Blomquist P, Siesjö BK: Intracellular pH in the brain following transient ischemia. *J Cereb Blood Flow Metab* 3:109–114, 1983.

63. Mahnensmith RL, Aronson PS: The plasma membrane sodium–hydrogen exchanger and its role in physiological and pathophysiological processes. *Circ Res* 56:773–788, 1985.

64. Mayer M: Two channels reduced to one [news]. *Nature* 324:480–481, 1987.

65. McCord JM: Oxygen-derived free radicals in postischemic tissue injury. *N Engl J Med* 312:159–163, 1985.

66. McNamara JO, Galloway MT, Rigsbee LC, et al: Evidence implicating substantia nigra in regulation of kindled seizure threshold. *J Neurosci* 4:2410–2417, 1984.

67. Miller JR, Myers RE: Neurological effects of systemic circulation arrest in the monkey. *Neurology* 20:715–724, 1970.

68. Moskowitz MA, Kiwak KJ, Hekiman K, et al: Synthesis of compounds with properties of leukotrienes C_4 and D_4 in gerbil brains after ischemia and reperfusion. *Science* 224:886–889, 1984.

69. Myers RE: Anoxic brain pathology and blood glucose (abstract). *Neurology* 26:345, 1976.

70. Myers RE: A unitary theory of causation of anoxic and hypoxic brain pathology. *Adv Neurol* 26:195–213, 1979.

71. Myers RE: Lactic acid accumulation as cause of brain edema and cerebral necrosis resulting from oxygen deprivation. In Korobkin R, Guilleminault G (eds): *Advances in Perinatal Neurology.* New York, Spectrum, 1979, pp 85–114.

72. Myers RE, Yamaguchi S: Effects of serum glucose concentration on brain response to circulatory arrest (abstract). *J Neuropathol Exp Neurol* 35:301, 1976.

73. Myers RE, Yamaguchi S: Nervous system effects of cardiac arrest in monkeys. *Arch Neurol* 34:65–74, 1977.

74. Nemoto EM, Bleyaert AL, Stezoski SW, et al: Global brain ischemia: A reproducible monkey model. *Stroke* 8:558–564, 1977.

75. Nicholson C: Dynamics of the brain cell microenvironment. *Neurosci Res Program Bull* 18:177–187, 1980.

76. Nilsson B, Norberg K, Nordström C-H, et al: Rate of energy utilization in the cerebral cortex of rats. *Acta Physiol Scand* 93:569–571, 1975.

77. Nordström C-H, Rehncrona S, Siesjö BK: Restitution of cerebral energy state after complete and incomplete ischemia of 30 minute duration. *Acta Physiol Scand* 97:270–272, 1976.

78. Nordström C-H, Rehncrona S, Siesjö BK: Effects of phenobarbital in cerebral ischemia. Part II: Restitution of cerebral energy state as well as of glycolytic metabolites, citric acid cycle intermediates and associated amino acids after pronounced incomplete ischemia. *Stroke* 9:335–343, 1978.

79. Nordström C-H, Siesjö BK: Effects of phenobarbital in cerebral ischemia. Part I: Cerebral energy metabolism during pronounced incomplete ischemia. *Stroke* 9:327–335, 1978.

80. Olney JW: Neurotoxicity of excitatory amino acids. In McGeer EG, Olney JW, McGreer PL (eds): *Kainic as a Tool in Neurobiology.* New York, Raven Press, 1978, pp 95–121.

81. Oyzurt E, Graham DI, McCulloch J, et al: The NMDA receptor antagonist MK-801 reduces focal ischemic brain damage in the cat. *J Cereb Blood Flow Metab* 7[Suppl 1]:S146, 1987.

82. Petito CK, Pulsinelli WA, Jacobson G, et al: Edema and vascular permeability in cerebral ischemia: Comparison between ischemic neuronal damage and infarction. *J Neuropathol Exp Neurol* 41:423–436, 1982.

83. Plum F: What causes infarction in ischemic brain? The Robert Wartenberg Lecture. *Neurology* 33:222–233, 1983.

84. Pouysségur J: The growth factor-activatable Na$^+$/H$^+$ exchange system: A genetic approach. *TIBS* 8:453–457, 1985.

85. Pulsinelli WA, Brierley JB, Plum F: Temporal profile of neuronal damage in a model of transient forebrain ischemia. *Ann Neurol* 11:491–498, 1982.

86. Pulsinelli WA, Duffy T: Regional energy balance in rat brain after transient forebrain ischemia. *J Neurochem* 40:1500–1503, 1983.

87. Pulsinelli WA, Waldman S, Rawlinson D, et al: Moderate hyperglycemia augments ischemic brain damage: A neuropathologic study in the rat. *Neurology* 32:1239–1246, 1982.

88. Raichle M: The pathophysiology of brain ischemia. *Ann Neurol* 13:2–10, 1983.

89. Rehncrona S, Mela L, Siesjö BK: Recovery of brain mitochondrial function in the rat after complete and incomplete cerebral ischemia. *Stroke* 10:437–446, 1979.

90. Rehncrona S, Rosén I, Siesjö BK: Excessive cellular acidosis: An important mechanism of neuronal damage in the brain. *Acta Physiol Scand* 110:435–437, 1980.

91. Rehncrona S, Rosén I, Siesjö BK: Brain lactic acidosis and ischemic cell damage: 1. Biochemistry and neurophysiology. *J Cereb Blood Flow Metab* 1:297–311, 1981.

92. Rehncrona S, Westerberg E, Åkesson B, et al: Brain cortical fatty acids and phospholipids during and following complete and severe incomplete ischemia. *J Neurochem* 38:84–93, 1982.

93. Roos A, Boron WF: Intracellular pH. *Physiol Rev* 61:296–434, 1981.

94. Rothman S: Synaptic release of excitatory amino acid neurotransmitter mediates anoxic neuronal death. *J Neurosci* 4:1884–1891, 1984.

95. Rothman SM, Olney JW: Glutamate and the pathophysiology of hypoxic-ischemic brain damage. *Ann Neurol* 19:105–111, 1986.

96. Safar P: Cerebral resuscitation after cardiac arrest: A review. *Circulation* 74(Suppl IV):138–153, 1986.

97. Safar P, Stezoski W, Nemoto EM: Amelioration of brain damage after 12 minutes' cardiac arrest in dogs. *Arch Neurol* 33:91–95, 1976.

98. Sano K, Asano T, Tanishima T, et al: Lipid peroxidation as a cause of cerebral vasospasm. *Neurol Res* 2:253–272, 1980.

99. Schlaepfer WW: Neurofilaments: Structure, metabolism and implications in disease. *J Neuropathol Exp Neurol* 46:117–129, 1987.

100. Schwartz R, Foster AC, French ED, et al: Excitotoxic models for neurodegenerative disorders. *Life Sci* 35:19–32, 1984.

101. Siemkowicz E, Hansen AJ: Clinical restitution following cerebral ischemia in hypo-, normo-, and hyperglycemic rats. *Acta Neurol Scand* 58:1–8, 1978.

102. Siemkowicz E, Hansen AJ: Brain extracellular ion composition and EEG activity following 10 minutes ischemia in normo- and hyperglycemic rats *Stroke* 12:236–240, 1981.

103. Siesjö BK: *Brain Energy Metabolism.* New York, John Wiley & Sons, 1978.

104. Siesjö BK: Cell damage in the brain: A speculative synthesis. *J Cereb Blood Flow Metab* 1:155–185, 1981.

105. Siesjö BK: Cerebral circulation and metabolism. *J Neurosurg* 60:883–908, 1984.

106. Siesjö BK: Acid–base homeostasis in the brain: Physiology, chemistry, and neurochemical pathology. *Prog Brain Res* 63:121–154, 1985.

107. Siesjö BK: Historical overview: Calcium, ischemia, and death of brain cells. *Ann NY Acad Sci* 522:638–661, 1988.

108. Siesjö BK, Bendek G, Koide T, et al: Influence of acidosis in lipid peroxidation in brain tissue in vitro. *J Cereb Blood Flow Metab* 5:253–258, 1985.

109. Siesjö BK, Wieloch T: Cerebral metabolism in ischemia: A neurochemical basis for therapy. *Br J Anaesth* 57:47–62, 1985.

110. Siesjö BK, Wieloch T: Epileptic brain damage: Pathophysiology and neurochemical pathology. *Adv Neurol* 44:813–847, 1986.

111. Simon RP, Swan JH, Griffith T, et al: Blockade of N-methyl-D-aspartate receptors may protect against ischemic damage in the brain. *Science* 226:850–852, 1984.

112. Sloper JJ, Johnson P, Powell TPS: Selective degeneration of interneurons in the motor cortex of infant monkeys following controlled hypoxia: A possible cause of epilepsy. *Brain Res* 198:204–209, 1980.

113. Smith M-L, Auer RN, Siesjö BK: The density and distribution of ischemic brain injury in the rat following two to ten minues of forebrain ischemia. *Acta Neuropathol (Berl)* 64:319–332, 1984.

114. Smith M-L, Hanwehr R von, Siesjö BK: Changes in extra- and intracellular pH in the brain during and following ischemia in hyperglycemic and in

moderately hypoglycemic rats. *J Cereb Blood Flow Metab* 6:574–583, 1986.

115. Smith M-L, Kalimo H, Warner DS, et al: Glucose pretreatment preceding forebrain ischemia causes substantia nigra damage. *J Cereb Blood Flow Metab* 7(Suppl 1):S73, 1987.

116. Smith M-L, Kalimo H, Warner DS, et al: Morphological lesions in the brain preceding the development of postischemic seizures. *Acta Neuropathol (Berl)* 76:253–264, 1988.

117. Smith M-L, Siesjö BK: Acidosis-related brain damage: Immediate and delayed events. In Somjen G (ed): *Mechanisms of Cerebral Hypoxia and Stroke.* New York, Plenum, 1988, pp 57–71.

118. Steen PA, Gisvold SE, Milde JH, et al: Nimodipine improves outcome when given after complete ischemia in primates. *Anesthesiology* 62:406–414, 1985.

119. Steenbergen C, Hill ML, Jennings RB: Volume regulation and plasma membrane injury in aerobic, anaerobic, and ischemic myocardium in vitro. *Circ Res* 57:864–875, 1985.

120. Vaagenes P, Cantadore R, Safar P, et al: Amelioration of brain damage by lidoflazine after prolonged ventricular cardiac arrest in dogs. *Crit Care Med* 12:846–855, 1984.

121. Van Harreveld A, Fifkova E: Swelling of dendritic spines in the fascia dentata after stimulation of the perforant fibers as a mechanism of post-tetanic potentiation. *Exp Neurol* 49:736–749, 1975.

122. Warner DS, Smith M-L, Siesjö BK: Ischemia in normo- and hyperglycemic rats: Effects on brain water and electrolytes. *Stroke* 18:464–471, 1987.

123. Watkins JC: Excitatory amino acids and central synaptic transmission. *TIPS* 5:373–380, 1984.

124. Wei EP, Kontos HA, Dietrich WD, et al: Inhibition by free radical scavengers and by cyclooxygenase inhibitors of pial arteriolar abnormalities from concussive brain injury in cats. *Circ Res* 48:95–103, 1981.

125. Welsh FA, Ginsberg MD, Budd WW: Deleterious effect of glucose pretreatment on recovery from diffuse cerebral ischemia in the cat. II. Regional metabolite levels. *Stroke* 11:355–365, 1980.

126. Wieloch T: Hypoglycemia-induced neuronal damage prevented by an N-methyl-D-aspartate antagonist. *Science* 230:681–683, 1985.

127. Wieloch T, Koide T, Westerberg E: Inhibitory neurotransmitters and neuromodulators as protective agents against ischemic brain damage. In Krieglstein J (ed): *Pharmacology of Cerebral Ischemia.* New York, Elsevier, 1986, pp 191–197.

128. Wieloch T, Lindvall O, Blomquist P, et al: Evidence for amelioration of ischaemic neuronal damage in the hippocampal formation by lesion of the perforant path. *Neurol Res* 7:24–26, 1985.

129. Wolfe LS: Eicosanoids: Prostaglandins, thromboxanes, leukotrienes, and other derivatives of carbon-20 unsaturated fatty acids. *J Neurochem* 38:1–14, 1982.

130. Yoshida Y, Busto R, Martinez E, et al: Regional brain energy metabolism after complete versus incomplete ischemia in the rat in the absence of severe lactic acidosis. *J Cereb Blood Flow Metab* 5:490–501, 1985.

131. Yoshida S, Ikeda M, Busto R, et al: Cerebral phosphoinositide, triacylglycerol, and energy metabolism in reversible ischemia: Origin and fate of free fatty acids. *J Neurochem* 47:744–757, 1986.

CHAPTER SIX

Ischemic Cerebral Edema

Jeffrey B. Randall, M.D.
Julian T. Hoff, M.D.

Edema is an important consequence of cerebral ischemia. Though mild edema may be asymptomatic, more severe cases cause signs of focal or generalized neuronal dysfunction. Localized or diffuse brain swelling may be demonstrated by computerized tomography or magnetic resonance imaging. In the most extreme instances, transtentorial cerebral herniation may result. Cerebral edema is the most common cause of death in patients with acute stroke (29).

Cerebral edema can be described as an increase in brain volume caused by an increase in sodium (Na^+) and water content. Its formation is dependent on a variety of factors, including intravascular hydrostatic pressure, capillary endothelial permeability, interstitial hydrostatic pressure, and metabolic factors, such as availability of substrates and the accumulation of toxins. Edema formation varies within a region of brain according to the depth and duration of ischemia, as well as the degree of reperfusion.

Since early in this century, investigators have understood that cerebral edema is not a single pathophysiologic entity. In 1904, Reichardt (25) made the distinction between *Hirnodem* (brain edema), in which the cut surface of the brain was wet, and *Hirnschwellung* (brain swelling), in which it was dry. These were felt to represent excess fluid in the extracellular and intracellular spaces, respectively. This distinction was further characterized by Klatzo (17) in his classic work on the neuropathology of edema. He termed the edema involving primarily cellular elements as *cytotoxic*. Edema located in the extracellular spaces (ECSs), resulting primarily from increased capillary permeability to plasma proteins, was referred to as *vasogenic*. A third type of edema, commonly known as *interstitial* (hydrocephalic) edema, was first described by Fishman (8). In interstitial edema, obstruction to the outflow of cerebral spinal fluid (CSF) causes accumulation of edema fluid in the interstitial spaces. *Ischemic* edema that accompanies impaired arteral perfusion is a combination of the first two forms, with cytotoxic edema occurring during the first few hours followed later by the vasogenic form. This chapter focuses on the current views of the pathophysiologic mechanisms accounting for clinical and experimental observations of ischemic cerebral edema.

FORMS OF EDEMA

Cytoxic (cellular) edema occurs when cell membrane permeability is disturbed, allowing abnormal amounts of protein-poor fluid to pass from the ECS into neurons and glia, causing them to swell and the surrounding ECS to shrink (17). This form occurs clinically after water intoxication, hypoxia, and other systemic insults. Cytotoxic edema has been created experimentally by treatment with ouabain, a specific inhibitor of the sodium–potassium adenosine triphosphatase (Na^+–K^+ ATPase)-catalyzed ion pump. With membrane pump failure, ionic gradients cannot be maintained. Sodium influx exceeds potassium (K^+) outflow and cells swell as interstitial water passively diffuses into them, with resultant shrinkage of the ECS.

Vasogenic edema occurs when brain blood vessels are damaged and become abnormally permeable, allowing protein-rich fluid to flow from the vascular compartment into the ECS. The ECS enlarges, the distance between cells increases, and on gross examination the brain parenchyma appears softened (17). The occurrence of vasogenic edema depends on the duration and severity of the ischemic insult (28). When cerebral blood flow (CBF) ceases, serum protein extravasation does not occur because there is no hydrostatic force to drive fluid from the vessels into the parenchyma (7, 13). Consequently, vasogenic edema does not form in the presence of complete ischemia, but it does develop during postischemic reperfusion.

Ischemic edema is a combination of the cytotoxic and vasogenic forms of brain edema. According to Klatzo (17), it results from a combination of insults which develop sequentially. First, cellular hypoxia occurs, triggering the onset of cytotoxic edema. Glial swelling can be detected within a few minutes of the onset of the hypoxic event. This response is usually not severe enough by itself to cause gross brain swelling and intracranial hypertension. Vasogenic edema then develops hours to days after the ischemic event and frequently is accompanied by progressive elevation of intracranial pressure (ICP) (23). The mechanism by which edema fluid accumulates in cells and in the interstitium after arterial occlusion as well as its time course are currently under investigation. How one form of edema affects the other is also a subject of interest.

Resolution of edema characteristically begins several days after the onset of ischemia, provided the subject survives the insult. However, in some cases ICP rises enough to compromise CBF further and a cyclical reaction develops involving CBF, ICP, and ischemic edema.

EDEMA THRESHOLDS

The threshold of regional CBF (rCBF) below which edema forms due to ischemia is about 20 ml/100/g/minute (1, 7, 30). Electrical conductivity of brain tissue is impaired at that same degree of ischemia. If rCBF falls to 10 to 15 ml/100 g/minute, cellular metabolism is compromised, the energy charge is impaired, and cellular ionic pumps fail. Intracellular potassium then passes from cells into the ECS while Na^+ and calcium (Ca^{2+}) move the opposite way. The loss of Na^+ and chloride

(Cl^-) from the ECS causes electrical impedance of cortical tissue to rise as the ECS shrinks. The accumulation of Na^+, Cl^-, Ca^{2+}, and other osmotically active products of metabolism (e.g. lactate, free fatty acids, neurotransmitters) results in an intracellular hyperosmolar state. Water is then imbibed to restore osmotic equilibrium and the cells swell to accommodate the increased fluid volume. However, the shift of fluids and electrolytes from extracellular to intracellular compartments does not completely explain the increase in total water and Na^+ content of the edematous area. Intravascular fluid and electrolytes may also contribute to the parenchymal shifts occurring between ECS and cells (28).

BLOOD–BRAIN BARRIER

Brain capillary endothelial cells are normally sealed together by tight junctions, forming a permeability barrier that restricts movement of most polar solutes into the brain (3). Compounds important for brain metabolism still enter brain tissue because of specific transport systems present in endothelial cell membranes. Despite an active process for limiting Na^+ flux into endothelial cells, small amounts of Na^+ do cross the capillary endothelial membranes. Na^+ is actively pumped out of endothelial cells into brain ECS by the Na^+–K^+ ATPase-catalyzed pump located on the antiluminal membrane (2). In most cells, two K^+ ions enter the cell for every three Na^+ ions pumped out. Thus, more Na^+ enters brain than K^+ exits; water accompanies Na^+ entry. These processes must involve fluid and electrolyte exchanges between blood and ECS; however, the exchanges occur at a time when the brain capillaries still form a barrier to the extravasation of proteins and sucrose (Fig. 6.1). In effect then, protein-poor fluid crosses the intact blood–brain barrier into the ECS during the cytotoxic phase of brain edema and later, protein-rich fluid crosses a disrupted blood–brain barrier during the vasogenic phase (22, 23).

The blood–brain barrier's impermeability to serum protein or small molecules remains nearly intact during the early stage

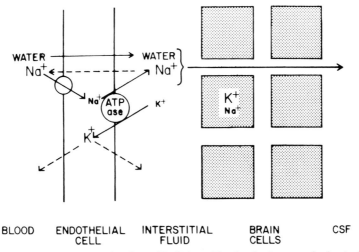

Figure 6.1. Proposed flow of water and sodium (Na$^+$) from blood to brain to cerebral spinal fluid (CSF). In the normal brain, Na$^+$ from plasma crosses the endothelial cells by sequential transport across the luminal and antiluminal membranes *(dashed line)*. This process occurs in exchange for potassium (K$^+$) in the interstitial fluid, which may then either enter the blood or be recycled back to the brain *(dashed line)*. Water follows to maintain osmotic equilibrium. Once Na$^+$ reaches the brain's interstitial space, it is cleared by bulk flow with water through the interstitial space, or it may possibly return to the blood if appropriate transport systems are present in the endothelial cells *(dashed line)*. ATP = adenosine triphosphatase.

of cerebral ischemia. A breakdown of the blood–brain barrier to both small and large molecules does develop in ischemic tissue 12 hours after occlusion of the middle cerebral artery (MCA). The increase in blood–brain barrier permeability to carbon-14-labeled sucrose correlates directly with the rise of water content within 72 hours of MCA occlusion, whereas iodine-125-labeled bovine serum albumin does not (14). This implies that accumulation of edema fluid is associated with blood–brain barrier disruption to small molecules during the later stages of ischemic brain edema formation.

DURATION AND SEVERITY OF ISCHEMIA

In a model of total ischemia in the cat, Schuier and Hossmann (27) found a 42% reduction in the ECS 1 hour after the onset of ischemia without any increase in total brain water. With ischemia lasting more than 1 hour, a net increase in brain Na$^+$ occurs with a resultant increase in brain water, though the blood–brain barrier still remains intact to plasma proteins (9). Because permeability of endothelial cells to

Na$^+$ is normally quite low, the mechanism of this Na$^+$ increase is not clear. Some investigators have proposed that, as ion pumps fail and Na$^+$ moves into cells, a gradient is created for the diffusion of Na$^+$ from blood to brain (13). Others, however, have found that Na$^+$ permeability is not increased after 3 hours of ischemia (16), suggesting that the reduction of interstitial spaces by swollen cells may inhibit the clearance of Na$^+$ and water by bulk flow into the CSF (Fig. 6.2).

While edema forms below a threshold for ischemia of 20 ml/100 g/minute (7, 30), the edema worsens with the duration of ischemia. In gerbils, Iannotti and Hoff (14) found that edema does not reverse if CBF of 10 ml/100 g/minute is maintained for 60 minutes.

The degree of blood–brain barrier breakdown is proportional to the duration of ischemia. The severity of the ischemic insult is similarly important. In a situation of profound global ischemia, using four-vessel occlusion in rats, Todd et al (32) found that no resolution of edema occurred beyond 15 minutes of ischemia. Restoration of circulation has been reported to both reduce (7, 14) and increase (13) edema. Worsening of edema may be

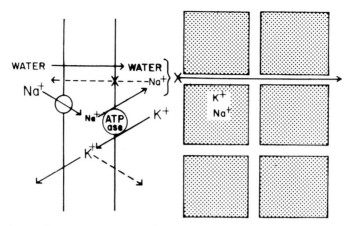

Figure 6.2. In ischemia, brain cells swell and reduce the size of the interstitial spaces. Consequently, the bulk flow of sodium (Na^+) and water into the cerebral spinal fluid is impeded and edema develops *(dashed line)*. Alternatively, Na^+ may accumulate in the brain if its return to the blood is blocked. In either case ischemic brain edema would result from reduced clearance of Na^+ and water secreted by the brain capillaries. Leakage of potassium (K^+) from the intracellular to the extracellular space also occurs *(dashed line)*. ATPase = adenosine triphosphatase.

related to the degree of postischemic hyperemia with its associated increase in hydrostatic pressure (33).

BLOOD PRESSURE

Blood flows to the periphery of ischemic regions through collateral circulation. Because these vessels tend to be maximally dilated, autoregulation is impaired. Symon et al (31) found autoregulation to be partially preserved if the postocclusion flow was greater than 40% of normal, but absent if the flow was less than 20% of normal. In these regions, a reduction in blood pressure can cause worsening of ischemia. Likewise, high blood pressure transmitted to dysautoregulated capillaries may precipitate the formation of significant edema.

Although rises in blood pressure usually increase CBF in ischemic brain, false autoregulation may occur. In such a situation, the presence of extracellular edema compresses capillaries, preventing their dilatation and the associated increase in CBF (18). Iannotti et al (15) provided evidence for increased tissue pressure early in ischemia, before the blood–brain barrier is compromised.

Although these factors suggest that extremes of blood pressure may be harmful, lesser fluctuations of blood pressure may

be worse. In a study of monkeys, Matakas et al (21) induced edema by balloon compression after which blood pressure was repeatedly raised with norepinephrine. With each dose, blood pressure, cerebral perfusion pressure, and ICP increased. Although blood pressure returned to normal between doses, ICP decreased less, resulting in an overall rise in ICP during the experiments.

HYDROSTATIC AND OSMOTIC GRADIENTS

The edema process in brain is modified by blood–brain barrier permeability, capillary hydraulic conductivity, hydrostatic differences, and osmotic pressure gradients. Hatashita and Hoff (11) recently demonstrated that a tissue pressure gradient develops within ischemic cortex and is associated with brain edema. The magnitude of the gradient is related to the severity of ischemic edema in that same tissue. In the initial stage of cerebral ischemia, low hydraulic conductivity and low compliance of ischemic tissue limit the accumulation of edema fluid and prevent rapid movement of that fluid. Later, as the ischemic injury progresses, edema fluid accumulates in highly compliant brain parenchyma, then migrates through highly

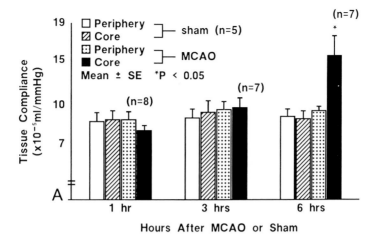

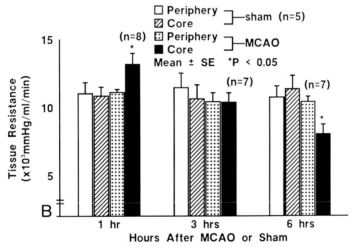

Figure 6.3. Brain tissue *A*, compliance and *B*, resistance in the core and periphery, 1, 3, and 6 hours after middle cerebral artery occlusion (MCAO) or sham operation. Tissue compliance increased markedly in the core 6 hours after MCAO. Tissue resistance increases 1 hour after occlusion and then decreases by 6 hours.

conductive tissue into CSF spaces, driven by the pressure gradient that develops between the edematous tissue and the CSF (Fig. 6.3).

An increase in osmolality of ischemic brain tissue is found 3 and 6 hours after MCA occlusion (12). The osmotic gradient between ischemic brain and blood is about 26 mOsm/kg. The increment in brain osmolality correlates with that of water content until water content increases to about 20 mg/g of brain. These findings indicate that the osmotic pressure gradient which develops between ischemic brain and blood

is a fundamental factor in the early accumulation of edema fluid after ischemic injury. A significant increase in tissue osmolality is not found 1 hour after MCA occlusion despite an increase in water content.

The accumulation of edema fluid is related to a hydrostatic pressure gradient which develops early after the onset of ischemia. Then an osmotic pressure gradient develops as the ischemic injury progresses. Further accumulation of edema fluid is associated with disruption of the blood–brain barrier to small molecules in the later stages of ischemic edema formation.

MEDIATORS OF ISCHEMIC EDEMA

Calcium

Large amounts of Ca^{2+} accumulate in the brain with ischemia. Though some Ca^{2+} is released from mitochondria, the total amount measured is many times greater than that available in preischemic brain. Evidence suggests that the continued influx of Ca^{2+} is along a concentration gradient caused by the precipitation of Ca^{2+} as it avidly binds to inorganic phosphates (24). The source of this Ca^{2+} must be blood or CSF.

Ca^{2+} activates phospholipases, which in turn break down membrane phospholipids. Influx of more Ca^{2+} continues this vicious cycle. The rise in intracellular Ca^{2+} may be a final common pathway leading to cell death (26). Magnesium may protect against ischemic damage by reducing Ca^{2+} influx or by stablizing membranes.

Arachidonic Acid

Release of free arachidonic acid from membranes occurs soon after the onset of ischemia. This release is mediated by the enzymatic action of phospholipase A_2, itself activated by Ca^{2+} ions and oxygen free radicals. Free arachidonic acid has direct damaging effects on the blood–brain barrier (4). This may be related to its effect on membrane function or to its role as a chemoattractant for leukocytes. Arachidonic acid exerts secondary effects through its conversion to prostaglandins through the cyclooxygenase pathway and to leukotrienes through the lipoxygenase pathway.

Leukotrienes have been studied as mediators of cerebral edema because concentrations are known to increase with ischemia. They cause a significant constriction of pial vessels. Their role in causing blood–brain barrier dysfunction and edema is unclear, though opening of the barrier has been seen in some experiments.

Free Radicals

Oxygen free radicals, produced by the single electron reduction of molecular oxygen, are highly reactive compounds which can cause peroxidation of lipid membranes and the release of arachidonic acid. These radicals, which include superoxide, hydrogen peroxide, and the hydroxyl radical, can be generated by the conversion of arachidonic acid to prostaglandins and by the enzymatic action of xanthine oxidase. The presence of free radicals has been demonstrated in situations of partial ischemia, postischemic reperfusion, and several other brain injury models. When brain capillaries are exposed to free radicals, a decrease in Na^+–K^+ ATPase activity is observed (19). Free radicals have been shown to increase capillary permeability to Evan's blue (6). Treatment with liposome-encapsulated superoxide dismutase, a scavenger of free radicals, has attenuated cold-induced edema in cats (5). Preliminary studies in rats suggest that infarct size is reduced by treatment with allopurinol, a specific xanthine oxidase inhibitor (20). Though evidence is incomplete, free radicals may be important mediators of ischemic brain edema—especially in situations where circulation of oxygen-rich blood is restored to ischemic regions.

Other Potential Mediators

Additional candidates which deserve discussion for their roles as mediators of ischemia include bradykinin, histamine, serotonin, and glutamate. Bradykinin can be formed intravascularly or in brain parenchyma and it increases in concentration with ischemia. The influence of bradykinin on edema has been studied. Unterberg and Baethmann (34) superfused cat cerebral cortex with bradykinin and showed increased permeability to Na^+-fluorescein. They believed this to be due to the opening of tight junctions. Bradykinin is also a potent dilator of cerebral arterioles—an effect which can be diminished by pretreatment with a B2 kininergic receptor antagonist.

Histamine increases cerebral capillary permeability and diameter. Its role in edema is unclear, however, because tissue concentrations have not been measured in conditions of ischemia (35). Serotonin opens the blood–brain barrier, but tissue levels of serotonin have not correlated with edema formation. The excitatory neurotransmitter glutamate can have neurotoxic actions and may promote neuronal swelling (10). Brain regions with high glutamate concentrations, such as cerebral cortex and hippocampus, are often preferentially damaged by ischemia.

PERSPECTIVE

Ischemic edema is a complex pathophysiologic state. Breakdown of cellular metabolism triggers a cascade of events influenced by a number of biochemical mediators including arachidonic acid, Ca^{2+}, and oxygen free radicals. Parameters vital to the extent of neuronal damage include not only depth and duration of ischemia, but also the rate at which it develops as well as the timing and effectiveness of the eventual reintroduction of blood flow.

During the later stages of ischemia, destruction of membranes and vasogenic edema cause largely irreparable damage. In the initial period of cytotoxic edema, however, cellular structure remains intact and ischemic changes are potentially reversible. A spatial continuum of edema exists for any area of ischemic brain. At present, no specific treatment is available to prevent or reverse ischemic edema. However, agents that improve CBF, reduce lipid peroxidation, or inhibit excitatory amino-acid release may secondarily relieve ischemic edema. Thus, therapeutic interventions, discussed in Chapters 18 to 29 of this volume, may be directed at restoring normal function to marginally perfused regions that are subject to reversible ischemic injury.

References

1. Astrup J, Siesjö B, Symon L: Thresholds in cerebral ischemia—The ischemic penumbra. *Stroke* 12:723–725, 1981.

2. Betz AL, Firth JA, Goldstein GW: Polarity of the blood–brain barrier: Distribution of enzymes between the luminal and antiluminal membranes of brain capillary endothelial cells. *Brain Res* 192:17–28, 1980.

3. Brightman MW, Klatzo I, Olsson Y, et al: The blood–brain barrier to proteins under normal and pathological conditions. *J Neurol Sci* 10:215–239, 1970.

4. Chan PH, Fishman RA: The role of arachidonic acid in vasogenic brain edema. *Fed Proc* 43:210–214, 1984.

5. Chan PH, Longar S, Fishman RA: Protective effects of liposome-entrapped superoxide dismutase on posttraumatic brain edema. *Ann Neurol* 21:540–547, 1987.

6. Chan PH, Schmidley JW, Fishman RA, et al: Brain injury, edema, and vascular permeability changes induced by oxygen-derived free radicals. *Neurology* 34:315–320, 1984.

7. Crockard HA, Lanotti F, Hunstock AT, et al: Cerebral blood flow and edema following carotid occlusion in the gerbil. *Stroke* 11:494–498, 1980.

8. Fishman RA: Brain edema. *N Engl J Med* 293:706–711, 1975.

9. Gotoh O, Asano T, Koide T, et al: Ischemic brain edema following occlusion of the middle cerebral artery in the rat. I. The time courses of the brain water, sodium, and potassium contents and blood–brain barrier permeability to 125I-albumin. *Stroke* 16:101–109, 1985.

10. Greenamyre JT: The role of glutamate in neurotransmission and in neurologic disease. *Arch Neurol* 43:1058–1063, 1986.

11. Hatashita S, Hoff JT: Biomechanics of brain edema in acute ischemia in cats. *Stroke* 19:91–97, 1988.

12. Hatashita S, Hoff JT, Salamat SM: Ischemic brain edema and the osmotic gradient between blood and brain. *J Cereb Blood Flow Metab* 8:552–559, 1988.

13. Hossmann KA: Pathophysiology of vasogenic and cytotoxic brain edema. In Hartmann A, Brock M (eds): *Treatment of Cerebral Edema*. Berlin, Springer-Verlag, 1982, pp 1–10.

14. Iannotti F, Hoff JT: Ischemic brain edema with and without reperfusion: An experimental study in gerbils. *Stroke* 14:562–567, 1983.

15. Iannotti F, Hoff JT, Schielke GP: Brain tissue pressure in focal cerebral ischemia. *J Neurosurg* 62:83–89, 1985.

16. Ki WD, Betz AL, Schielke GP, et al: Transport of sodium from blood to brain in ischemic brain edema. *Stroke* 18:150–157, 1987.

17. Klatzo I: Neuropathological aspects of brain edema. *J Neuropathol Exp Neurol* 26:1–14, 1967.

18. Little JR: Microvascular alterations and edema in focal cerebral ischemia. In Pappius HM, Feindel W (eds): *Dynamics of Brain Edema*. Berlin, Springer-Verlag, 1976, pp 236–243.

19. Lo WD, Betz AL: Oxygen free-radical reduction of brain capillary rubidium uptake. *J Neurochem* 40:394–398, 1986.

20. Martz D, Rayos G, Schielke G, et al: Allopurinol limits infarct size in partial ischemia. In Hoff JT, Betz AL (eds): *Intracranial Pressure VII*. Berlin, Springer-Verlag, 1989, in press.

21. Matakas F, Waechter R von, Eibs G: Relation

between cerebral perfusion pressure and arterial pressure in brain edema. *Lancet* 1:684, 1972.

22. O'Brien MD: Ischemic cerebral edema. In Hartmann A, Brock M (eds): *Treatment of Cerebral Edema*. Berlin, Springer-Verlag, 1982, pp 19–23.

23. Olsson Y, Crowell RM, Klatzo I: The blood–brain barrier to protein tracers in focal cerebral ischemia and infarction caused by occlusion of the middle cerebral artery. *Acta Neuropathol* 18:89–102, 1971.

24. Rappaport ZH, Young W, Flamm ES: Regional brain calcium changes in the rat middle cerebral artery occlusion model of ischemia. *Stroke* 18:760–764, 1987.

25. Reichardt M: Zur Entstehung des Hirndrocks. *Dtsch Z Nervenheilk* 28:306, 1904.

26. Schanne FAX, Kane AB, Young EE, et al: Calcium dependence of toxic cell death: A final common pathway. *Science* 206:700–702, 1979.

27. Schuier FJ, Hossmann KA: Experimental brain infarcts in cats. II. Ischemic brain edema. *Stroke* 11:593–601, 1980.

28. Siesjö BK: Cerebral circulation and metabolism. *J Neurosurg* 60:883–908, 1984.

29. Silver FL, Norris JW, Lewis AJ, et al: Early mortaility following stroke: A prospective view. *Stroke* 15:492–496, 1984.

30. Symon L, Branston NM, Chikovani O: Ischemic brain edema following middle cerebral artery occlusion in baboons: Relationship between regional cerebral water content and flow at 1 to 2 hours. *Stroke* 10:184–191, 1979.

31. Symon L, Branston NM, Strong AJ: Autoregulation in acute focal ischemia. *Stroke* 7:547–554, 1976.

32. Todd NV, Picozzi P, Crockard HA, et al: Duration of ischemia influences the development and resolution of ischemic brain edema. *Stroke* 17:466–471, 1986.

33. Todd NV, Picozzi MD, Crockard HA, et al: Reperfusion after cerebral ischemia: Influence of duration of ischemia. *Stroke* 17:460–466, 1986.

34. Unterberg A, Baethmann AJ: The kallikrein-kinin system as mediator in vasogenic brain edema. Part 1. Cerebral exposure to bradykinin and plasma. *J Neurosurg* 61:87–96, 1984.

35. Wahl M, Unterberg A, Baethmann A, et al: Mediators of blood–brain barrier dysfunction and formation of vasogenic brain edema. *J Cereb Blood Flow Metab* 8:621–634, 1988.

CHAPTER SEVEN

Relevance of Experimental Models to Clinical Stroke

Julio H. Garcia, M.D.

Neurologic injury as a result of insufficient blood flow (ischemia) is the most frequent cause of organic neurologic disease. Ischemic injury to the brain is of two types: *global ischemia*, produced by systemic alterations in blood pressure or by conditions that simultaneously affect the perfusion pressure of the entire cerebrum; and *focal* or *regional ischemia*, resulting in localized neurologic deficits, generically called *ischemic strokes*. Most strokes are caused by arterial occlusions (14).

Global and focal ischemic injuries share the same underlying cause: reduced blood flow and availability of the metabolic substrates and diminished clearance of toxic metabolites. The histopathologic features of the resulting brain lesions are similar, which is probably why it is generally assumed that, in both conditions, brain tissue necrosis develops by an identical process. Although the validity of this assumption has not been established, the following concepts regarding ischemia are accepted by most investigators:

1. Loss of cerebral function may be entirely reversible under certain circumstances following reperfusion of the tissue (10, 19, 26). The local cerebral blood flow (CBF) values associated with loss of neuronal function (i.e., the ischemic thresholds) are well defined (22), but how long the central nervous system can tolerate ischemia with no impairment of functional recovery and structural preservation is unknown, except in very general terms (20, 30).
2. Ischemia first injures neurons, as opposed to glia and other cells, and among specific neuronal groups (e.g. those in the CA1 sector of the hippocampus),

some neurons are more susceptible than their neighbors to the same ischemic conditions. This variability is known as *selective vulnerability* (17).

3. The morphologic expressions of structural abnormalities that are thought to be indicative of irreversible neuronal injury (or cellular necrosis) develop over a period of minutes, hours, or even days after the initial ischemic injury (24). This "maturation," or the length of time after the ischemic insult that it takes for brain tissue examined pathologically to demonstrate ischemic necrosis, depends on the methods of tissue preparation used (15, 18, 35). For example, electron microscopy and special histochemical stains performed after perfusion fixation or in vivo freezing are the most sensitive methods for visualizing ischemic neuronal damage.

The possibility that, peripheral to a brain infarction, there is an area of sublethal ischemic brain injury in which functional impairment and tissue alteration may be reversed by reperfusion has spurred renewed interest in exploring therapeutic and prophylactic approaches that may prevent thrombosis from propagating and ischemic injury from spreading. This peripheral area where less severe circulatory alterations are detectable has been called the *ischemic penumbra* (2). However, laboratory testing of therapeutic regimens, which have been based on the attempted blockade of various reactions believed to be responsible for ischemic cell injury, have often produced inconclusive results (3). For example, Sauter and Rudin (31) reported that treatment with a calcium antagonist before or after middle cerebral artery (MCA) occlusion in rats resulted in a substantial reduction of infarct size, as determined by magnetic resonance (MR) imaging at 24, 48, and 72 hours after the occlusion of the vessel. In contrast, Barnett et al (5) reported that infusion of nimodipine, a calcium entry blocker, did not reduce brain infarct size in adult cats subjected to MCA occlusion. These and similar seemingly contradictory results concerning the treatment of focal ischemia with various therapeutic means have been analyzed extensively by Baethmann and Jansen (3), who commented that the disparate results may reflect the lack of an appropriate experimental model in which hemodynamic parameters (specifically, local CBF) could be maintained at steady-state conditions (i.e. conditions preventing spontaneous CBF variations) during the experiment. We have analyzed some of the advances made in the identification of neurophysiologic and neuropathologic abnormalities induced by ischemia that is produced experimentally by single-artery occlusion (16), and Molinari (25) and Welch et al (35) have examined the clinical relevance of various experimental stroke models.

REGIONAL ISCHEMIA

One major objective of experiments that study regional ischemia has been to induce brain lesions, either focal or generalized, in a reproducible manner. Investigations generally are aimed either at limiting the size of the lesion (based on the assumption that the brain lesions would have a predictable size and distribution) or at ameliorating the severity of the neurologic deficit. Attempts to attain these objectives have focused on reperfusing the ischemic territory or administering, either before or after the onset of ischemia, drugs purported to halt one or more of the deleterious neurochemical effects of brain ischemia.

The effects of varying the duration of temporary cerebral vascular occlusion have also been evaluated (10, 11), but there are considerable variations in the size and location of the ischemic lesions produced by MCA occlusion and these variations may be independent of the duration of the arterial occlusion. In three well-studied animal species (subhuman primates, cat, and rat), occluding the MCA for identical periods of time yields lesions that vary widely, within each species, in size and location (19). Such variability in the infarct size and location can be attributed to anatomic variations in collateral arterial channels that determine the compensatory responses of microcirculatory CBF in areas peripheral to the occluded vessel (29). These variations probably reflect circulatory adjustments made possible by flow through the anastomoses between branches of the MCA and of the anterior and posterior cerebral arteries. The wide individual variations in the anatomic configuration of these vessels and the adjustments of the autonomic vascular responses may further explain why it has not been possible to generate lesions of a predictable size by means of a single artery occlusion (25). Several reasons can be cited for changing microcirculatory conditions, including function of the collateral anastomotic channels, development of microthrombi, adhesion of leukocytes to the endothelial walls, vascular responses to drugs administered as anesthetics or for treatment, altered vascular autonomic responses, effects of local tissue swelling, and other as yet undetermined factors.

Numerous and ingenious modifications to surgical procedures designed to occlude one or more intracranial arterial branches have recently been used in attempts to influence the size and location of brain infarctions (37). In some instances, previously implanted intraorbital devices have been used to occlude a vessel in the awake cat in order to avoid the potential protection provided the ischemic brain by barbiturates or other anesthetics (34). Other surgical methods induce lesions of different types, depending on where a surgical clip is placed in the circle of Willis (7). As an alternative approach, selective and delayed hippocampal neuronal necrosis has been induced in gerbils simply by transient (5 minutes) unilateral carotid artery occlusion (23). Other investigators have attempted to use microsurgical techniques to create reproducible ischemic lesions after proximal MCA occlusion in rats with more standardized infarct areas or volumes (32). Combining distal MCA occlusion in rats with permanent right carotid artery ligation and 60-minute temporary left carotid artery occlusion yielded a focal cortical ischemic lesion in which the maximum cross-sectional area of infarction measured 10.4 ± 1.1 mm^2 (9). By use of a model with such a small range of variation in infarct size, the effects of pharmacologic or physiologic manipulations could easily be demonstrated. Other methods of extracranial vascular occlusion have been developed in rats to produce lesions due to temporary regional ischemia that are more variable in size but permit evaluation of the effects of reperfusion (4, 38).

In one study of transient regional ischemia in unanesthetized cats, the MCA was temporarily occluded with an implanted, externally controlled device. The occlusion was reversed to allow reperfusion of the MCA territory after 2 to 24 hours of ischemia. The results of this study showed, as did comparable observations in humans (27) and subhuman primates (19), that the size and location of an ischemic cerebral lesion may be governed by both the severity and duration of the reduction of local CBF. Occlusion of a single artery in the brain does not create uniform changes in the corresponding arterial region; rather, the area destined to become infarcted can be characterized initially as a veritable patchwork of different zones where local CBF measured sequentially may be high, low, or normal and where the microcirculatory conditions fluctuate over time as a function of both local and systemic circulatory parameters (35).

GLOBAL ISCHEMIA

A widely used model of global ischemia based on four-vessel occlusion in rats (28) has characterized two different types of neuronal response: reversible injury in the cerebral cortex and irreversible necrosis in the caudate–putamen. Owing to differences in collateral circulation and difficulties with the occlusion of the vertebral arteries, however, the outcome for individual animals remains unpredictable. The ganglion blocker nitroprusside has been introduced as an adjuvant agent administered simultaneously with occlusion of the carotid arteries to produce hypotension in order to facilitate the creation of steady-state ischemic brain conditions (21).

In other experiments, global ischemia in dogs has been created with hypotension by withdrawal or reinfusion of arterial blood through an arterial catheter and the metabolism of high-energy phosphates monitored simultaneously with in vivo MR spectroscopy (1). Hemodynamic conditions have been difficult to reproduce in each experiment, however, because of fluctuations in cerebral perfusion pressure brought about by fluctuations in systemic blood pressure. Two other significant physiologic determinants of cerebral ischemic injury are intracranial pressure and vascular reactivity. Animal models in which the influence of these factors is measured and the ischemic conditions are both constant and within the penumbra, or range of potential reversibility, can begin to provide answers to questions concerning metabolic and neurochemical factors such as the role that calcium flux and free-radical generation, among other mechanisms, may have in the pathogenesis of ischemic cell necrosis. (18).

ALTERNATIVE APPROACHES

Several other experimental preparations have been developed to more reliably control parameters of ischemic brain injury. Segmental ischemia of undetermined severity has been induced in the lumbar spinal cord of rabbits by temporary ligation of the corresponding segment of the abdominal aorta (39). More reproducible results that are comparable to those of brain ischemia are observed. Localized microvascular thrombosis can be induced in the brain in rats injected with rose Bengal dye by shining an argon laser beam through the intact dura; the authors have suggested that the microcirculatory and structural alterations induced by this ischemic injury to a well-defined site of the brain are identical to those occurring in the early stages of a brain infarct (12).

In attempts to standardize the degree of ischemia in an experimental lesion, Boehme et al (8) developed a computer-regulated system to lower cerebral perfusion pressure that creates cerebral ischemia of a predictable severity and duration at various sites in the brain. This animal model begins to address the investigator's need to establish a pathophysiologic steady state by maintaining CBF at a constant level of ischemia and by selecting a specific percentage decrease of CBF from control levels. Clearly, study of changes in CBF that are either too mild to produce neurologic deficit (more than 23 ml/100 g/minute) or too severe to allow functional recovery of cell membranes (less than 10 ml/100 g/minute) would afford no useful data. The ideal levels of ischemia to be investigated, because of their potential reversibility, are those found in areas of ischemic penumbra (12 to 24 ml/100 g/minute) as defined by Astrup et al (2). In order to take into account the issue of selective neuronal vulnerability, circulatory conditions should be maintained within the ischemic penumbra at constant levels throughout the course of an experiment. The rat model described by Boehme et al (8) would be significantly improved in this respect if the computer were to respond to a local CBF signal rather than to a signal based on carotid arterial flow.

Finally, an objective, quantifiable method to measure the extent and type of early ischemic cellular injury neuropathologically is needed. Eke et al (13) have recently completed an analysis of a light-microscopic method that allows typing and counting of neurons injured by ischemia; the overall grading results for cell damage ranged between 4.7% and 17.3%, depending on the degree of ischemia. This quantitative method is well suited to evaluate the effect of treatment regimens on ischemic neuronal damage. Previously described cerebral spinal fluid enzyme determinations, such as those reported by Vaagenes et al (33), may lack the necessary reproducibility to draw statistically valid conclusions.

Enzyme histochemical and immunohistochemical stains (14) have been used to provide more sensitive methods for identification of early ischemic neuronal damage in acute ischemia experiments (6, 36). Such methods may also provide the ability to distinguish reversible ischemic cellular injury from intracellular alterations that herald the ultimate occurrence of necrosis and infarction.

Acknowledgment—This work was supported in part by a grant in aid from the Department of Pathology, University of Alabama at Birmingham, and by U.S. Public Health Service grant NS-08802.

References

1. Anderson ML, Garcia JH, Smith DS, et al: Experimental brain ischemia: NMR and histologic evaluation (abstract). *J Neuropathol Exp Neurol* 46:403, 1987.
2. Astrup J, Siesjö BK, Symon L: Thresholds in cerebral ischemia—the ischemic penumbra. *Stroke* 12:723–725, 1981.
3. Baethmann A, Jansen M: Possible role of calcium entry blockers in brain protection. *Eur Neurol* 25:102–113, 1986.
4. Bannister CM, Chapman SA: Ischemia and revascularization of the middle cerebral territory of the rat brain by manipulation of the blood vessels in the neck. *Surg Neurol* 21:351–357, 1984.
5. Barnett GH, Bosi B, Little JR, et al: Effects of nimodipine on acute focal cerebral ischemia. *Stroke* 17:884–890, 1986.
6. Bederson JB, Pitts LH, Germano SM, et al: Evaluation of 2,3,5-triphenyltetrazolium chloride as a stain for detection and quantification of experimental cerebral infarction in rats. *Stroke* 17:1304–1308, 1986.
7. Bederson JB, Pitts LH, Tsuji M, et al: Rat middle cerebral artery occlusion: Evaluation of the model and development of a neurologic examination. *Stroke* 17:472–476, 1986.
8. Boehme RJ, Conger KA, Anderson ML: Computer-regulated constant pressure ischemia in the rat: The animal model. *J Cereb Blood Flow Metab* 8:236–243, 1988.
9. Chen ST, Hsu CY, Hogan EL, et al: A model of focal ischemic stroke in the rat: Reproducible extensive cortical infarction. *Stroke* 17:738–743, 1986.
10. Crowell RM, Olsson Y, Klatzo I, et al: Temporary occlusion of the middle cerebral artery in the monkey: Clinical and pathological observations. *Stroke* 1:439–448, 1970.
11. Del Zoppo GJ, Copeland BR, Harker LA: Experimental acute thrombotic stroke in baboons. *Stroke* 17:1254–1265, 1986.
12. Dietrich WD, Ginsberg MD, Busto R, et al: Photochemically induced cortical infarction of the rat.

1. Time course of hemodynamic consequences. *J Cereb Blood Flow Metab* 6:184–194, 1986.

13. Eke A, Conger KA, Anderson M, et al: Enhanced grading of ischemic neuronal injury by light microscopic evaluation of nuclear features. *Stroke,* in press.

14. Ferrante RJ, Kowall NW, Beal MF, et al: Selective sparing of a class of striatal neurons in Huntington's disease. *Science* 230:561–563, 1985.

15. Garcia JH: Ischemic injuries of the brain. Morphologic evolution. *Arch Pathol Lab Med* 107:157–161, 1983.

16. Garcia JH: Experimental ischemic stroke: A review. *Stroke* 15:5–14, 1984.

17. Garcia JH: Circulatory disorders of the brain. In Davis RL, Robertson D (eds): *Textbook of Neuropathology.* Baltimore, Williams & Wilkins, 1985, pp 548–631.

18. Garcia JH, Anderson ML: Physiopathology of cerebral ischemia. *Crit Rev Neurobiol* 4:303–324, 1989.

19. Garcia JH, Mitchem HL, Briggs L, et al: Transient focal ischemia in subhuman primates: Neuronal injury as a function of local cerebral blood flow. *J Neuropathol Exp Neurol* 42:44–60, 1983.

20. Grennell RG: Central nervous system resistance. I. The effects of temporary arrest of cerebral circulation for periods of two to ten minutes. *J Neuropathol Exp Neurol* 5:131–154, 1946.

21. Grogaard B, Gerdin B, Arfors KE: Forebrain ischemia in the rat. Relation between duration of ischemia, use of adjunctive ganglionic blockade and long-term recovery. *Stroke* 17:1010–1015, 1986.

22. Heiss WD: Flow thresholds of functional and morphological damage of brain tissue. *Stroke* 14:329–331, 1983.

23. Kirino T, Tamura A, Sano K: A reversible type of neuronal injury following ischemia in the gerbil hippocampus. *Stroke* 17:455–459, 1986.

24. Lindenberg R: Patterns of CNS vulnerability in acute hypoxaemia including anesthesia accidents. In Schadé JP, McMenemey WH (eds): *Selective Vulnerability of the Brain in Hypoxaemia.* Oxford, Blackwell Scientific, 1963, pp 189–193.

25. Molinari GF: Clinical relevance of experimental stroke models. In Price TR, Nelson E (eds): *Cerebrovascular Diseases* (Transactions of the Eleventh [Princeton] Conference). New York, Raven Press, 1979, pp 19–33.

26. Nemoto EM, Bleyaert AL, Stezoski SW, et al: Global brain ischemia: A reproducible monkey model. *Stroke* 8:558–564, 1977.

27. Olsen TS: Regional cerebral blood flow after occlusion of the middle cerebral artery. *Acta Neurol Scand* 73:321–337, 1986.

28. Pulsinelli WA, Brierley JB: A new model of bilateral hemispheric ischemia in the unanesthetized rat. *Stroke* 10:267–272, 1979.

29. Ratcheson RA, Ferrendelli JA: Regional cortical metabolism in focal ischemia. *J Neurosurg* 52:755–763, 1980.

30. Rossen R, Herman K, Anderson JP: Acute arrest of cerebral circulation in man. *Arch Neurol Psychiatry* 50:510–528, 1943.

31. Sauter A, Rudin M: Calcium antagonists reduce the extent of infarction in middle cerebral artery occlusion model as determined by quantitative magnetic resonance imaging. *Stroke* 17:1228–1234, 1986.

32. Tamura A, Graham ID, McCulloch J, et al: Focal cerebral ischemia in the rat. *J Cereb Blood Flow Metab* 1:53–69, 1981.

33. Vaagenes P, Safar P, Diven W, et al: Brain enzyme levels in CSF after cardiac arrest and resuscitation in dogs: Markers of damage and predictors of outcome. *J Cereb Blood Flow Metab* 8:262–275, 1988.

34. Weinstein PR, Anderson GG, Telles DA: Neurological deficit and cerebral infarction after temporary middle cerebral artery occlusion in unanesthetized cats. *Stroke* 17:318–324, 1986.

35. Welch KMA, Levine SR, Ewing JR: Viewing of stroke pathophysiology: An analysis of contemporary methods. *Stroke* 17:1071–1077, 1986.

36. Yamamoto K, Yoshimine T, Yanagihara T: Cerebral ischemia in rabbit: A new experimental model with immunohistochemical investigation. *J Cereb Blood Flow Metab* 5:529–536, 1985.

37. Yoshimine T, Yanagihara T: Regional cerebral ischemia by occlusion of the posterior communicating artery and the middle cerebral artery in gerbils. *J Neurosurg* 58:362–367, 1983.

38. Zea Longa E, Weinstein PR, Carlson S, et al: Reversible middle cerebral artery occlusion without craniectomy in the rat. *Stroke* 20:84–91, 1989.

39. Zivin JA, Degirolami U: Spinal cord infarction: A highly reproducible stroke model. *Stroke* 11:200–202, 1984.

CHAPTER EIGHT

Imaging Methods: CT, MR, Xenon-Enhanced CT, and SPECT

Richard E. Latchaw, M.D.
Elizabeth A. Eelkema, M.D.
Stephen T. Hecht, M.D.

Therapy and prognosis differ depending on whether cerebral ischemia is acute, subacute, or chronic (12). The goals of different imaging methodologies likewise differ for acute and chronic stroke. The diagnosis of acute ischemia and infarction of the brain is primarily a clinical one, with imaging techniques providing collaborative evidence. In a case of acute stroke, the goals of imaging are to: (a) confirm the anatomic localization of the infarct that is suggested clinically; (b) determine the anatomic extent of the ischemia; (c) exclude hemorrhage, the presence of which alters the medical management; (d) exclude other entities masquerading as acute ischemia, such as a focal intracerebral or extracerebral mass lesion; and (e) determine how much tissue is receiving blood flow of less than 18 ml/100 g/minute—the approximate threshold for prolonged ischemia to produce infarction (21)—in order to distinguish between brain tissue that is dead or will surely die and that which might be salvageable.

In the subacute or chronic condition, the goals of imaging, in addition to defining the anatomic localization and extent of the lesion, are to distinguish infarcted from ischemic regions and to determine whether there is low flow to tissue because there is a physiologic need for the flow but an inadequate supply, or whether there is simply low demand for flow because of either necrosis from previous infarction in the region or a decreased cellular metabolic rate owing to any of a variety of causes. Flow augmentation procedures might be of value to increase blood flow to viable ischemic brain tissue, but they are of little value and may be harmful if the affected brain is already irreversibly damaged.

The two most common methods of visualizing the brain anatomically are computerized tomography (CT) and magnetic resonance (MR) imaging. MR imaging is the more sensitive of the two techniques, but CT is the more readily available. In order to visualize the dynamics of cerebral perfusion with CT, it is necessary to inject the patient with a tracer material or some type of contrast agent. The xenon-CT method is a relatively new method that uses stable (nonradioactive) xenon rather than xenon-133. Single photon emission CT (SPECT) similarly to xenon-133 CT or positron emission tomography (PET), uses an injected radioactive tracer. SPECT uses tomographic imaging methods and principles of interpretation that were developed for CT. Each of these techniques has its goals, advantages, and disadvantages.

COMPUTERIZED TOMOGRAPHY

The appearance of ischemia and infarction on CT scans is familiar (13, 16, 17). The new generation of scanners have better contrast and spatial resolution, allowing us to visualize acute ischemia and infarction earlier and with better definition of boundaries than did the older machines. Today, large areas of infarction can be visualized within a few hours after the ictus, although the findings may be subtle, such as effacement of sulci, loss of the normal distinction between gray and white

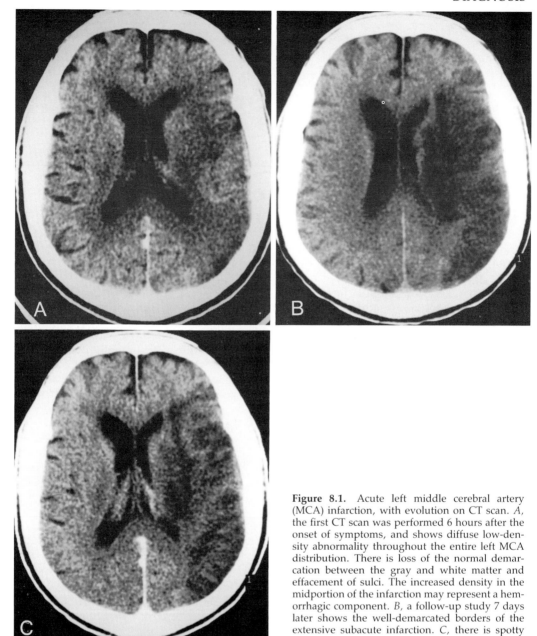

Figure 8.1. Acute left middle cerebral artery (MCA) infarction, with evolution on CT scan. *A,* the first CT scan was performed 6 hours after the onset of symptoms, and shows diffuse low-density abnormality throughout the entire left MCA distribution. There is loss of the normal demarcation between the gray and white matter and effacement of sulci. The increased density in the midportion of the infarction may represent a hemorrhagic component. *B,* a follow-up study 7 days later shows the well-demarcated borders of the extensive subacute infarction. *C,* there is spotty contrast enhancement of this infarct.

matter, and a subtle overall decrease in the density of tissue (Figs. 8.1 and 8.2) (32). For less severe strokes or those situated in the posterior fossa, a region in which scans are likely to show artifacts, it may take up to 24 hours or more before the signs of ischemia are visualized (Fig. 8.3). In our experience, the earlier the visualization, the more ominous is the prognosis for the extent and severity of infarction and the degree of cerebral swelling. Unfortunately, even if acute ischemia or infarction can be visualized with a high-quality CT scanner within hours after the event, it may already be too late to initiate therapy necessary to prevent cell death.

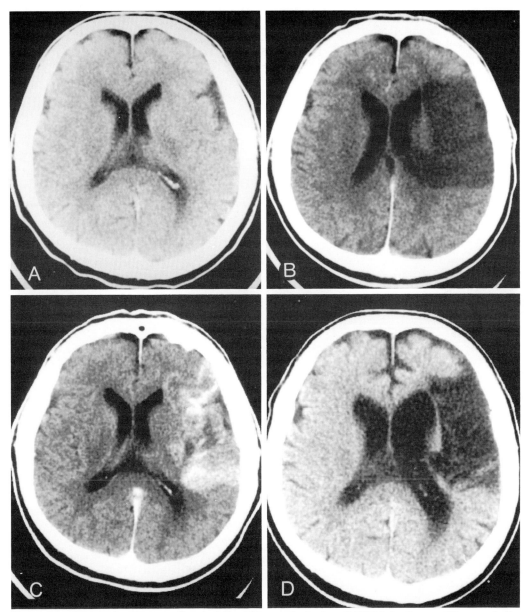

Figure 8.2. Progressive changes of acute left middle cerebral artery (MCA) infarction on CT scan. *A,* the initial scan, performed within hours after the acute onset of right-sided weakness, shows focal areas of volume loss but is otherwise unremarkable in this 64-year-old man. *B,* an enhanced CT scan made 1 day later shows the extensive left MCA distribution infarction and the effacement of the enlarged sulci noted on the earlier scan. There is no evidence of enhancement. *C,* a follow-up scan made 2 weeks later shows extensive enhancement throughout much of the left MCA distribution. *D,* a scan made 18 months later shows the sharp demarcation of the infarct and the secondary volume loss in the left hemisphere.

A contrast-enhanced study that demonstrates leakage of the iodinated contrast material through the damaged blood–brain barrier may not become positive for up to 24 hours after onset of neurologic deficit (Figs. 8.1 and 8.2) (22). Contrast enhancement of acute ischemic lesions also suggests a poor prognosis due to infarction since the early stages of potentially reversible ischemic edema are not associated with

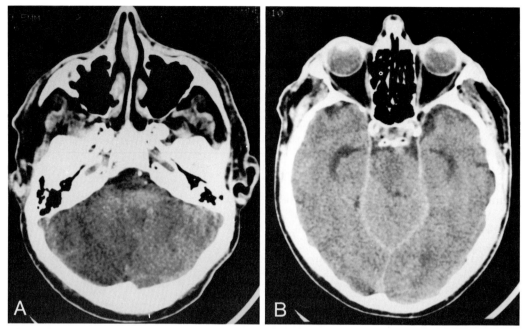

Figure 8.3. Right cerebellar and brain stem infarction on CT scan. This 60-year-old man presented with acute onset of confusion, progressing to stupor over 24 hours, and physical findings of right cerebellar and brain stem dysfunction. *A,* an unenhanced scan through the mid-cerebellum, made 24 hours after onset of confusion, shows extensive low-density abnormality involving the right cerebellar hemisphere with effacement of the fourth ventricle. *B,* a scan through the mid-pons shows infarction involving the right side of the brain stem. There is also dilatation of the temporal horns, indicative of obstructive hydrocephalus from the cerebellar swelling. The patient required emergency ventriculostomy and right cerebellar decompression.

blood–brain barrier damage. Therefore, we do not use the contrast study in patients whom we see within the first 24 hours after the ictus. Usually, only an unenhanced study is performed in order to exclude hemorrhage that would preclude anticoagulation therapy. CT is the most sensitive imaging modality for visualizing acute hemorrhage. It can accurately exclude hemorrhage in a 10- to 15-minute procedure. It is also easier to monitor a confused patient suffering from acute ischemia if CT is used rather than MR imaging.

If the unenhanced CT scan suggests the presence of a focal intracerebral or extracerebral mass, then a contrast-enhanced CT scan is extremely valuable. It is also of value if the clinical picture is confusing. However, neither plain CT nor static contrast-enhanced images provides any information regarding the dynamics of cerebral blood flow (CBF). There has been work with dynamic CT, a method in which

a bolus injection of contrast media passes through the cerebral vasculature while a rapid series of CT images is obtained in order to detect decreased circulation time (20, 28, 30). Unfortunately, most scanners in use require at least 1 to 2 seconds of scanning time and several seconds for incremental table movements—too slow a process in which to obtain serial images at multiple levels to evaluate vascular hemodynamics. A single level must be selected in order for a rapid series of sectional images to be obtained which will allow a measurement of intravascular circulation times. In the patient with acute stroke whose plain CT scan appears normal or is equivocal, one must either predict the appropriate level at which to image the brain on the basis of clinical findings or be rather arbitrary in selecting the level to image for a dynamic CT study. Most of the work done with dynamic CT has been performed to examine stroke in the subacute stage, where an apparent abnormality on either the plain or enhanced scan has guided the selection of an appropriate scanning level for the dynamic series. A new scanner that has been recently introduced operates at subsecond speeds. Such scanners offer the possibility of even more rapid dynamic CT, the usefulness of which remains to be demonstrated.

In the patient with subacute to chronic stroke, CT is useful for demonstrating the extent and location of the low-density infarct lesion (13, 16, 17). The contrast-enhanced study is likewise very good for demonstrating breakdown of the blood–brain barrier in order to determine the extent and distribution of the ischemic process (13, 16, 17). Ischemia in the white matter is more difficult to visualize than ischemia in other brain regions because white matter is lower in density than gray matter on normal CT scans, and the changes caused by ischemia and infarction must be more severe in order to be visualized. Small lacunar infarctions may also be difficult to visualize on CT (4). An apparently normal CT scan does not exclude lacunar infarction because many technical factors, such as the thickness of the slice made and partial-volume effects, compromise the ability to detect small low-density lesions.

MAGNETIC RESONANCE IMAGING

MR imaging is significantly more sensitive for detecting ischemic alterations in brain tissue and is also more capable of detecting early cerebral edema than is CT (Fig. 8.4) (2). Imaging of animal brains after acute vascular occlusion suggests that MR imaging may be capable of detecting acute ischemic edema much earlier than CT—between 30 minutes and a few hours after the ictus (3). Unfortunately, little work has been done with MR imaging in patients who present very acutely, to determine how soon after the ictus an acute infarction can be consistently visualized. Even with a more sensitive technology, it may not be possible consistently to demonstrate ischemia in its very early stages— and early detection of ischemia or infarc-

tion is of consequence only if it is early enough that management of the patient can be altered. Early confirmation of ischemia by MR imaging may be helpful, particularly if new thrombolytic agents such as tissue plasminogen activator prove to be of value and can be administered soon after onset of the ischemic event. Such visualization may be helpful in selecting patients for treatment and monitoring response to the drug.

The MR imaging procedure takes substantially longer than CT, increasing the possibility of the patient's moving, which degrades image quality. It is difficult to monitor the patient who is encased deeply within a magnet, and therefore the acute stroke patient, like the acute trauma patient, is generally referred to a CT scanner rather than to the MR imaging suite.

It is also more difficult to visualize acute hemorrhage with MR imaging than with CT (1, 5). The findings of acute hemorrhage are far more subtle with MR imaging than with CT, and consist of a subtle decrease of intensity on the T_2-weighted images using high-field systems. The more characteristic high signal intensity on both the T_1- and T_2-weighted images of acute hemorrhage is not demonstrated until several days after the ictus (Fig. 8.5) (9, 13, 39).

Gadolinium diethylenetriamine pentaacetic acid (Gd-DTPA), a paramagnetic contrast agent, does not facilitate the visualization of ischemia that began less than 16 hours before MR imaging (19, 27). Although MR imaging is a more sensitive technique than CT for detecting changes in the tissues, the poor perfusion to the area of ischemia, and hence the lack of delivery of the contrast agent to the ischemic tissues, together with the time required for the development of collateral circulation and breakdown of the blood–brain barrier, all reduce the usefulness of Gd-DTPA in cases of acute ischemia. Like contrast-enhanced CT, MR imaging with Gd-DTPA enhances infarcted tissues in the late acute and subacute phases (Fig. 8.6) (31).

The distinction on MR imaging between ischemic infarction, with a subtle mass effect, and infection can be difficult. In large

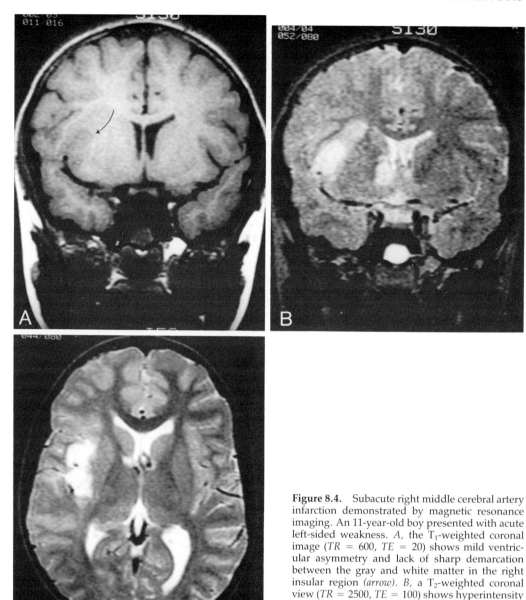

Figure 8.4. Subacute right middle cerebral artery infarction demonstrated by magnetic resonance imaging. An 11-year-old boy presented with acute left-sided weakness. *A,* the T_1-weighted coronal image ($TR = 600$, $TE = 20$) shows mild ventricular asymmetry and lack of sharp demarcation between the gray and white matter in the right insular region *(arrow).* *B,* a T_2-weighted coronal view ($TR = 2500$, $TE = 100$) shows hyperintensity in the insular region and in the right basal ganglia. *C,* the axial T_2-weighted image ($TR = 2500$, $TE = 100$) shows hyperintensity in the same regions.

measure, it is still necessary to depend on the distribution of the ischemic process and the medical history as aids to the interpretation of the image.

As yet, there are no clinically available MR imaging techniques to evaluate cerebral perfusion. Pulsing sequences to quantitate CBF and to distinguish perfusion from diffusion are in their infancy (6, 33).

The use of an injectable or inhaled contrast agent to quantitate blood flow with MR imaging is purely conjectural at this time.

For evaluating stroke in the subacute to chronic state, MR imaging is exquisitely sensitive in detecting the edema, demyelination, and gliosis of ischemia and infarction. It is also useful for visualizing subacute and chronic hemorrhage. Sub-

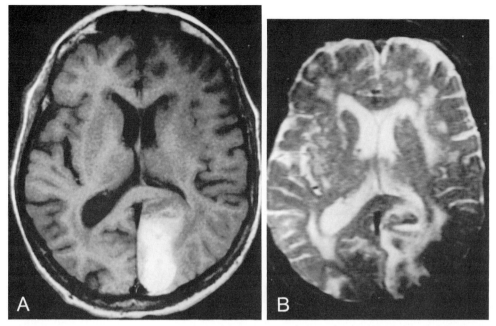

Figure 8.5. Subacute left parietal–occipital hemorrhagic infarction. This 83-year-old woman had the acute onset of left homonymous hemianopsia. *A,* the T_1-weighted magnetic resonance image ($TR = 600$, $TE = 20$) shows a large area of hyperintensity involving the left occipital lobe. *B,* the T_2-weighted image ($TR = 2500$, $TE = 100$) shows a mixed pattern of hyperintensity, isointensity, and hypointensity throughout the parietal and occipital lobes indicative of subacute hemorrhage and infarction. There are also multiple areas of hyperintensity involving the basal ganglia and deep white matter, consistent with chronic changes of infarction.

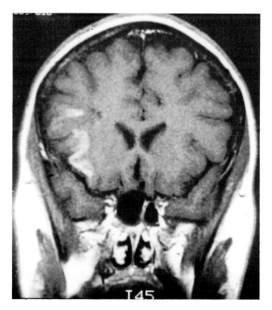

Figure 8.6. Gadolinium-enhanced magnetic resonance image demonstrating middle cerebral artery (MCA) infarction. This 35-year-old woman with ovarian carcinoma had presented 3 days previously with acute left-sided weakness. The coronal image following the injection of gadolinium-DTPA shows enhancement of the cortical and subcortical infarction in the right MCA distribution.

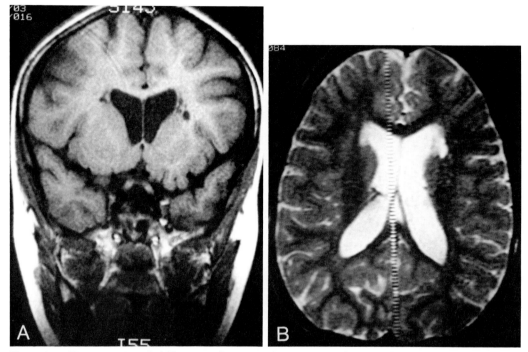

Figure 8.7. Demonstration of old lacunar infarcts on MR imaging. *A*, the coronal T_1-weighted image (TR = 600, TE = 20) shows multiple hypointense foci around both frontal horns. *B*, the axial T_2-weighted image (TR = 3000, TE = 100) demonstrates the hyperintensities of these lacunar infarcts.

acute hemorrhage is characterized by a relative hyperintensity on both T_1- and T_2-weighted images (Fig. 8.5), while hemosiderin in chronic extracellular blood collections has a markedly hypointense appearance on both T_1- and T_2-weighted images (9, 13). MR imaging is the best technique available for visualizing subacute to chronic lacunar infarctions (Fig. 8.7) (4). It is far more sensitive for evaluating ischemic edema and infarction in the white matter than is CT (Fig. 8.8) (26). The ability of MR to image the brain directly in multiple planes without reformation artifacts makes this technique extremely valuable for anatomic localization. Its ability to show differences between tissues allows demonstration of the diverse pathologic manifestations of infarction, such as the difference between microcystic and macrocystic changes (26). However, the significance of these differences for therapeutic management is unknown. Lastly, blood vessel morphology and gross flow patterns are far better demonstrated with

MR imaging than with contrast-enhanced CT. Distinction can be made between rapid and slow flow, and gross vessel occlusion (Fig. 8.9) and subintimal hemorrhage or dissection can be detected (8).

There is some interest in using MR imaging to image the distribution of sodium in brain in an effort to diagnose and determine the extent of ischemia, edema, and infarction (14). The extracellular sodium concentration is altered during ischemia, and MR imaging may be able to detect these changes as indications of ischemia far earlier than other imaging methods. However, there are problems with this methodology. Sodium is present at 1/4,000th the concentration in the body as is hydrogen, which is used for standard MR imaging. Therefore, the signal available is inherently smaller than that available for hydrogen imaging, requiring extremely long imaging times which increases the possibility of artifact due to patient motion. Because of the lower signal, spatial resolution is likewise less than with

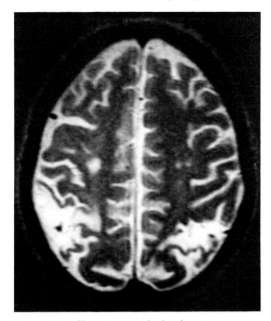

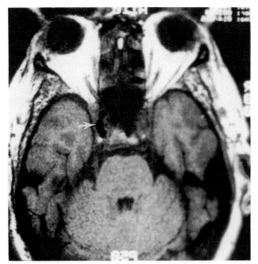

Figure 8.9. Thrombosed left internal carotid artery shown on magnetic resonance imaging. The 55-year-old man had had a diagnosis of acute right-sided weakness 5 days previously, but the symptoms had resolved. The T_1-weighted axial view at the level of the cavernous sinuses shows the hypointensity (signal void) characteristic of rapid blood flow through the normal right internal carotid artery *(arrow)*. The occluded left internal carotid artery is visualized.

Figure 8.8. Chronic watershed infarction on magnetic resonance imaging. A heavily T_2-weighted image (*TR* = 2500, *TE* = 100) shows bilateral, high-convexity, parietal, chronic watershed infarctions between the distributions of the middle cerebral artery and posterior cerebral artery. There are also small areas of infarction involving the deep white matter.

hydrogen imaging. Additional studies are needed before the clinical applicability of this technique can be determined.

XENON-ENHANCED COMPUTERIZED TOMOGRAPHY

The xenon-CT method uses inhaled stable xenon as a contrast agent (35, 38). Xenon, like iodine, is a radiographic contrast agent. Unlike iodinated contrast agents in which iodine is attached to macromolecules, the small xenon molecule dissolved in blood passes easily through the blood–brain barrier into the cerebral parenchyma. The molecule is small, lipophilic, and nonionic, and therefore is an excellent perfusion agent because there is no impediment to its rapid passage into the cerebral parenchyma in either normal or diseased states.

A series of four xenon-CT scans are performed over 4.3 minutes at any level studied. Baseline scans obtained before the inhalation of xenon are subtracted from subsequent xenon-enhanced images in order to determine the progressive increase in tissue density due to the presence of xenon in the tissue. A close approximation of the intraarterial concentration of xenon is obtained by determining the pulmonary end-tidal xenon concentration as measured in the exhaled air. By knowing the intraarterial concentration and the buildup of xenon concentration in the tissue over time (as determined by the rate of increase in CT number), CBF is computed for each image pixel and the values are depicted as image density in order to construct a blood flow map.

The number of levels studied is determined by the heating capacity and cooling time of the scanner's x-ray tube. At our institution, we use a GE 9800 scanner (General Electric Corporation, Schenectady, NY), which allows up to three levels to be studied in each patient. The selection of levels to be imaged is determined by the clinical situation. Solid-state detector

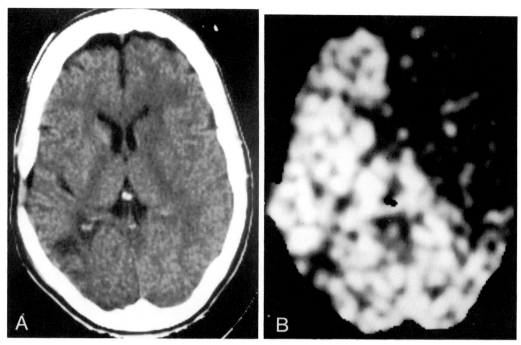

Figure 8.10. Acute left frontotemporal infarction invisible on plain CT but demonstrated on a xenon-CT cerebral blood flow study. The 66-year-old woman had undergone partial resection of a left cavernous sinus meningioma, and demonstrated right-sided weakness in the recovery room. *A*, the baseline CT scan is unremarkable in the left frontal and temporal regions (note the preexisting right parietotemporal infarct and craniotomy defect). *B*, a xenon-enhanced CT scan, obtained minutes later with the patient still on the CT table, shows the markedly decreased flows in the left frontal and temporal regions, ranging from 7 to 9 ml/ 100 g/minute.

systems are now available which, in comparison with other CT scanners, provide either twice the information at the same x-ray dose or the same information at half the x-ray dose (and hence half the x-ray tube power demand and heating). Future investigations will focus on increasing the number of levels that can be studied and reducing the concentration of xenon necessary to perform a diagnostic study.

The xenon-CT technique is more sensitive to the extent and degree of ischemia than either CT or MR imaging in the patient with acute stroke (Fig. 8.10) (18, 36). The CBF data it provides permit one to define the extent and severity of the ischemic lesion and to be sure of the diagnosis in confusing clinical situations. Although there may be a lack of coupling of blood flow to metabolism in acute infarction, which may result in some limitations for interpretation of the information obtained with xenon-CT, the usefulness of

this technique is not compromised in assessing acute stroke. For example, CBF may be elevated despite infarction if reperfusion of an ischemic lesion has already occurred (*see* Chapter 2, this volume).

The xenon-CT method provides reasonably good spatial resolution, on the order of 6 mm (34). This resolution is certainly the best of any afforded by the other CBF modalities now available. Because it uses a CT scanner, the technique is potentially widely available. It is a procedure that is quick and relatively easy to perform. After obtaining a static CT scan, the physician can simply place the inhalation mask on the patient's face, or connect the inhalation tubing to the endotracheal tube of an intubated patient, for performance of a blood flow study requiring approximately 20 additional minutes of CT time. Computer processing for a three-level study requires approximately 20 more minutes.

Adverse reactions to inhalation of stable

xenon are minimal, certainly less severe than the sensitivity reactions observed to intravenously injected contrast agents (24). Although it has been argued that xenon is a vasodilator and therefore provides spuriously high blood flow values, this vasodilatory property actually could be viewed as a pharmacologic challenge; that is, if blood flow values remain low, even in the face of xenon-induced vasodilation, proximal vascular occlusion and distal vasoparalysis must have already occurred. One problem with the technique is the patient's motion. In the confused patient, motion may be a significant problem that produces misregistration artifacts. Even with well-designed head holders, motion degrades approximately 10% of studies. Xenon produces a sensation of intoxication even in the neurologically intact patient. Such a reaction may be disturbing to an already confused ischemic patient, leading to inadvertent motion during scanning. Motion artifact may be decreased with the use of solid state detectors, which may allow a significant decrease in the concentration of administered xenon and therefore a reduction in the intoxicating effect.

A lesser problem is the radiation dosage to the patient. Four xenon-enhanced CT scans plus two baseline scans produce a total radiation dose of 18 to 20 rads to a single point in the irradiated field. We avoid the most sensitive organ in the head, the eye. The brain is relatively radiation resistant. By comparison, however, cerebral angiography gives up to 60 rads to the eye. The radiation dose would only be a hazard if multiple studies were performed through the same imaging plane.

In the patient with subacute or chronic ischemia, the xenon-CT method also accurately defines the distribution of blood flow associated with the lesion (Fig. 8.11). The technique is quantitative, and regions of interest of any size can be selected for quantitative measurement of CBF (Figs. 8.10 and 8.11). Levels of blood flow (ml/100 g/minute) can be determined for gray matter, white matter, or any combination of tissues. The error is approximately 12% for a 2-cm voxel, making it a relatively accurate technique as compared to other CBF methods (10, 38).

In the chronic state of ischemia, CBF may be coupled to metabolism, so that a determination of blood flow parallels cellular metabolism. However, simply measuring a single blood flow value does not determine whether there is a decreased supply of blood with normal demand or a decreased level of cellular metabolism requiring less flow. Such decreased metabolism may result from deafferentation of input from an area of infarction located in the vicinity or at some distance (diaschisis) but not actually involving tissues in the region of interest or from previous ischemia or other metabolic processes that affected the tissue directly, such as those occurring in a number of the degenerative disorders. If both blood flow and metabolic rates were measured simultaneously, such as can be accomplished with PET scanning, this problem would be solved. An extremely expensive and difficult technology, PET is considered to be a research tool rather than a practical clinical tool at this time. Moreover, PET scanning affords only a limited direct anatomic correlation with flow and metabolism from transmission images as compared to the xenon-CT technique, which uses the anatomic distribution of the lesion obtained from preliminary CT images as the basis for selecting levels of interest and constructing the blood flow map.

In order to overcome the problem of the lack of metabolic data with the xenon-CT method, we use "double studies" in most of our xenon-CT examinations. For patients who potentially may undergo sacrifice of one of their carotid arteries, for example, from skull base tumor surgery or carotid occlusion for giant aneurysm, a xenon study before and after balloon occlusion of the internal carotid artery is performed in order to assess the patient's collateral flow potential (Fig. 8.12) (7). In order to assess autoregulation and to determine the appropriate level of hypocarbia in posttraumatic patients with cerebral edema, a baseline study at the respiratory rate and PCO_2 level being maintained and a repeat study 15 minutes later after decreasing the PCO_2 by 10 torr (23). Finally, in the ischemic patient, we perform a xenon-CT blood flow study before and after

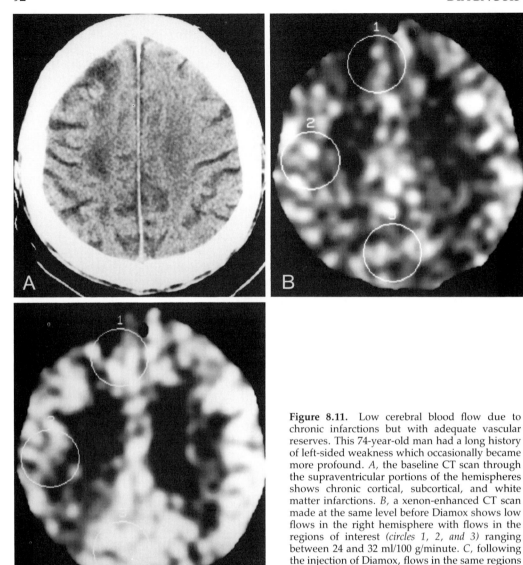

Figure 8.11. Low cerebral blood flow due to chronic infarctions but with adequate vascular reserves. This 74-year-old man had a long history of left-sided weakness which occasionally became more profound. *A*, the baseline CT scan through the supraventricular portions of the hemispheres shows chronic cortical, subcortical, and white matter infarctions. *B*, a xenon-enhanced CT scan made at the same level before Diamox shows low flows in the right hemisphere with flows in the regions of interest (*circles 1, 2, and 3*) ranging between 24 and 32 ml/100 g/minute. *C*, following the injection of Diamox, flows in the same regions of interest increased to between 61 and 87 ml/100 g/minute. These findings indicate low flows due to low need but adequate vascular reserves.

the intravenous administration of 1 g of acetazolamide (Diamox, Lederle Laboratories, Wayne, NJ) (29). Diamox is a potent vasodilator that increases blood flow in those patients and brain regions with adequate vascular reserves. Therefore, in an area where CBF is low because of the lack of need for more flow, CBF will increase with the administration of Diamox (Fig. 8.11). In low-flow areas with more need than supply, flows will not increase (Fig.

8.13). This test, therefore, quickly and accurately defines areas which may benefit from flow augmentation procedures. No blood flow data of this type were available during an extracranial–intracranial arterial bypass study which may have failed to define a small population of patients who were truly suffering from a low-flow state (11). This technique requires prospective evaluation to determine whether it might help to select those patients who could

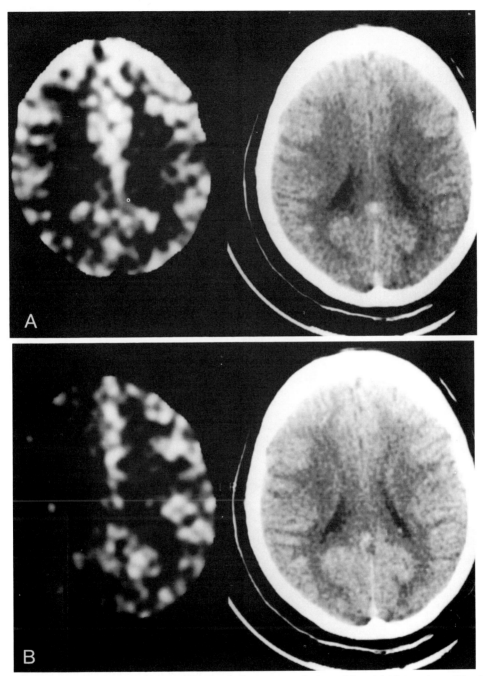

Figure 8.12. Low cerebral blood flow following balloon test occlusion of the right internal carotid artery. This 65-year-old woman was to undergo an extensive resection at the base of the right side of the skull for squamous cell carcinoma. In order to test for adequacy of collateral during a potential right carotid occlusion at surgery, a Swan-Ganz balloon catheter was inflated in the right internal carotid artery. Neurologic testing for 15 minutes showed no evidence of neurologic deficit. The baloon was deflated and the patient underwent xenon-enhanced CT. *A,* with the balloon deflated, a xenon-CT scan through the high convexities showed normal and symmetrical flows bilaterally. *B,* with the balloon inflated, there was a marked decrease of flow to the right cerebral hemisphere (mean, 18 ml/100 g/minute). Although the patient was still asymptomatic, these flows were on the threshold for infarction and might have caused infarction if prolonged. The study indicated the high risk of right cerebral hemispheric infarction if carotid occlusion had to be performed during surgery.

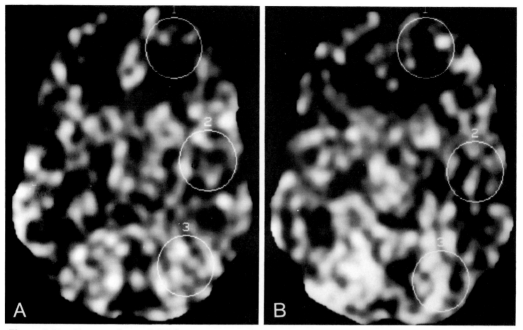

Figure 8.13. Xenon-enhanced CT demonstration of inadequate vascular reserves in the anterior portions of the cerebral hemispheres. The 59-year-old man presented with syncope and was found angiographically to have bilateral carotid occlusions. *A,* the xenon-CT study before the injection of Diamox shows relatively low flows in the frontal regions (28 ml/100 g/minute in region one), with normal flows in regions two and three (range, between 40 and 55 ml/100 g/minute). *B,* following the injection of Diamox, flows in the frontal regions increased to 34 ml/100 g/minute, while there was no significant increase in the middle cerebral distributions. There was a dramatic increase of flows in the occipital regions. Angiography showed collateral flow to all portions of the brain from the vertebral basilar circulation. Xenon-CT study showed that the collateral circulation was maximally vasodilated. There was a greater need for blood flow and vascular reserves were inadequate, prompting extracranial–intracranial vascular bypass.

benefit from such flow augmentation procedures (37).

SINGLE PHOTON EMISSION COMPUTERIZED TOMOGRAPHY

Although SPECT has been available as a nuclear medicine technique for a number of years, iodine-123 iodoamphetamine compounds that may be used in assessing CBF have only recently become generally available in this country. These compounds are initially distributed in the brain in concentrations proportional to local CBF. Although they are said to pass rather easily across the blood–brain barrier, change of the partition coefficient in the diseased state may influence their rate of passage (15). Iodoamphetamines bind to a variety

of receptors, the alteration of which in the pathologic state may also lead to spurious results regarding the status of CBF (15, 25). In short, the iodoamphetamine compounds measure both CBF and receptor availability, and it will be necessary to develop methodologies to isolate the flow component if this technique is to become accurate for the quantitative evaluation of CBF

It is difficult to quantitate CBF with SPECT/iodoamphetamine because of constraints related to both biologic factors and instrumentation (15). Rather, it generally is necessary to evaluate relative flows by comparing similar areas in the normal and abnormal hemispheres (Fig. 8.14) (15). Spatial resolution is significantly poorer with SPECT than with the xenon-CT technique. It is not known at this time whether this is a significant limitation in obtaining the diagnostic information needed for the

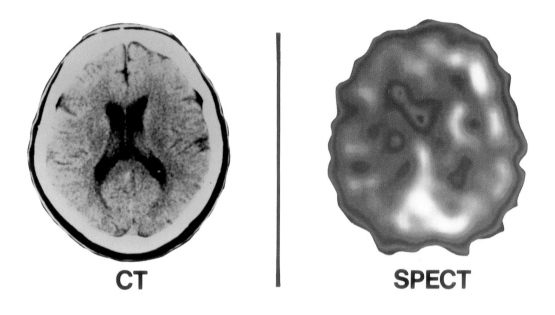

Figure 8.14. Single photon emission CT (SPECT)-iodoamphetamine study demonstrating low right hemispheric uptake with an accompanying normal CT scan. This patient had acute left-sided weakness, and a CT scan of the head made a few hours after his admission to the hospital showed no abnormalities. A SPECT study 48 hours later showed low uptake involving the entire right cerebral hemisphere, lowest in the right frontal periventricular white matter. (Courtesy of Medi-Physics, Inc. [a Division of Roche Pharmaceuticals], Emeryville, CA.)

types of therapeutic regimens currently available to treat ischemia. There is no high-resolution anatomic correlate with SPECT as there is with xenon-CT, which uses the anatomic CT image paired with the physiologic flow map.

As discussed earlier in relation to xenon-CT, a single determination of CBF says nothing about low need verses low supply; a double study or physiologic challenge is necessary to make that determination. Recirculation of tracer initially sequestered in other parts of the body and a total body washout time of 24 hours (15) limit the accuracy that can be achieved in sequential studies. Conceivably, two studies could be done on consecutive days after manipulating a physiologic parameter such as blood pressure. Because the radiation dose is low, multiple studies could be performed safely.

Clearly there needs to be direct comparison of the SPECT-iodoamphetamine CBF technique with xenon-CT, xenon-133 CBF studies and PET scanning in order to determine the relative accuracy and efficacy of these tomographic techniques (*see* Chapters 2 and 9, this volume). Although the SPECT-iodoamphetamine CBF technique may offer the advantage of avoiding the intoxicating effects of xenon, therefore reducing the potential for motion artifact, nonetheless questions of tracer distribution and kinetics in both the normal and diseased states, the inability to easily and accurately quantitate CBF, and the lack of an anatomic correlate all suggest that the SPECT-iodoamphetamine CBF technique must be considered less advantageous than other methodologies.

PERSPECTIVE

Acute cerebral ischemia is a clinical diagnosis. The main value of CT scanning without use of a contrast agent is to rapidly and effectively demonstrate ischemic edema and exclude the presence of hematoma or other focal mass lesion. The presence of ischemia and infarction can be confirmed rapidly using the xenon-CT CBF technique, which requires additional time in relation to plain CT but which can be compromised by motion from the patient in about 10% of cases. CT is readily available and reasonably accurate, and the studies are rapidly acquired. MR imaging is more sensitive for the visualization of early ischemic edema and infarction. As yet, it is not known whether the consistent demonstration of early ischemia by MR imaging, combined with new and effective treatment regimens, will improve the patient's outcome. MR imaging technology is more expensive than CT and interpretation of the images more difficult than with CT. Better clinical results are necessary to justify its use in patients with acute stroke. The role of sodium imaging in the diagnosis of early stroke remains to be determined.

In the patient with chronic ischemia, MR imaging is more sensitive than CT to areas of ischemic edema and infarction. An unanswered question is whether MR imaging can distinguish infarcted from ischemic but viable tissue that may benefit from treatment. If not, then the less expensive CT scan may remain the basic screening modality for static imaging; MR imaging may be used only for aiding in the resolution of confusing cases.

The xenon-CT methodology using a physiologic or pharmacologic challenge technique may help define the role of flow augmentation procedures and treatment regimens for subacute or chronic ischemia. The role of SPECT-CBF methods in the evaluation of ischemia and infarction remains to be determined.

References

1. Bradley WG, Schmidt PG: Effect of methemoglobin formation on the MR appearance of subarachnoid hemorrhage. *Radiology* 156:99–103, 1985.
2. Brant-Zawadzki M, Norman D (eds): *Magnetic Resonance Imaging of the Central Nervous System.* New York, Raven Press, 1987, pp 221–234.
3. Brant-Zawadzki M, Pereira B, Weinstein P, et al: MR imaging of acute experimental ischemia in cats. *AJNR* 7:7–11, 1986.
4. Brown JJ, Hesselink JR, Rothrock JF: MR and CT of lacunar infarcts. *AJNR* 9:477–482, 1988.
5. De La Paz RL, New PFJ, Buonanno FS, et al: NMR imaging of intracranial hemorrhage. *J Comput Assist Tomogr* 8:599–607, 1984.
6. Dumoulin CL, Hart HH: Magnetic resonance angiography. *Radiology* 161:717–720, 1986.
7. Erba SM, Horton JA, Latchaw RE, et al: Balloon test occlusion of the internal carotid artery with stable xenon/CT cerebral blood flow imaging. *AJNR* 9:533–538, 1988.
8. Goldberg HI, Grossman RI, Gomori JM, et al: Cervical internal carotid artery dissecting hemorrhage: Diagnosis using MR. *Radiology* 158:157–161, 1986.
9. Gomori JM, Grossman R, Goldberg HI, et al: Intracranial hematomas: Imaging by high-field MR. *Radiology* 157:87–93, 1985.
10. Good WF, Gur D, Yonas H, et al: Errors in cerebral blood flow determination by xenon-enhanced computed tomography due to estimation of arterial xenon concentration. *Med Phys* 14:377–381, 1987.
11. Gur D, Yonas H: Extracranial–intracranial arterial bypass. *N Engl J Med* 314:1192, 1986.
12. Haughton VM: Vascular diseases. In Williams AL, Haughton VM (eds): *Cranial Computed Tomography.* St. Louis, CV Mosby, 1985, pp 88–147.
13. Hecht-Leavitt C, Gomori JM, Grossman RI: High-field MRI of hemorrhagic cortical infarction. *AJNR* 7:581–585, 1986.
14. Hilal SK, Maudsley AA, Simon HE, et al: In vivo NMR imaging of tissue sodium in the intact cat before and after acute cerebral stroke. *AJNR* 4:245–249, 1983.
15. Holman BL, Hill TC: Perfusion imaging with single-photon emission computed tomography. In Wood JH (ed): *Cerebral Blood Flow.* New York, McGraw-Hill, 1987, pp 243–256.
16. Horton JA: Cerebral infarction. In Latchaw RE (ed): *Computed Tomography of the Head, Neck, and Spine.* Chicago, Year Book, 1985, pp 101–115.
17. Houser OW, Campbell JK, Baker HL, et al: Radiologic evaluation of ischemic cerebrovascular syndromes with emphasis on computed tomography. *Radiol Clin North Am* 20:123–142, 1982.
18. Hughes RL, Yonas H, Gur D, et al: Stable xenon-enhanced CT in the first eight hours of cerebral infarction. *Stroke* 18:283, 1987.
19. Imakita S, Nishimura T, Naito H, et al: Magnetic resonance imaging of human cerebral infarction: Enhancement with Gd-DTPA. *Neuoradiology* 29:422–429, 1987.
20. Jinkins JR: Dynamic CT of micro- and macroan-

giopathic states of the cerebrum. *Neuroradiology* 30:22–30, 1988.

21. Jones TH, Morawetz RB, Crowell RM, et al: Thresholds of focal cerebral ischemia in awake monkeys. *J Neurosurg* 54:773–782, 1981.

22. Kuroiwa T, Seida M, Tomida S, et al: Discrepancies among CT, histological, and blood–brain barrier findings in early cerebral ischemia. *J Neurosurg* 65:517–524, 1986.

23. Latchaw RE, Yonas H, Darby JM, et al: Xenon/CT cerebral blood flow determination following cranial trauma. *Acta Radiol* 369(Suppl):370–373, 1986.

24. Latchaw RE, Yonas H, Pentheny S, et al: Adverse reactions to xenon-enhanced CT cerebral blood flow determination. *Radiology* 163:251–254, 1987.

25. Lee RGL, Hill TC, Holman L, et al: Predictive value of perfusion defect size using N-isopropyl-(I-123)-p-iodoamphetamine emission tomography in acute stroke. *J Neurosurg* 61:449–452, 1984.

26. Marshall VG, Bradley WG Jr, Marshall CE, et al: Deep white matter infarction: Correlation of MR imaging and histopathologic findings. *Radiology* 167:517–522, 1988.

27. McNamara MT, Brant-Zawadzki M, Berry I, et al: Acute experimental cerebral ischemia: MR enhancement using Gd-DTPA. *Radiology* 158:701–705, 1986.

28. Norman D, Axel L, Berninger WH, et al: Dynamic computed tomography of the brain: Techniques, data analysis, and applications. *AJR* 136:759–770, 1981.

29. Rogg J, Rutigliano M, Yonas H, et al: The acetazolamide challenge: Imaging techniques to evaluate cerebral blood flow reserve. *AJNR* 10:803–810, 1989.

30. Traupe H, Heiss WD, Hoeffken W, et al: Hyperperfusion and enhancement in dynamic computed tomography of ischemic stroke patients. *J Comput Assist Tomogr* 3:627–632, 1979.

31. Virapongse C, Mancuso A, Quisling R: Human brain infarcts: Gd-DTPA-enhanced MR imaging. *Radiology* 161:785–794, 1986.

32. Wall SD, Brant-Zawadzki M, Jeffrey RB, et al: High frequency CT findings within 24 hours after cerebral infarction. *AJR* 138:307–311, 1982.

33. Wedeen VJ, Rosen BR, Chesler D, et al: MR velocity imaging by phase display. *J Comput Assist Tomogr* 9:530–536, 1985.

34. Yonas H: Xenon-enhanced CT: Evaluating cerebral blood flow. *Diagn Imaging* 10:88–94, 1988.

35. Yonas H, Good WF, Gur D, et al: Mapping cerebral blood flow by xenon-enhanced computed tomography: Clinical experience. *Radiology* 152:435–442, 1984.

36. Yonas H, Gur D, Glaassen D, et al: Stable xenon-enhanced computed tomography in the study of clinical and pathologic correlates of focal ischemia in baboons. *Stroke* 19:228–238, 1988.

37. Yonas H, Gur D, Good BC, et al: Stable xenon-CT blood flow mapping for evaluation of patients with extracranial–intracranial bypass surgery. *J Neurosurg* 62:324–333, 1985.

38. Yonas H, Gur D, Latchaw RE, et al: Xenon computed tomographic blood flow mapping. In Wood JH (ed): *Cerebral Blood Flow.* New York, McGraw-Hill, 1987, pp 220–242.

39. Zimmerman RD, Heier LA, Snow RB, et al: Acute intracranial hemorrhage: Intensity changes on sequential MR scans at 0.5 T. *AJR* 150:651–661, 1988.

CHAPTER NINE

Positron Emission Tomography

William J. Powers, M.D.

For many years, the use of radiotracers in clinical investigation was hampered by the lack of an accurate, noninvasive method for localizing and accurately measuring the internal distribution of radioactive molecules. In the late 1970s, application of the principles of computerized tomography (CT) to this problem resulted in the development of positron emission tomography (PET). By taking advantage of the physical properties of certain radioactive nuclides that release positrons as they decay, PET can provide quantitatively accurate tomographic images of regional radioactivity distribution in vivo. When combined with appropriate positron-emitting radiotracers and mathematical models, PET can be used to make a variety of physiologic measurements in the brain and other organs, including cerebral blood flow (CBF), cerebral blood volume (CBV), and cerebral metabolic rate of oxygen ($CMRO_2$). The technical aspects of PET and its practical applications have been well described (18, 30).

During the past decade, considerable research has been done with PET in the study of patients with cerebral vascular disease, and much of this work has been reviewed (2, 10, 19, 28). This chapter concerns only those observations which are directly relevant to defining the role of PET in the clinical evaluation of patients with transient cerebral ischemia and acute ischemic stroke.

CEREBRAL ISCHEMIA: ASSESSMENT OF HEMODYNAMIC FACTORS

Determining the role that hemodynamic factors play in the pathogenesis, prognosis, and choice of treatment for patients with cerebral ischemia and infarction requires a method to evaluate accurately the hemodynamic status of the cerebral circulation in awake subjects under normal conditions. Direct measurement of the perfusion pressure in the distal arterial bed of the cerebral circulation is clearly impracticable, but an indirect and accurate assessment can be made by evaluating the compensatory responses of the brain to reductions in cerebral perfusion pressure (CPP). Such an approach is possible with PET, but the assessment must be based on a thorough understanding of the changes that occur within the cerebral circulation as CPP declines.

As CPP falls, CBF is maintained initially by dilation of precapillary resistance vessels (autoregulation). As a result, both CBV and the CBV/CBF ratio increase. $CMRO_2$ and the oxygen extraction fraction (OEF; normally about one-third of the total arterial oxygen content) remain constant. Once vasodilation has reached its maximal effectiveness, cerebral autoregulation fails and CBF begins to fall. CBV may decrease as vessels collapse, but the CBV/CBF remains elevated. Because CBV/CBF is mathematically equivalent to the mean vascular transit time for red blood cells through the cerebral vessels, an increase in this ratio indicates slowing of the cerebral circulation (22). A progressive increase in OEF then maintains $CMRO_2$. Once OEF increases to its maximum possible level, further decline in blood flow causes disruption of normal cellular metabolism and infarction may result (15, 19, 28) (Fig. 9.1).

The development of PET in combination with appropriate radiotracers and mathematical models has made it practical to measure regional CBF (rCBF), CBV, and OEF in human subjects. On the basis of a

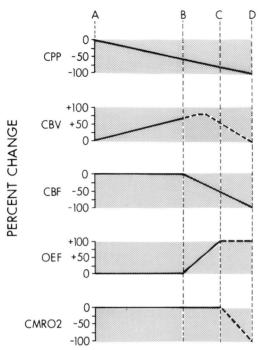

Figure 9.1. Compensatory responses to reduced cerebral perfusion pressure (CPP). As CPP falls, cerebral blood flow (CBF) is initially maintained by dilation of precapillary resistance vessels. As a result, both cerebral blood volume (CBV) and CBV/CBF ratio (not shown) increase. When vasodilation can no longer compensate, cerebral autoregulation fails and blood flow begins to fall (B); this occurs before maximal vasodilation. As CPP continues to fall, CBV may decrease as vessels collapse, but the CBV/CBF ratio will remain elevated. A progressive increase in the oxygen extraction fraction (OEF) now maintains cerebral metabolic rate of oxygen ($CMRO_2$). Once this mechanism becomes maximal (C), further declines in blood flow cause disruption of normal cellular metabolism and function. *Dashed lines* indicate conditions for which data are inadequate to draw firm conclusions. (From Powers WJ, Press GA, Grubb RL Jr, et al: The effect of hemodynamically significant carotid artery disease on the hemodynamic status of the cerebral circulation. *Ann Intern Med* 106:27–35, 1987.)

combination of these measurements and the physiologic information just described, it is possible to categorize regional cerebral hemodynamics in individual patients as: *(a)* normal; *(b)* reduced CPP with normal CBF (increased CBV/CBF, normal OEF); or *(c)* reduced CBF relative to the local metabolic rate (increased OEF) (2, 10, 11, 23, 24, 27) (Fig. 9.2). It is immediately apparent that measurement of these multiple

physiologic variables is necessary to assess cerebral hemodynamics accurately. Measurements of CBF alone are inadequate for this purpose because they cannot detect reductions in CPP when CBF is maintained by compensatory vasodilation, nor can they differentiate decreased CBF caused by reduced blood supply from that caused by reduced metabolic demands (Figs. 9.2 and 9.3).

Gibbs et al (11) have described 32 patients with internal carotid artery occlusion in whom PET measurements of uninfarcted brain tissue were made. They found small but significant decreases in both CBF and $CMRO_2$ distal to the occlusion associated with significant increases in both CBV and OEF. They suggested that CBF/CBV, which is the reciprocal of mean vascular transit time, was the best index of abnormal hemodynamic status because patients with clinical features suggesting hemodynamic perfusion failure (such as border zone infarcts or hemispheric ischemic symptoms precipitated by sudden standing) and bilateral carotid occlusion had the lowest values for this ratio. Samson et al (32) have used PET to study 37 patients with internal carotid artery occlusion. A relative increase in OEF distal to the occlusion was found in 15 of those patients. In 27 patients who underwent four-vessel angiography to assess collateral circulation, an increase in OEF was associated either with ophthalmic collaterals or collateral circulation through the circle of Willis originating from a stenosed artery.

We have investigated the relation of PET measurements of cerebral hemodynamics to arteriographic findings in 19 patients with predominantly unilateral carotid artery disease of greater than 67% diameter reduction, so-called hemodynamically significant lesions (27). These patients had no clinical or CT evidence of cerebral infarction. The 19 patients were categorized on the basis of their PET studies into three groups: *(a)* normal (Stage 0), with normal CBV/CBF and normal OEF; *(b)* low CPP (Stage I), with increased CBV/CBF and normal OEF; and *(c)* low CBF (Stage II), with increased OEF (Fig. 9.2). In the middle cerebral artery (MCA) territory distal to the

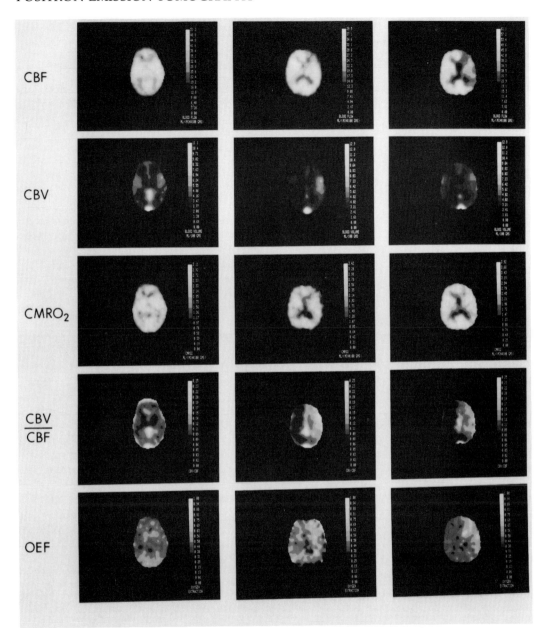

Figure 9.2. Positron emission tomography (PET) of regional cerebral hemodynamics and metabolism in three patients with right internal carotid artery occlusion. Each of the panels shows one tomographic slice depicting a different physiologic measurement. Note that the right cerebral hemisphere is on the right and the front of the brain is at the top. PET measurements from a 59-year-old woman with episodes of transient blindness in her right eye (*left column*) show normal cerebral blood flow (CBF), cerebral blood volume (CBV), cerebral metabolic rate of oxygen ($CMRO_2$), CBV/CBF, and oxygen extraction fraction (OEF). PET studies of a 65-year-old woman with episodes of transient left-sided weakness (*center column*) show elevated CBV and CBV/CBF in the right hemisphere. Both CBF and $CMRO_2$ are slightly and proportionately decreased in the right frontal region, as evidenced by a uniform OEF throughout the brain. PET studies of a 69-year-old man who had had one episode of transient left-sided weakness 6 weeks earlier (*right column*): Right hemispheric CBF is reduced relative to $CMRO_2$. CBV, CBV/CBF, and OEF are all increased in the right hemisphere. (From Powers WJ, Press GA, Grubb RL Jr, et al: The effect of hemodynamically significant carotid artery disease on the hemodynamic status of the cerebral circulation. *Ann Intern Med* 106:27–35, 1987.)

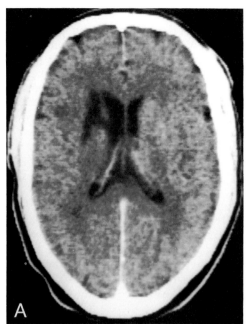

Figure 9.3. Positron emission tomography (PET) and x-ray computerized tomography (CT) scans from a 62-year-old man who suffered a left hemisphere infarct 2 months earlier. Note that the right cerebral hemisphere is on the right and the front of the brain is at the top. Carotid arteriography showed severe stenosis at the origin of the left internal carotid artery. *A*, x-ray CT shows a subcortical infarct with structurally normal overlying cortex. *B*, the preoperative PET study *(upper row)* shows reduced cerebral blood flow (CBF) *(far left)* and cerebral metabolic rate of oxygen *(center left)* in the area of the infarct as well as in overlying cortex that is structurally normal by CT. Cerebral blood volume *(center right)* and oxygen extraction fraction *(far right)* are normal in this region of cortex, indicating that the reduction in CBF is not caused by reduced flow through the stenotic carotid artery but is secondary to reduced metabolic demand from disruption of afferent and efferent pathways by the subcortical infarct. Following left carotid endarterectomy *(lower row)*, there was no change in any of the PET measurements, confirming the nonhemodynamic nature of the abnormalities.

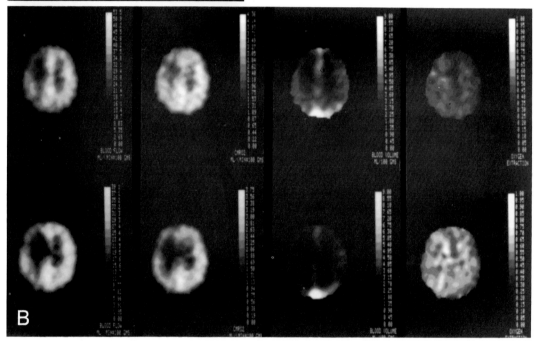

hemodynamically significant carotid artery stenosis, PET demonstrated normal cerebral hemodynamics (Stage 0) in seven patients, reduced CPP with normal CBF (Stage I) in eight, and both reduced CPP and reduced CBF (Stage II) in four. There was no significant relation between the hemo-

dynamic status of the cerebral circulation as measured by PET and either the percent carotid stenosis or the diameter of the residual carotid lumen in millimeters. There was, however, a highly significant relation between the three PET categories of cerebral hemodynamics and the pattern of collateral flow. Collateral circulation to the middle cerebral artery (MCA) through meningeal anastomoses from the ipsilateral anterior cerebral artery was present only in patients with reduced CBF (three of four patients in Stage II), and not in patients with normal CBF (0 of 15 patients in Stages 0 and I, $p<0.005$). Collateral circulation through the ipsilateral ophthalmic artery was observed only in patients with reduced CPP (seven of 12 patients in Stages I and II) and not in patients with normal hemodynamics (zero of seven patients in Stage 0, $p<0.02$.)

These three studies showed that neither the presence nor severity of a carotid artery lesion is a reliable indicator of the hemodynamic status of the cerebral circulation in the ipsilateral hemisphere. The primary determinant of cerebral hemodynamics in cases of a carotid artery lesion is the adequacy of collateral circulatory pathways. The arteriographic pattern of abnormal collateral circulation through ophthalmic or meningeal vessels is a specific, but not a sensitive, indicator of abnormal cerebral hemodynamics. Thus, PET permits the classification of patients who are otherwise homogeneous with respect to clinical and arteriographic findings into different categories based on the hemodynamic status of the cerebral circulation.

This use of PET to define hemodynamic status has been applied to patients undergoing superficial temporal artery-to-middle cerebral artery (STA-MCA) bypass surgery to monitor the circulatory and metabolic effects of surgery and to try to define, within an otherwise homogeneous population, subgroups who might respond differently to treatment (4, 5, 12, 13, 23, 25, 29). In general, these studies have yielded similar results. Patients with focal increases in OEF in noninfarcted brain preoperatively have increased CBF to that area following surgery (4, 5, 25, 31). Accompanying the increase in CBF there is a significant decrease in OEF, implying that increased local extraction of oxygen had served as a compensatory mechanism preoperatively. No significant change in $CMRO_2$ occurs postoperatively, indicating that the compensation has been adequate. There is also no postoperative change in CBV, suggesting that although the bypass improves blood flow, perfusion pressure is still below the autoregulatory limit and maximal vasodilation is still present (Fig. 9.4). In other patients who do not have regions of increased OEF preoperatively, the predominant effect of surgery is to reduce CBV with little change in CBF or $CMRO_2$; it appears that these patients have not reached the limit of autoregulation preoperatively. Surgery improves CPP, reducing the amount of vasodilation necessary to maintain flow.

A report of 12 patients undergoing STA-MCA bypass by Samson et al (31) noted, in contrast to earlier experience, that a relative increase in hemispheric OEF preoperatively was not a reliable indication that there would be a postoperative increase in CBF. Moreover, they found bilateral postoperative increases in $CMRO_2$, but no change in OEF, occurring in patients with carotid occlusion and severe contralateral stenosis. They proposed that reversal of a chronic ischemic depression of oxygen metabolism would explain the latter observation. The clinical correlate, if any, of these metabolic changes has yet to be determined.

ROLE OF POSITRON EMISSION TOMOGRAPHY IN CLINICAL MANAGEMENT

Does the assessment of cerebral hemodynamics with PET provide information that is valuable in the clinical management of individual patients? At first, it seems that the answer to this question must be yes. Accurate knowledge of cerebral hemodynamics should permit the identification of a subgroup of patients who are at high risk for stroke on hemodynamic grounds (either spontaneously or secondary to hypotensive episodes occurring during major cardiovascular surgery) and who, therefore, need surgical revascularization by STA-MCA bypass or carotid endarterectomy to reduce this risk. Although these are plausible hypotheses, they remain to be proved. A longitudinal study to evaluate the risk of stroke in individuals with

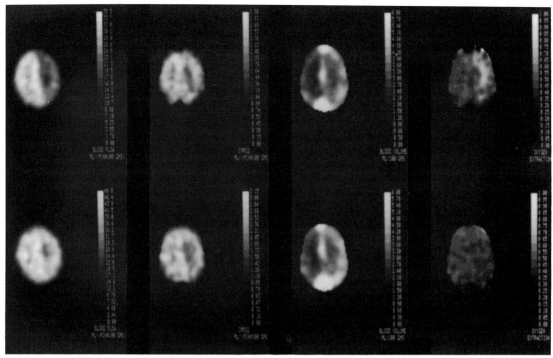

Figure 9.4. Preoperative and postoperative positron emission tomography scans from a 65-year-old woman who underwent superficial temporal artery-to-middle cerebral artery bypass anastomosis on the right side. She had had several episodes of visual blurring in the right eye followed by numbness and weakness of the left arm and leg. Note that the right cerebral hemisphere is on the right and the front of the brain is at the top. Carotid arteriography showed total occlusion of the right internal carotid artery with collateral flow through the right ophthalmic and anterior cerebral arteries. Preoperatively *(upper row)*, the right hemisphere showed markedly lower cerebral blood flow (CBF; *far left*), slightly lower cerebral metabolic rate of oxygen (CMRO$_2$; *center left*), higher cerebral blood volume (CBV; *center right*) and higher oxygen extraction fraction (OEF; *far right*). Postoperatively *(lower row)*, there was a relative increase in right hemisphere CBF *(far left)*, no change in CMRO$_2$ or CBV *(center left and right)*, and OEF became symmetrical *(far right)*.

normal or abnormal PET studies is needed, as is a randomized, controlled trial of surgical versus medical treatment in patients who show PET evidence of reduced CPP.

We have recently completed a nonrandomized, retrospective 2-year follow-up evaluation of 56 patients with symptomatic occlusion or intracranial stenosis of the carotid–middle cerebral arterial system who were studied by PET: 27 patients subsequently underwent STA-MCA bypass, and 29 did not (23, 24, 29). At the time of PET, the two groups were similar with respect to age, sex, and arteriographic lesions and the percentage with hypertension, diabetes, and transient ischemic attacks. For the nonoperated group, the rate of stroke at 1 year was two of 29 patients (6.9%) and at 2 years, five of 29 (17.2%).

In comparison, for the operated group, the stroke rate at 1 year was five of 27 patients (18.5%) and at 2 years, also five of 27 (18.5%). No new strokes occurred in the second year. For patients who showed PET evidence of abnormal hemodynamics (Stages I and II), the stroke rate in the nonoperated group was one of 20 patients (5%) at 1 year and four of 20 (20%) at 2 years; and in the operated group, was four of 22 patients (18.2%) at 1 year and 2 years. Among the 14 patients who had the most severe hemodynamic abnormalities manifested by focal increases in OEF (Stage II), the stroke rate at 2 years was two of five patients in the nonoperated group and two of nine in the operated group.

Although the results of this study are not definitive because of its retrospective, nonrandomized design and the small number of patients in the series, our data do not support the hypothesis that measurement of cerebral hemodynamics can identify a subgroup of patients at high risk for early stroke who can be helped by STA-MCA bypass. Unless further studies show results to the contrary, prognostic or therapeutic significance cannot be attributed to PET findings of cerebral hemodynamic compromise.

Acute Ischemic Stroke

Positron Emission Tomography Findings in Ischemic Brain

PET studies of CBF and metabolism in patients with acute ischemic stroke have provided information about the evolution of acute cerebral infarction that is remarkably consistent across all reported series (3, 6, 8, 14, 16, 33). In the affected region of brain, both CBF and $CMRO_2$ are reduced. During the first 24 hours, two different patterns are seen with regard to the relationship between CBF and $CMRO_2$. In approximately one-half of patients, the reduction in CBF exceeds that in $CMRO_2$, resulting in increased OEF. In the other half, $CMRO_2$ is reduced as much as or more than CBF and OEF is low or normal. Because $CMRO_2$ varies little, this variability in OEF is primarily a result of differences in CBF (8). Within the next few days following the ictus, $CMRO_2$ usually changes little but in some patients it may increase or decrease substantially. CBF usually increases and, as a result, OEF decreases. During the first week, CBF increases further with little or no change in $CMRO_2$, causing OEF to decrease even further. This CBF increase peaks at 1 to 2 weeks and then declines. By 1 month, CBF and $CMRO_2$ are relatively matched and OEF is normal or slightly decreased.

The correct interpretation of the changes in CBF, $CMRO_2$, and OEF that occur within these first few days is uncertain. The initial period of increased OEF seen in some patients has been interpreted as indicating a state of "critical perfusion" in nonfunc-tional but still viable brain tissue. Irreversible infarction is believed to take place hours to days later, when OEF decreases (16, 33). Spontaneous reperfusion occurs, but usually too late to save the damaged tissue. This reperfusion usually exceeds the metabolic requirements of the tissue ("luxury" perfusion), resulting in a further reduction in OEF. This hypothesis suggests that there is a period of time after an acute ischemic stroke during which neurons potentially can be salvaged by reperfusion and that a local increase in OEF, as measured by PET, may identify these salvageable neurons. Owing to the phenomenon of luxury perfusion in irreversibly infarcted tissue, it is unlikely that PET measurements of CBF alone would be adequate to reliably identify regions of brain in which ischemia is reversible. Because cellular metabolism is nearly normal when neuronal electrical failure occurs during ischemia (1, 9, 17), the concurrent measurement of $CMRO_2$ and CBF might provide sufficient information to identify ischemic tissue that is nonfunctional but viable.

With these ideas in mind, Baron et al (6, 8) studied 25 patients from days 2 to 38 after acute ischemic stroke. Regional data on CBF, $CMRO_2$, and OEF were taken from brain sites that remained viable and from sites later shown by CT to be infarcted. Neither CBF nor OEF proved to be generally useful in discriminating viable from nonviable tissue. A minimum threshold value for $CMRO_2$ of 1.5 to 1.7 ml/100 g/minute for viable tissue provided good differentiation. However, in none of the patients was an attempt made to reperfuse brain tissue; the natural evolution of acute ischemic stroke was simply allowed to run its course. Wise et al (33) did attempt to forestall permanent infarction in a patient with acute ischemic stroke who had persistent elevation of regional OEF on day 4. The systemic blood pressure was raised by angiotensin infusion, resulting in increased blood flow to the ischemic area. OEF decreased but $CMRO_2$ did not change and there was no clinical improvement. The case report suggests that irreversible neuronal damage with loss of autoregulation had occurred and that the increased

OEF was simply helping to maintain oxygen metabolism at a reduced level.

We have studied the CBF and $CMRO_2$ requirements for human cerebral function and viability with PET in 24 normal subjects, 24 patients with severe carotid artery disease who had normal neurologic function and no evidence of cerebral infarction, and 10 patients with established cerebral infarcts that had occurred from 8 days to 3 years earlier (21). Minimum values for CBF and $CMRO_2$ in the 48 subjects who had normal neurologic function and no infarction were 19 ml/100 g/minute for CBF and 1.3 ml/100 g/minute for $CMRO_2$. In the 10 subjects with cerebral infarcts, CBF ranged from 7 to 44 ml/100 g/minute and $CMRO_2$ from 0.1 to 2.6 ml/100 g/minute. Truly reversible symptomatic cerebral ischemia has, to my knowledge, been studied with PET in only three patients (7, 20), all of whom underwent PET when they had focal clinical neurologic deficits. They then went on to make a clinical recovery with no evidence of cerebral infarction in the affected area of brain, as shown by follow-up CT scan. The PET measurements were taken from relatively large areas of ischemic brain: CBF ranged from 13 to 16 ml/100 g/minute and $CMRO_2$ was 1.3 to 2.6 ml/100 g/minute; OEF in two patients was quite high (0.95 and 0.99), and in the third was within the normal range (0.49) but higher than in the rest of the brain.

Taken together, all of these studies suggest that the combination of CBF in the range of 13 to 18 ml/100 g/minute and $CMRO_2$ above 1.3 ml/100/minute observed with PET may identify nonfunctional but viable cerebral tissue (26). This combination of PET findings exists in some patients studied within a few days of having an acute stroke (6, 8, 33), again suggesting that there may be a critical period during which ischemic damage could be reversed by reperfusion. Proof of such a period of reversibility requires PET studies of patients during periods of acute cerebral ischemia to document that tissue reperfusion and reoxygenation occurs with therapeutic intervention. PET measurements during the subsequent clinical course must then be correlated with the initial PET measurements. Such studies have not been performed and this clinical application of PET, although attractive, remains theoretical.

Identification of the Ischemic Penumbra

All of the data and conclusions discussed so far derive from PET measurements of relatively large areas of ischemic brain. Experimental studies of acute focal ischemia have shown that viable but electrically inactive tissue forms a ring, an "ischemic penumbra," around the more densely ischemic center in which both energy failure and ion pump failure have occurred. Methodologic limitations greatly reduce the accuracy of PET in detecting a small penumbral region around an area of infarcted tissue.

In a PET image, the radioactivity from a region of interest in the object under study is redistributed over a larger area. Consequently, a specific region in the reconstructed image, regardless of its size, contains only a portion of the radioactivity actually within that region in the original structure—the remainder has been redistributed into surrounding regions of the image. Similarly, some radioactivity from surrounding regions has been redistributed to the region of interest. Owing to such partial-volume averaging, PET measurements of rCBF and $CMRO_2$ at the edge of an infarct are influenced both by values within the infarct and by values in the surrounding brain tissue.

We have investigated the effect of partial-volume averaging on the detection of an ischemic penumbra by performing computer simulations of cerebral infarction with and without an ischemic penumbra (26). In the case of infarction without penumbra, we assumed that there was an abrupt reduction in CBF and $CMRO_2$ levels from normal to the values found in infarcted tissue. Because of partial-volume averaging, this abrupt decrease is imaged by PET as a gradual transition (Fig. 9.5). Regional values for CBF and $CMRO_2$ within the penumbral range will be detected in this transition zone even when no actual regions with these values exist in the brain.

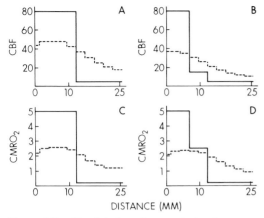

Figure 9.5. Simulated positron emission tomography (PET) measurements of cerebral blood flow (CBF) and cerebral metabolic rate of oxygen ($CMRO_2$) in ml/100 g/minute. *Solid lines* represent the true values and *dashed lines* represent values measured by PET. Values measured by PET in the area surrounding the infarct are approximately the same whether or not there is a penumbra. *A,* cerebral infarct without penumbra. True CBF in normal brain surrounding the infarct is 80 ml/100 g/minute and abruptly changes to a value of 5 ml/100 g/minute within the infarct. *B,* cerebral infarct with penumbra. True CBF in normal brain is 80 ml/100 g/minute, penumbral flow is 15 ml/100 g/minute, and infarct flow is 5 ml/minute. *C,* cerebral infarct without penumbra demonstrates an abrupt decrease in true $CMRO_2$ from 5 ml/100 g/minute (normal brain) to 0.2 ml/100 g/minute (infarct). *D,* cerebral infarct with penumbra shows true $CMRO_2$ of 5 ml/100 g/minute in normal brain, 2.5 ml/100 g/minute in penumbra, and 0 in the infarct. (From Powers WJ, Mintun MA: The role of positron tomography in identification of the ischemic penumbra. In Powers WJ, Raichle ME (eds): *Cerebrovascular Diseases* (Transactions of the Fifteenth Research [Princeton] Conference). New York, Raven Press, 1987, pp 273-281.)

When a penumbral region surrounds the infarct (Fig. 9.5), PET measurements will again show a gradual transition that is a little different from that seen in the infarcted region without penumbra. Thus, a transitional zone of flow and metabolism around an infarct will always be detected with PET whether or not there is a true physiologic or anatomic penumbra (Fig. 9.6). This problem is common to all emission CT and occurs with single photon emission CT estimates of CBF, as well as with PET. Scanners with improved resolution will merely reduce the size of the

apparent transitional zone; they cannot eliminate it entirely.

Does this mean that PET is useless for demonstrating existence of a periinfarct penumbra? Not necessarily. In association with the CBF and $CMRO_2$ values that occur in the physiologic penumbra there is an increase in OEF. Because the OEF in the penumbral region surrounding an infarct should be greater than that in both normal brain and established infarction, an elevated OEF cannot appear as an artifact of partial-volume averaging due to the contribution of both these tissues. The sensitivity of PET in detecting a region of increased OEF surrounding an infarct depends on the size of the penumbral region, the magnitude of the increase in OEF, and the spatial resolution of the scanner. Our simulations, based on a final reconstructed image resolution of 18 mm, have shown that a 2.7-mm or 5.4-mm penumbral ring with OEF of 1.0 was detected reliably. Penumbral regions with OEF of 0.6 were not detected if they were 2.7 mm wide, and were sometimes seen if they were 5.4 mm wide. Because of partial-volume averaging, these penumbral rings did not appear as distinct rings on the PET image but rather as larger, ill-defined areas (Fig. 9.7).

As noted earlier, large regions with CBF and $CMRO_2$ in the penumbral range and high OEF have been seen within the first day in approximately 50% of patients with acute stroke. Whether these regions represent penumbral rings distorted by the PET reconstruction process or larger more homogenous areas remains to be determined. To my knowledge, no region of increased OEF surrounding an area of established cerebral infarction more than a few days old has been observed with PET. This failure to find a penumbral ring with PET in patients with established infarcts suggests that (*a*) a chronic penumbra does not occur in human beings; (*b*) the penumbra exists in at least some patients, but is less than a few millimeters in size and is therefore unlikely to be clinically important; or (*c*) the assumption of increased OEF within the penumbra is incorrect. It should be stressed that the simple demonstration of a region of increased oxygen

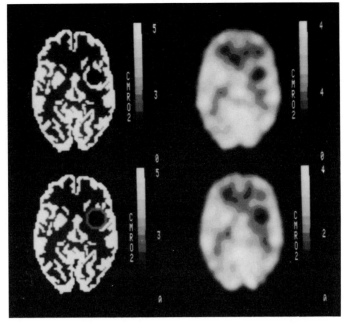

Figure 9.6. Simulated positron emission tomography (PET) images corresponding to cerebral metabolic rate of oxygen ($CMRO_2$) data shown in Figure 9.5. Note that the right cerebral hemisphere is on the right and the front of the brain is at the top. Digitized brain slices simulate true $CMRO_2$ values from a right Sylvian infarct without penumbra *(upper left)* and with penumbra *(lower left)*. Simulated PET reconstructions of the digitized data show no obvious difference between infarct without penumbra *(upper right)* and with penumbra *(lower left)* except that the latter appears slightly larger. (From Powers WJ, Mintun MA: The role of positron tomography in identification of the ischemic penumbra. In Powers WJ, Raichle ME (eds): *Cerebrovascular Diseases* (Transactions of the Fifteenth Research [Princeton] Conference). New York, Raven Press, 1987, pp 273–281.)

extraction bordering an infarct would not prove the existence of a region of non-functional but viable tissue. The OEF simply reflects the balance between blood supply and oxygen demand. Increases in OEF can be caused by any of a variety of combinations of CBF and $CMRO_2$, including those that are seen in poorly perfused but functional tissue as well as in irreversibly damaged tissue.

PERSPECTIVE ON POSITRON EMISSION TOMOGRAPHY AND ISCHEMIA

What can be said about PET's ability to differentiate tissue in which ischemia is reversible from tissue that is irreversibly infarcted in the patient with ischemic stroke? PET's role in detecting large re-gions of nonfunctional but viable tissue using combined measurements of CBF and $CMRO_2$ is promising, although still not established. Its role in the detection of very small regions—in specific, the penumbral ring—is more problematic at this time.

PET measurements in patients with acute ischemia are potentially of value in selecting candidates for therapeutic intervention and in monitoring the cerebral circulatory and metabolic consequences of the intervention. Accurate measurement of rCBF and $CMRO_2$, currently possible only with PET, is indispensable for determining if therapeutic measures designed to improve oxygenation of ischemic areas actually achieve that end. With such information, rational adjustment of both intensity and duration of treatment can be carried out to ensure therapeutic benefit and minimize side effects. These are exciting possibilities, but before such clinical applica-

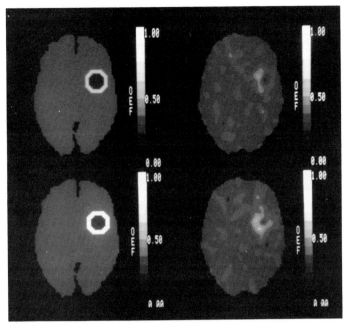

Figure 9.7. Simulated positron emission tomography (PET) images of oxygen extraction fraction (OEF) in cerebral infarction with penumbra. Note that the right cerebral hemisphere is on the right and the front of the brain is at the top. Digitized brain slices simulate true OEF of 0.60 *(upper left)* and 1.0 *(lower left)* in a penumbra 2 pixels (5.4 mm) wide. Simulated PET reconstruction of digitized data shows a 2 pixel (5.4 mm) penumbra with OEF of 0.6 *(upper right)* and 1.0 *(lower left)*. (From Powers WJ, Mintun MA: The role of positron tomography in identification of the ischemic penumbra. In Powers WJ, Raichle ME (eds): *Cerebrovascular Diseases* (Transactions of the Fifteenth Research [Princeton] Conference). New York, Raven Press, 1987, pp 273–281.)

tions can be justified evidence is needed to prove that PET's adjuvant use would reduce morbidity and mortality. Thus, although PET has a major role in clinical research, its application to the care of patients with cerebral vascular disease remains uncertain.

Acknowledgment—This work was supported by U.S. Public Health Service grants no. NS06833, AG03991, HL13851 from the National Institutes of Health and by the McDonnell Center for the Study of Higher Brain Function, at Washington University School of Medicine, St. Louis, MO.

References

1. Astrup J, Siesjö B, Symon L: Thresholds in cerebral ischemia—the ischemic penumbra. *Stroke* 12:723–725, 1981.
2. Baron JC: Positron tomography in cerebral ischemia. *Neuroradiology* 27:509–516, 1985.
3. Baron JC, Bousser MG, Comar D, et al: Non-invasive tomographic study of cerebral blood flow and oxygen metabolism in vivo. *Eur Neurol* 20:273–284, 1981.
4. Baron JC, Bousser MG, Rey A, et al: Reversal of focal "misery-perfusion syndrome" by extra–intracranial arterial bypass in hemodynamic cerebral ischemia. *Stroke* 12:454–459, 1981.
5. Baron JC, Rey A, Guillard A, et al: Non-invasive tomographic imaging of cerebral blood flow and oxygen extraction fraction in superficial temporal artery to middle cerebral artery anastomosis. In Meyer JS, Lechner H, Reivich M, et al (eds): *Cerebral Vascular Disease, 3* (Proceedings of the 10th International Salzburg Conference. International Congress Series No. 532). Amsterdam, Excerpta Medica, 1981, pp 58–64.
6. Baron JC, Rougemont D, Bousser MG, et al: Local CBF, oxygen extraction fraction and CMRO$_2$: Prognostic value in recent supratentorial infarction. *J Cereb Blood Flow Metab* 3 [Suppl 1]:S1–S2, 1983.
7. Baron JC, Rougemont D, Bousser M, et al: Caracteristiques de la perfusion de misere a la phase aigue de l'infarctus cerebral. In Lassen NA, Symon L, Baron JC (eds): *Penombre et Ischemie Cerebrale*. Paris, John Libbey, 1986, pp 25–30.
8. Baron JC, Rougemont D, Lebrun-Grandie P, et al: Measurement of local blood flow and oxygen consumption in evolving irreversible cerebral in-

farction: An in vivo study in man. In Meyer JS, Lechner H, Reivich M, et al (eds): *Cerebral Vascular Disease, 4* (Proceedings of the World Federation of Neurology 11th International Salzburg Conference. International Congress Series No. 616). Amsterdam, Excerpta Medica, 1983, pp 205–212.

9. Crockard HA, Gadian DG, Frackowaik RSJ, et al: Acute cerebral ischemia: Concurrent changes in cerebral blood flow, energy metabolites, pH, and lactate measured with hydrogen clearance and ^{31}P and ^{1}H nuclear magnetic resonance spectroscopy. II. Changes during ischemia. *J Cereb Blood Flow Metab* 7:394–402, 1987.

10. Frackowiak RSJ: The pathophysiology of human cerebral ischemia: A new perspective obtained with positron tomography. *Q J Med* 57:713–727, 1985.

11. Gibbs JM, Wise RJS, Leenders KL, et al: Evaluation of cerebral perfusion reserve in patients with carotid-artery occlusion. *Lancet* 1:310–314, 1984.

12. Gibbs JM, Wise RJS, Thomas DJ, et al: Cerebral haemodynamic changes after extracranial–intracranial bypass surgery. *J Neurol Neurosurg Psychiatry* 50:140–150, 1985.

13. Leblanc R, Tyler JL, Mohr G, et al: Hemodynamic and metabolic effects of cerebral revascularization. *J Neurosurg* 66:529–535, 1987.

14. Lenzi GL, Frackowiak RSJ, Jones T: Cerebral oxygen metabolism and blood flow in human cerebral ischemic infarction. *J Cereb Blood Flow Metab* 2:321–335, 1982.

15. Mackenzie ET, Farrar JK, Fitch W, et al: Effects of hemorrhagic hypotension on the cerebral circulation. 1. Cerebral blood flow and pial arteriolar caliber. *Stroke* 10:711–718, 1979.

16. Marchal G, Evans A, Dagher A, et al: The evolution of cerebral infarction with time: A PET study of the ischemic penumbra (abstract). *J Cereb Blood Flow Metab* 7 [Suppl 1]:599, 1987.

17. McPherson RW, Zeger S, Traystman RJ: Relationship of somatosensory evoked potentials and cerebral oxygen consumption during hypoxic hypoxia in dogs. *Stroke* 17:30–36, 1986.

18. Phelps ME, Mazziotta JC, Schelbert HR (eds): *Positron Emission Tomography and Autoradiography: Principles and Applications for the Brain and Heart.* New York, Raven Press, 1986.

19. Powers WJ: Positron emission tomography in cerebrovascular disease—clinical applications? In Theodore WH (ed): *Clinical Neuroimaging.* New York, Alan R. Liss, 1988, pp 49–74.

20. Powers WJ, Grubb RL Jr, Baker R, et al: Regional cerebral blood flow and metabolism in reversible ischemia due to vasospasm. *J Neurosurg* 62:539–546, 1985.

21. Powers WJ, Grubb RL Jr, Darriet D, et al: Cerebral blood flow and cerebral metabolic rate of oxygen requirements for cerebral function and viability in humans. *J Cereb Blood Flow Metab* 5:600–608, 1985.

22. Powers WJ, Grubb RL Jr, Raichle ME: Physiologic responses to focal cerebral ischemia in humans. *Ann Neurol* 16:546–552, 1984.

23. Powers WJ, Grubb RL Jr, Raichle ME: Clinical results of extracranial–intracranial bypass surgery in patients with hemodynamic cerebrovascular disease. *J Neurosurg* 70:61–67, 1989.

24. Powers WJ, Grubb RL Jr, Tempel LW, et al: Cerebral hemodynamics and 2-year stroke risk (abstract). *J Cereb Blood Flow Metab* 9[Suppl 1]:356, 1989.

25. Powers WJ, Martin WRW, Herscovitch P, et al: Extracranial–intracranial bypass surgery: Hemodynamic and metabolic results. *Neurology* 34:1168–1174, 1984.

26. Powers WJ, Mintun MA: The role of positron tomography in identification of the ischemic penumbra. In Powers WJ, Raichle ME (eds): *Cerebrovascular Diseases* (Transactions of the Fifteenth Research [Princeton] Conference). New York, Raven Press, 1987, pp 273–281.

27. Powers WJ, Press GA, Grubb RL Jr, et al: The effect of hemodynamically significant carotid artery disease on the hemodynamic status of the cerebral circulation. *Ann Intern Med* 106:27–35, 1987.

28. Powers WJ, Raichle ME: Positron emission tomography and its application to the study of cerebrovascular disease in man. *Stroke* 16:361–376, 1985.

29. Powers WJ, Tempel LW, Grubb RL Jr: Influence of cerebral hemodynamics on stroke risk: One year follow-up of 30 medically treated patients. *Ann Neurol* 25:325–330, 1989.

30. Reivich M, Alavi A (eds): *Positron Emission Tomography.* New York, Alan R. Liss, 1985.

31. Samson Y, Baron JC, Bousser MG, et al: Effects of extra–intracranial arterial bypass on cerebral blood flow and oxygen metabolism in humans. *Stroke* 16:609–616, 1985.

32. Samson Y, Baron JC, Bousser MG, et al: Cerebral haemodynamic and metabolic changes in carotid artery occlusion: A PET study. In Meyer JS, Lechner H, Reivich M, et al (eds): *Cerebrovascular Disease, 5* (Proceedings of the World Federation of Neurology 12th International Salzburg Conference. International Congress Series No. 687). Amsterdam, Excerpta Medica, 1985, pp 128–135.

33. Wise RJS, Bernardi S, Frackowiak RSJ, et al: Serial observations on the pathophysiology of acute stroke. *Brain* 106:197–222, 1983.

CHAPTER TEN

Magnetic Resonance Spectroscopy in Brain Ischemia

Philip R. Weinstein, M.D.
Robert Vink, Ph.D.

Magnetic resonance (MR) spectroscopy has great but as yet unrealized potential for the study of biologic systems. Although other biologic applications of MR spectroscopy were developed in the 1950s, it was not until surface coil techniques were introduced in 1980 (1) that the technology was successfully used to study organ biochemistry in vivo. Since then, in vivo organ metabolism has been investigated extensively with MR spectroscopy. In this chapter, we present a brief overview of MR spectroscopy as it pertains to the study of brain ischemia, including current efforts to determine whether MR spectroscopy can be applied clinically to assess tissue viability, distinguish reversible ischemia from infarction, and select or monitor therapy. The principles of MR spectroscopy instrumentation (12, 21) will not be discussed here.

MR techniques use the magnetic properties of various tissue nuclei, such as protons (^1H), phosphorus (^{31}P), and carbon, to examine biologic events in vivo. MR studies are noninvasive and can provide either anatomic or metabolic information. MR imaging takes advantage of the high concentration and magnetic sensitivity of protons to create images of the body based on the different biophysical characteristics of various tissues (see Chapter 8, this volume). MR spectroscopy, on the other hand, detects the much weaker signals from ^{31}P, carbon, and other nuclei to provide information regarding metabolic pathways, bioenergetics status, and tissue viability based on changes in the tissue levels of various metabolites. The nuclei used most often for MR spectroscopy studies of brain ischemia have been ^{31}P and ^1H.

MAGNETIC RESONANCE SPECTRA

Phosphorus-31 Spectrum

The spectrum obtained by ^{31}P MR spectroscopy of brain typically consists of eight peaks representing the relative concentrations of metabolites resonating at different frequencies (29). Each peak occurs at a specific location in the radiofrequency spectrum known as the chemical shift. The chemical shift is a dimensionless number, usually expressed in parts per million (ppm), that is used to quantitate resonance frequencies relative to a known standard compound, such as 85% orthophosphoric acid or phosphocreatine (PCr). The values of the chemical shift depend on the properties of the metabolite in question and on the local ionic environment.

Figure 10.1 shows ^1H and ^{31}P spectra acquired from rat brain during ischemia and reperfusion. The peaks represent phosphomonoesters (e.g. phosphoethanolamine, fructose-1, 6-diphosphate, etc.), inorganic phosphate (P_i), phosphodiesters (glycerophosphoethanolamine, glycerophosphocholine, etc.), PCr, and the three phosphates of adenosine triphosphate (ATP). The γ- and α-ATP peaks share the same chemical shift as several other metabolites, including the phosphate groups of adenosine diphosphate (ADP). The eighth peak is a broad resonance, thought to arise from bone and phospholipid (14), that underlies all of the other peaks; it is usually subtracted from the spectrum before analysis so that individual peaks can be integrated more accurately

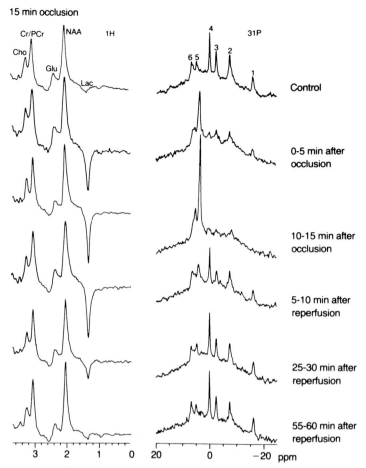

Figure 10.1. In vivo ^{1}H and ^{31}P magnetic resonance spectra from a rat brain during 15 minutes of complete ischemia and 1 hour of reperfusion after ischemia. Temporary bilateral common carotid artery occlusion was accomplished using vessel snares after microsurgical occlusion of the basilar artery and all extracranial carotid artery branches to produce immediate flattening of the electroencephalogram. Cho = choline; Cr/PCr = creatine/phosphocreatine; Glu = glutamate; NAA = N-acetylaspartate; Lac = lactate; 1, 2, 3 = β, α, γ, phosphates of adenosine triphosphate; 4 = creatine phosphate, 5 = inorganic phosphate; 6 = phosphomonoesters; ppm = parts per million. (From Shirane R, Chang L-H, Weinstein PR, et al: Sequential changes of brain metabolism during temporary global ischemia in the rat detected by simultaneous ^{1}H and ^{31}P MRS. In Suzuki J (ed): *Advances in Surgery for Cerebral Stroke*. Tokyo, Springer-Verlag, 1988, pp 633–637.)

The integrated area of each peak is proportional to the concentration of that metabolite, while the chemical shift reflects ionic concentration in the tissue. For example, the chemical shift of P_i is a weighted average of the chemical shifts of all molecules and $H_2PO_4^-$, which varies according to tissue pH and which has a proton dissociation constant of 6.88. This peak can therefore serve as an indicator of intracellular pH (26, 28). Similarly, the chemical shift of the β-ATP peak at any given pH is determined by the relative tissue concentration of magnesium (Mg^{2+})-bound and Mg^{2+}-free ATP and can therefore be used to determine the intracellular concentration of free Mg^{2+} (16, 35). In contrast, compared with other metabolites, PCr is relatively insensitive to physiologic changes in ionic concentration and is commonly used as an internal reference (0.00 ppm). Since PCr is reduced and P_i increased during ischemia, the PCr/P_i ratio is often calculated from recorded spectra as an indicator of tissue viability and bioenergetic state of the cell (8).

Hydrogen-1 Spectrum

The typical ^{1}H MR spectrum of brain and other tissues is dominated by a single intense water signal that makes less concentrated metabolites extremely difficult to detect. Using new techniques to suppress the water peak, it is now possible to monitor such metabolites, including creatine, PCr, amino acids (e.g. glutamate, aspartate, and glutamine), N-acetylaspartate (NAA), lactate, and lipids (Fig. 10.1). However, many of the peaks overlap significantly. Therefore, methods have been developed to "edit out" the signals of individual metabolites from the ^{1}H spectrum (18, 31, 38). Signal editing permits continuous monitoring of a particular metabolite without problems due to overlap of peaks (36); isolating the lactate signal is especially important for studies of brain ischemia. The resolution between adjacent peaks can be further increased by applying a stronger magnetic field.

EXPERIMENTAL STUDIES OF ISCHEMIA AND HYPOXIA

In the early 1980s, several investigators showed that MR spectroscopy could be used to investigate metabolic events in vivo during experimental ischemia (11, 27, 34). The initial ^{31}P MR spectroscopy studies from our laboratory evaluated the metabolic response of ventilated, physiologically monitored rats to 8, 15, and 30 minutes of incomplete forebrain ischemia followed by 60 minutes of reperfusion (2). The P_i peak area increased by 25% to 240% within 1 to 3 minutes after onset of ischemia, while PCr decreased by 15% to 75% and ATP decreased by 20% to 100%. Intracellular pH fell from 7.3 to 6.9 ± 0.6 in all 12 rats. The extent of metabolic recovery during reperfusion varied. In rats that failed to recover, the average PCr/ATP peak ratio 3 minutes after occlusion was 0.8; in rats that did recover, the ratio was 1.4. In a subsequent study, we found that when the lactate/NAA peak ratio was greater than 1.3 within 10 minutes after onset of ischemia, the lactate peak did not recover during reperfusion and the rats did not

survive the ischemic insult. Rats that had lower lactate/NAA peak ratios recovered metabolically and survived the 60-minute reperfusion period (30). Correlation of in vivo MR spectroscopy data with the results of an in vitro lactate dehydrogenase assay showed that when the lactate/NAA ratio was 1.5, the lactate concentration was 30 μmol/g (9).

In later studies (33), less variable results were obtained using a model that produced more complete transient global ischemia. A double-tuned surface coil was used to acquire ^{31}P and ^{1}H spectra simultaneously. Rats previously subjected to basilar and external carotid artery occlusion were placed in the spectrometer, and temporary bilateral common carotid artery occlusion was induced by remote control (33). The electroencephalogram (EEG) flattened immediately, PCr and ATP decreased by 90% to 100%, and P_i increased by up to 300%; intracellular pH dropped to approximately 6.3 within 5 minutes, while lactate increased to approximately 20 μmol/g (Fig. 10.2). However, the lactate concentration increased more slowly than pH decreased, reaching maximum levels 10 to 20 minutes after occlusion. Recovery of high-energy phosphates and reversal of lactic acidosis were complete within 30 to 60 minutes after both the 15- and 30-minute occlusions but were incomplete after the 60-minute occlusion, even after 2 hours of reperfusion. After 30 minutes of transient global ischemia, spectra obtained during recovery remained stable for up to 6 hours except for a slight elevation of the P_i peak. However, despite the return of normal energy and metabolite levels, histologic evidence of infarction becomes apparent in vulnerable areas of the hippocampus and basal ganglia beginning 6 hours after occlusion. The rats did not recover neurologically after 30 minutes of transient global ischemia and did not regain consciousness after 60 minutes of transient global ischemia. Thus, surface coil MR spectroscopy can detect the cortical metabolic response but may not detect irreversible metabolic derangement in subcortical structures that are perhaps "invisible" to present surface coil MR spectroscopy techniques; alternatively, mitochondrial func-

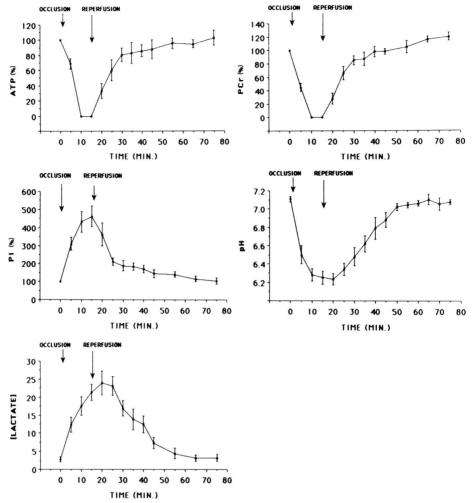

Figure 10.2. Time course of the percentage changes from control levels of adenosine triphosphate (ATP), phosphocreatine (PCr), inorganic phosphate (P_i), pH, and lactate concentration during 5 to 15 minutes of ischemia and 20 to 80 minutes of reperfusion after ischemia. Lactate levels are calculated concentrations (μmol/g). All values are mean $\pm$ standard error. (From Shirane R, Chang L-H, Weinstein PR, et al: Sequential changes of brain metabolism during temporary global ischemia in the rat detected by simultaneous ^{1}H and ^{31}P MRS. In Suzuki J (ed): *Advances in Surgery for Cerebral Stroke*. Tokyo, Springer-Verlag, 1988, pp 633–637.)

tion may recover despite irreversible ischemic cellular injury.

In other studies, however, metabolic thresholds of irreversible ischemic brain damage have been defined by correlating histologic, neurochemical, and neurologic findings with the rate and severity of lactic acidosis and depletion of high-energy phosphates determined by in vivo MR spectroscopy. In gerbils subjected to unilateral or bilateral carotid artery occlusion (10), reduction of local cerebral blood flow

(CBF) to 20 ml/100 g/minute (measured by the hydrogen clearance technique) caused a 20% to 30% reduction in ATP, a 0.6 unit drop in pH, and a significant but variable increase in the lactate/NAA ratio. Reducing CBF to 10 ml/100 g/minute increased the lactate/NAA ratio by 100% to 200%.

The effects of lactate accumulation on the development and resolution of acidosis and on energy metabolism have been studied with simultaneous ^{31}P and ^{1}H MR spectroscopy during global ischemia and hypoxia in cats (17). The capacity of brain tissue to buffer acids produced during ischemia was calculated as 29 μmol/g/pH unit, and the increases in lactate correlated with the decreases in intracellular pH. The recovery of PCr levels after the ischemic insult may have been delayed by the effect of metabolic acidosis on the creatine kinase reaction rather than by delayed recovery of the ATP/ADP ratio. The rate of lactate clearance showed zero-order kinetics ($k = 0.36$ μmol/g/minute), perhaps as a result of both lactate oxidation and efflux from cells (17).

Several MR spectroscopy studies have evaluated the effects of hypoxia and hypercarbia on cerebral energy metabolism. Rats and rabbits made hypoxic by inhalation of 4% to 12% oxygen had reversible increases in lactate and P_i, but the depletion of PCr and ATP was less rapid and severe than the increases in lactate and P_i despite the reduction of pH to 6.5 (4, 9, 15). In another study, respiratory acidosis was induced in rats by inhalation of carbon dioxide (CO_2) (25). Energy metabolism was not adversely affected even though the cerebral intracellular pH was 6.5 and the arterial CO_2 tension was 500 torr. pH recovered completely after reversal of hypoxia or hypercarbia, which suggests that hypoxia or acidosis alone without ischemia did not irreversibly impair mitochondrial function.

The additive effects of regional ischemia and hypoxia in rats have also been evaluated with ^{31}P MR spectroscopy (13). When hypoxia ($FiO_2 = 14\%$)* was superimposed upon ischemia produced by ligating the middle cerebral artery (MCA) and the carotid artery, the acidosis was more severe and the PCr/P_i ratio decreased further than during ischemia alone. High-energy phosphate levels did not change during hypoxia alone. As in the studies cited previously, infarction occurred even though the metabolite levels eventually returned to normal in both the permanent ischemia and the ischemia-hypoxia groups.

In cats subjected to temporary MCA occlusion, ^{31}P MR spectroscopy changes cor-

related in severity with the ischemic EEG changes and could therefore distinguish mild from severe strokes (22). In cats with severe strokes, the pH dropped from 7.1 to 6.2 to 6.3, ATP decreased by 57% to 79%, and the PCr/P_i ratio decreased by 60% to 70%. Neither pH nor ATP recovered during 4 hours of reperfusion, and the EEG remained depressed. In cats with mild strokes, the PCr/P_i ratio decreased only 40% in the first 10 minutes of occlusion and recovered spontaneously to a 10% to 30% decrease by the end of the ischemic period; pH did not decrease.

We have used MR imaging and MR spectroscopy in combination to study the effects of permanent and temporary regional ischemia in cats after MCA occlusion (23). The PCr/P_i ratio in the ischemic hemisphere decreased from 2.23 ± 0.40 to 0.68 ± 0.04 after permanent occlusion; at 12 hours, the ratio had recovered by 27%. MR imaging, however, showed a progressive increase in the signal intensity from the lesion over 3 to 12 hours. This finding suggests that while ischemic edema increased progressively, energy metabolism was recovering because of collateral flow development; alternatively, the PCr/P_i ratio improved because of washout of P_i. In some cats, MR imaging showed that the severity of the lesions increased during reperfusion after 2 hours of occlusion; both T_1- and T_2-weighted relaxation times increased. In other cats, lactic acidosis also increased, but high-energy phosphates recovered after blood flow was restored.

The findings in cats subjected to MCA occlusion (23), as well as the results of Germano et al (13) during regional ischemia in rats, suggest that MR spectroscopy data obtained with current localization techniques at a single time point that is delayed following the onset of experimental cerebral ischemia may not reliably indicate tissue viability or the severity of brain injury. Nonetheless, such observations illustrate the potential of using MR spectroscopy (especially with localization techniques described below) for sequential monitoring of cerebral metabolites in vivo to study the metabolic response to cerebral vascular occlusion.

---

*FiO_2 = fraction of oxygen inspired.

CLINICAL STUDIES OF ISCHEMIA

Localization

Perhaps the greatest difficulty in clinical MR spectroscopy studies of brain ischemia is localizing the tissue from which the spectra arise. Because of anatomic and pathophysiologic heterogeneity in the response to cerebral ischemia, both the volume and the location of the tissue must be known for the information to be clinically relevant. Several techniques have been developed to identify the source of the signal with reasonable accuracy (3, 5). With B_0 techniques, a magnetic field gradient is applied across the sample in much the same way as in MR imaging, whereas with B_1 techniques, the field profile of the surface coil is used. B_0 and B_1 techniques may also be used in combination in order to improve spatial resolution. Another promising method is to identify abnormal regions with MR imaging (19); metabolic information can then be acquired by MR spectroscopy from surface coils placed over that region.

Initially, clinical MR spectroscopy was restricted to the study of newborn infants (7, 20, 39). Large whole-body magnets were not available, and without depth resolution methods, MR spectroscopy could only be performed in infants because of their thin skull, scalp, and muscle layers. Neonates suffering asphyxia at birth during complicated deliveries demonstrated depletion of high-energy phosphates, elevated P_i, and a slight acidosis compared with normal controls (20). It was proposed that the PCr/P_i ratio correlated with the neurologic outcome in these infants, although later studies showed that these differences largely disappeared as the infant matured (39).

The first clinical ^{31}P MR spectroscopy studies that used spatial localization techniques in adults compared nine healthy subjects with four chronic stroke patients 10 weeks to 7 years after cerebral infarction (6). Surface coils 6.5 cm in diameter were placed over lesions identified by MR im-

aging, and depth resolution techniques were used to localize the signal. High-energy metabolites, P_i, and pH were not altered significantly, but the total ^{31}P MR spectroscopy signal was as much as 40% less in the infarct zone than in normal brain. The PCr/ATP and PCr/P_i ratios and pH levels did not change. MR spectroscopy in seven patients with acute strokes (32 to 72 hours after the onset of cerebral infarction) showed a lower PCr/P_i ratio in the affected hemisphere than in the homologous area of the opposite hemisphere or in normal controls (37). A relative alkalosis was seen in the infarct zone. There were no differences in any other metabolite ratios between the infarct zone and contralateral homologous area or normal controls. The differences in the PCr/P_i ratio disappeared by 7 days after infarction, and the alkalosis resolved within 10 days.

The results of studies in both infants and adults suggest that MR spectroscopy may be useful in predicting the extent of irreversible metabolic disturbance that may lead to brain necrosis in patients with acute strokes, as well as in determining the amount of infarcted tissue in patients with completed strokes. Further investigation of the clinical applications of MR spectroscopy is in progress, although the complex logistics involved and the time required to complete MR imaging/spectroscopy studies (about 2 hours) are disadvantages.

EVALUATION OF DRUG THERAPY

Sequential monitoring of cerebral metabolism with MR spectroscopy appears to be well suited for determining the effectiveness of drug therapies designed to protect the brain from the effects of ischemia. Although only a few such studies have been performed, they have provided some interesting results.

Calcium Channel Blockers

MR spectroscopy has been used to study the protective effects of several calcium blockers, including verapamil (32), gallopamil (24), nimodipine,† and the dihydro-pyridine calcium antagonists PY 108-068 and PN 200-110 (32). Although none of these drugs prevented energy depletion during global ischemia, nimodipine and the dihydropyridine antagonists retarded the rate at which high-energy phosphates were depleted. The rate of PCr depletion was not significantly affected by treatments that slowed the rate of ATP depletion. None of the calcium antagonists had beneficial effects on the development of acidosis after ischemia or on lactate metabolism after reperfusion. Another study has shown that gallopamil reduced the extent of acidosis by increasing the capacity of the brain to buffer acids produced during ischemia but did not affect the rate of lactate formation (24).

Barbiturates

In rats subjected to global ischemia, prophylactic administration of pentobarbital significantly slowed the depletion of high-energy phosphates but did not prevent depletion of energy metabolites (32). Pentobarbital had no effect on the extent of acidosis or the rate at which it developed. Other barbiturates have not been studied for possible protective benefit in ischemia.

Opiate Antagonists

Studies of ischemia and reperfusion in rats have shown that prophylactic administration of the TRH analogue DN-1417 (which, like other TRH analogues, has opiate antagonist properties) or the opiate antagonist nalmefene‡ enhanced the recovery of high-energy phosphates and intracellular pH after 30 or 60 minutes of global ischemia. ^{1}H MR spectroscopy studies of rats given nalmefene before the on-

set of ischemia have shown enhanced recovery and more rapid normalization of lactate levels during reperfusion.

CORRELATIONS WITH OTHER TECHNIQUES

Because it permits repeated measurements in a single animal, MR spectroscopy can be used to measure the rate of metabolic deterioration and recovery after ischemia or therapeutic intervention. The metabolic information obtained by MR spectroscopy can then be correlated with histologic data regarding tissue survival and with the results of neurologic or neurochemical studies in the same animal. In studies completed to date, therapies that improved metabolic status after ischemia and reperfusion as determined by MR spectroscopy also improved tissue survival (34). Furthermore, the recovery of energy state demonstrated by MR spectroscopy after global ischemia in rats treated prophylactically with TRH analogue DN-1417 was associated with enhanced local cerebral glucose utilization as determined by autoradiography.§ Thus, it would seem that MR spectroscopy compares favorably with alternative techniques in the investigation of tissue survival after ischemia.

FUTURE DIRECTIONS

Several MR spectroscopy techniques currently being developed have potential for the investigation of brain ischemia. Fluorine MR spectroscopy promises to be a particularly exciting technique because it may be able to monitor concurrently changes in intracellular ion concentrations, notably calcium and magnesium, which are critical cations in the regulation of cell metabolism. ^{1}H MR spectroscopy has already provided a method by which

---

†NEP Deutz, WMMJ Bovee, RAFM Chamuleau, et al: The effects of a calcium blocker on alterations in cortical electrical activity and brain energy state, studied by EEG-spectral analysis and ^{31}P-NMR spectroscopy, during transient cerebral ischemia in the conscious rat (abstract). Proceedings of the 4th Annual Meeting of the Society of Magnetic Resonance in Medicine, 1985, p 266.

‡PR Weinstein, unpublished data.

§Y Nagai, A Nagaoka, Y Nagawa, et al: Effects of DN-1417 (an analog of TRH) on ^{31}P NMR spectrum of rat brains and local cerebral glucose utilization (abstract). Proceedings of the 5th Annual Meeting of the Society of Magnetic Resonance in Medicine: Works in Progress, 1986, p 209.

lactate levels can be monitored sequentially. With carbon MR spectroscopy, it may be possible to determine fluxes of glucose from tissue glycogen or blood glucose to lactate. Lactate editing is now being used more extensively, and other editing techniques are being developed for continuous monitoring of levels of amino acids, such as aspartate and glutamate. Thus, MR spectroscopy may be useful for studying the excitotoxic theory of neuronal damage. MR spectroscopy performed with surface coils tuned to acquire spectra from several nuclei simultaneously promises to be an even more powerful tool for studying the pathophysiology of cerebral ischemia than the double-tuned coils currently in use.

References

1. Ackerman JJH, Grove TH, Wong GG, et al: Mapping of metabolites in whole animals by ^{31}P NMR using surface coils. *Nature* 283:167–170, 1980.
2. Andrews BT, Weinstein PR, Keniry M, et al: Sequential in vivo measurement of cerebral intracellular metabolites with phosphorus-31 magnetic resonance spectroscopy during global cerebral ischemia and reperfusion in rats. *Neurosurgery* 21:699–708, 1987.
3. Aue WP: Localization methods for in vivo nuclear magnetic resonance spectroscopy. *Rev Magn Reson Med* 1:21–72, 1986.
4. Behar KL, Hollander JA den, Stromski ME, et al: High-resolution ^{1}H nuclear magnetic resonance study of cerebral hypoxia in vivo. *Proc Natl Acad Sci USA* 80:4945–4948, 1983.
5. Bendall MR: Surface coil techniques for in vivo NMR. *Bull Magn Reson* 8:17–42, 1986.
6. Bottomley PA, Drayer BP, Smith LS: Chronic adult cerebral infarction studied by phosphorus NMR spectroscopy. *Radiology* 160:763–766, 1986.
7. Cady EB, Costello AM de L, Dawson MJ, et al: Noninvasive investigation of cerebral metabolism in newborn infants by phosphorus nuclear magnetic resonance spectroscopy. *Lancet* 1:1059–1062, 1983.
8. Chance B, Eleff JS, Leigh JS: Noninvasive, nondestructive approaches to cell bioenergetics. *Proc Natl Acad Sci USA* 77:7430–7434, 1980.
9. Chang LH, Pereira BM, Weinstein PR, et al: Comparison of lactate concentration determinations in ischemic and hypoxic rat brains by in vivo and in vitro ^{1}H NMR spectroscopy. *Magn Reson Med* 4:575–581, 1987.
10. Crockard HA, Gadian DG, Frackowiak RSJ, et al: Acute cerebral ischemia: Concurrent changes in cerebral blood flow, energy metabolites, pH, and lactate measured with hydrogen clearance and ^{31}P and ^{1}H nuclear magnetic resonance spectros-

11. Delpy DT, Gordon RE, Hope PL, et al: Noninvasive investigation of cerebral ischemia by phosphorus nuclear magnetic resonance. *Pediatrics* 70:310–313, 1982.
12. Gadian DG: *Nuclear Magnetic Resonance and Its Applications to Living Systems.* New York, Oxford University Press, 1982.
13. Germano IM, Pitts LH, Berry I, et al: High energy phosphate metabolism in experimental permanent focal cerebral ischemia: An in vivo ^{31}P magnetic resonance spectroscopy study. *J Cereb Blood Flow Metab* 8:24–31, 1988.
14. Gonzalez-Mendez R, Litt L, Koretsky AP, et al: Comparison of ^{31}P NMR spectra of in vivo rat brain using convolution difference and saturation with a surface coil: Source of the broad component in the brain spectrum. *J Magn Reson* 57:526–533, 1984.
15. Gonzalez-Mendez R, McNeill A, Gregory GA, et al: Effects of hypoxic hypoxia on cerebral phosphate metabolites and pH in the anesthetized infant rabbit. *J Cereb Blood Flow Metab* 5:512–516, 1985.
16. Gupta RK, Gupta P, Moore RD: NMR studies of intracellular metal ions in intact cells and tissues. *Annu Rev Biophys Bioeng* 13:221–246, 1984.
17. Gyulai L, Schnall M, McLaughlin AC, et al: Simultaneous ^{31}P-and ^{1}H-nuclear magnetic resonance studies of hypoxia and ischemia in the cat brain. *J Cereb Blood Flow Metab* 7:543–551, 1987.
18. Hetherington HP, Avison MJ, Shulman RG: ^{1}H homonuclear editing of rat brain using semiselective pulses. *Proc Natl Acad Sci USA* 82:3115–3118, 1985.
19. Hollander JA den, Luyten PR: Image-guided localized ^{1}H and ^{31}P NMR spectroscopy of humans. *Ann NY Acad Sci* 508:386–398, 1987.
20. Hope PL, Cady EB, Tofts PS, et al: Cerebral energy metabolism studied with phosphorus NMR spectroscopy in normal and birth-asphyxiated infants. *Lancet* 2:366–370, 1984.
21. James TL, Margulis AR (eds): *Biomedical Magnetic Resonance.* San Francisco, Radiology Research and Education Foundation, 1984.
22. Komatsumoto S, Nioka S, Greenberg JH, et al: Cerebral energy metabolism measured in vivo by ^{31}P NMR in middle cerebral artery occlusion in the cat—relation to severity of stroke. *J Cereb Blood Flow Metab* 7:557–562, 1987.
23. Levy RM, Berry I, Moseley ME, et al: Combined magnetic resonance imaging (MRI) and bihemispheric magnetic resonance spectroscopy (MRS) in acute experimental focal cerebral ischemia. *Acta Neuroradiol*, in press.
24. Ligeti L, Osbakken MD, Subramanian HV, et al: ^{31}P and ^{1}H NMR spectroscopy to study the effects of gallopamil on brain ischemia. *Magn Reson Med* 4:441–451, 1987.
25. Litt L, Gonzalez-Mendez R, Severinghaus JW, et al: Cerebral intracellular changes during supercarbia: An in vivo ^{31}P nuclear magnetic resonance study in rats. *J Cereb Blood Flow Metab* 5:537–544, 1985.
26. Moon RB, Richards JH: Determination of intra-

cellular pH by 31-P magnetic resonance. *J Biol Chem* 248:7276–7278, 1973.

27. Naruse S, Takada S, Koizuka I, et al: In vivo ^{31}P NMR studies of experimental cerebral infarction. *Jpn J Physiol* 33:19–28, 1983.

28. Petroff OAC, Prichard JW, Behar KL, et al: Cerebral intracellular pH by ^{31}P nuclear magnetic resonance spectroscopy. *Neurology* 35:781–788, 1985.

29. Prichard JW, Shulman RG: NMR spectroscopy of brain metabolism in vivo. *Annu Rev Neurosci* 8:61–85, 1986.

30. Richards TL, Keniry MA, Weinstein PR, et al: Measurement of lactate accumulation by in vivo proton NMR spectroscopy during global cerebral ischemia in rats. *Magn Reson Med* 5:353–357, 1987.

31. Rothman DL, Behar KL, Hetherington HP, et al: Homonuclear ^{1}H double-difference spectroscopy of the rat brain in vivo. *Proc Natl Acad Sci USA* 81:6330–6334, 1984.

32. Sauter A, Rudin M: Effects of calcium antagonists on high-energy phosphates in ischemic rat brain measured by ^{31}P NMR spectroscopy. *Magn Reson Med* 4:1–8, 1987.

33. Shirane R, Chang LH, Weinstein PR, et al: Sequential changes of brain metabolism during temporary global ischemia in the rat detected by simultaneous ^{1}H and ^{31}P MRS. In Suzuki J (ed): *Advances in Surgery for Cerebral Stroke.* Tokyo, Springer-Verlag, 1988, pp 633–638.

34. Thulborn KR, du Boulay GH, Duchen LW, et al: A ^{31}P nuclear magnetic resonance in vivo study of cerebral ischemia in the gerbil. *J Cereb Blood Flow Metab* 2:299–306, 1982.

35. Vink R, McIntosh TK, Demediuk P, et al: Decline in intracellular free $Mg2^+$ is associated with irreversible tissue injury after brain trauma. *J Biol Chem* 263:757–761, 1988.

36. Vink R, McIntosh TK, Faden AI: Nonedited ^{1}H NMR lactate/n-acetyl aspartate ratios and the in vivo determination of lactate concentration in brain. *Magn Reson Med* 7:95–99, 1988.

37. Welch KMA, Levine SR, Helpern JA, et al: A serial study of acute human stroke by ^{31}P NMR spectroscopy. *Neurology* 37(Suppl 1):249, 1987.

38. Williams SR, Gadian DG, Proctor E: A method for lactate detection in vivo by spectral editing without the need for double irradiation. *J Magn Reson* 66:562–567, 1986.

39. Younkin DP, Delivoria-Papadopoulos M, Leonard JC, et al: Unique aspects of human newborn cerebral metabolism evaluated with phosphorus nuclear magnetic resonance spectroscopy. *Ann Neurol* 16:581–586, 1984.

CHAPTER ELEVEN

Electrophysiologic Evaluation: Electroencephalography, Evoked Potentials, and Magnetoencephalography

Marc R. Nuwer, M.D., Ph.D.

In the past decade, the microcomputer revolution has altered the field of electroencephalography. The electroencephalogram (EEG) can now be quantitated, permitting numerical comparisons to normative data or to patients' previous baseline data. Evoked potential (EP) testing has become simpler, more automated, more readily available, and less expensive. New, extremely sensitive superconducting magnetic detectors have permitted dynamic measurements of the brain's magnetic fields. Especially for quantitative EEG and EPs, considerable basic and clinical scientific efforts have been made toward elucidating the physiology of cerebral ischemia. This review outlines the salient studies in these several expanding fields of electrophysiology.

Quantitative EEG and EP techniques have good sensitivity for identifying abnormalities in patients with cerebral vascular disease. In some studies, these modalities have detected abnormalities in most of the patients with transient ischemia attack (TIA) and almost all of the stroke patients evaluated. Rates of false-positive findings among age-matched subjects are low, usually less than 5%. The tests, however, do not distinguish between ischemia and other focal brain lesions, such as tumors. Whereas they lateralize the lesion in most cases, they may not provide exact localization; however, certain EEG or EP features can help distinguish deep from superficial lesions. Changes in the test results over time may reflect alterations in the patient's clinical state. These evaluations may even be used to monitor patients in the intensive care unit (ICU) or operating room. Computer-processed information can be presented in ways that are difficult or impossible to visualize in routine EEGs. Computers also are able to present more clearly some of the subtle features that are easily overlooked on routine EEGs.

Many quantitative techniques have been proposed for use in detecting and monitoring ischemia and similar cerebral vascular disorders, but there is no consensus about which particular technique is the most sensitive. Quantitative EEG evaluation is likely never to equal the exquisite localization achievable with magnetic resonance (MR) imaging or cerebral computerized tomography (CT), but EEG can provide information about physiology that is not readily available from such purely anatomic tests. Moreover, EEG and EP are usually less costly than those neuroimaging techniques, involve no use of radiation, cause no claustrophobia, and can be done using a portable unit or continuously in an ICU or operating room. EEG examination can also detect those physiologic abnormalities, such as epileptic spikes, that have no correlate in neuroimaging studies. Overall, modern quantitative EEG and EP tests provide information that is complementary to the findings provided by CT or MR imaging.

ELECTROENCEPHALOGRAPHY

Techniques

Traditional EEG relies on measurements of the momentary fluctuations in scalp electrical potentials. Ischemic abnormalities may be revealed because they cause EEG activity that is excessively slow and focal compared to the patient's own contralateral EEG and to values obtained in normal patients of the same age range. Reduced amplitude of normal background fast activity may also indicate an area of possible ischemia. Routine EEG analysis shows abnormalities in 40% to 70% of patients with stroke, although a careful, unblinded review may yield a higher rate of detected abnormality.

In contrast, quantitative EEG techniques assess the amount and distribution of various frequency components of the EEG, usually by means of Fourier transform analysis, to yield spectral or frequency analysis data. Results of these analyses, in turn, may be compared with age-matched normative data to more readily reveal abnormal activity than that found with routine EEG evaluation. Left–right asymmetries of frequency content can also be distinguished. Ratios computed among the various EEG frequency bands, such as delta plus theta divided by alpha plus beta, can detect subtle degrees of change. One technique, known as the *relative frequency content*, entails obtaining a ratio between each of the common frequency bands—delta, theta, alpha, and beta—using the sum of all four bands as the denominator of the ratio; in this technique, a band is usually referred to as a percentage of total, for example, "percent delta" or "relative delta." Other specific, quantitative EEG features considered to provide sensitive assessment of cerebral vascular status include the peak frequency in the alpha band and the decrease or blocking of alpha upon eye opening. Such techniques have been applied in basic research and in certain specific clinical uses, such as for cerebral vascular disease, epilepsy, and other neurologic disorders (13, 24, 30, 32, 34). They have also been used in studies of dementia, depression, dyslexia, and schizophrenia, but have not yet proved to have a definite clinical use.

Substantial technical problems exist in the field of quantitative EEG, however (31). Electrical artifacts from heart, muscle, head movement, eye movement, blinks, and myriad other sources occur at the scalp. All of these artifacts are picked up by the EEG equipment, and only with great difficulty can they be distinguished from electrical potentials of cerebral origin—such a distinction generally must be made by a trained electroencephalographer. As yet, there is no standardization for specific recording techniques, such as filter settings, or for frequency divisions between the named frequency bands that are commonly used. The particular algorithms used in the computing functions are not standardized either, which may cause considerable confusion in trying to compare separate studies. Quantitative signal processing can also produce very large numbers of statistical tests on data, leading to confusion regarding interpretation of apparently, but not truly, statistically significant results when thousands of such statistical tests have been performed. Because of these technical and other related problems, the American Electroencephalographic Society (2) has urged caution in this field. The society recommends that quantitative EEG testing be regarded as an adjunct to traditional EEG recording, when done for clinical purposes. Among a variety of further precautions and recommendations, it is particularly important to note that recordings should be read by an electroencephalographer who is trained in both traditional EEG methods and the new quantitative methods.

Sensitivity and Specificity

Several investigators have reported data on the sensitivity and specificity of quantitative EEG in patients with cerebral vascular disease. The multiparametric asymmetry score used by Köpruner and Pfurtscheller (22) is a single scalar value based on a weighted combination of asymmetries in theta/beta ratio, central mu peak frequency, relative delta power, relative theta power, and alpha blocking. Those investigators tested their method on 32 patients and 50 normal subjects. The score correctly classified patients with cerebral vascular disease versus normal subjects in 93% of the study group. There were a few inaccurate scores, mainly in patients with

TIAs; otherwise, this EEG technique discriminated very well between normal subjects and patients with various degrees of cerebral vascular disease, including TIA, mild stroke, and severe stroke. These sensitivity and specificity rates may be higher than would be seen in routine practice because the subjects used to derive the score initially were the same as those used for testing the power of the score.

Comparison to standard age-matched normative data was used by Jonkman et al (20) to classify 64 normal control subjects and 94 patients. The patient group included 54 patients with completed or partial, nonprogressive stroke and 40 patients with TIA or reversible ischemic neurologic deficit. Neurometrics classification was used, a technique based on statistical testing of 168 specific EEG features (19). The quantitative EEG was considered abnormal in 90% of the patients and 3% of the normal control population. Significant overall asymmetry was found in 82% of patients but only 2% of controls on quantitative EEG. In contrast, 60% of all patients showed abnormalities on routine EEG traces assessed with traditional visual assessment techniques. Routine visual EEG assessment suggested abnormalities not seen by the quantitative testing in only 2% of patients. By comparison, the Neurometrics method revealed abnormalities in 84% of the patients whose routine EEG was normal according to routine visual assessment. Although excellent sensitivity and specificity were achieved in this study, the quantitative techniques used are complex and must be interpreted cautiously. Overall, the findings clearly indicate the advantages achieved by complex electrophysiologic methods in a population of patients with cerebral vascular disease.

Sainio et al (37) used a set of 24 quantitative EEG parameters to study 15 stroke patients; these included several ratios of various frequency bands, the absolute and relative powers in six frequency bands, and the mean frequencies of the alpha band and of the whole spectrum. The quantitative EEG tests correctly predicted the lateralization of the lesion in 87% of the patients, whereas routine EEG assessment was able to lateralize the lesion in

only 54% of the records. Normal control subjects were not included in this study.

Twenty patients with TIAs or mild stroke were studied by Van Huffelen et al (40). All 20 patients had normal EEGs according to routine visual assessment. Quantitative EEG techniques distinguished these patients from 50 normal control subjects with an 80% specificity and 70% test sensitivity. The most accurate quantitative EEG parameters in this study were: (a) the alpha peak frequency asymmetry with the subject's eyes closed; (b) the alpha peak frequency asymmetry change when the eyes were subsequently open; (c) mu asymmetry with the eyes open; (d) asymmetry of alpha with the eyes closed; and (e) alpha blocking. Overall, this study shows how quantitative EEG testing can discriminate relatively mild degrees of cerebral vascular disease, even in patients with EEGs that appear normal on routine testing.

We have assessed simple quantitative EEG testing in 20 patients who had mild stroke (33). Asymmetries of absolute power in the four EEG frequency bands traditionally used were assessed after determining normal asymmetry limits in 20 age-matched control subjects. Abnormally large asymmetric increases in delta and decreases in alpha activity were seen in 85% of the stroke patients and in none of the normal subjects. The scalp area localized by this technique in each case correlated with the patients' signs, symptoms, and neuroimaging studies. Routine EEG showed abnormalities in only six of the 20 patients and was less accurate in predicting the location or lateralization of the lesion. CT or MR imaging showed abnormalities in only nine of 19 patients.

Two situations accounted for the discrepancy between normal findings on CT or MR imaging and abnormal findings on quantitative EEG testing. First, in some cases CT was performed within the first 2 to 3 days after the acute onset of stroke. The EEG changes, of course, occur immediately at the onset of the acute event rather than after several days' delay (Fig. 11.1). Second, in some patients the symptoms were quite mild and waxed and waned over time, suggesting a marginal degree of ischemia insufficient to cause frank in-

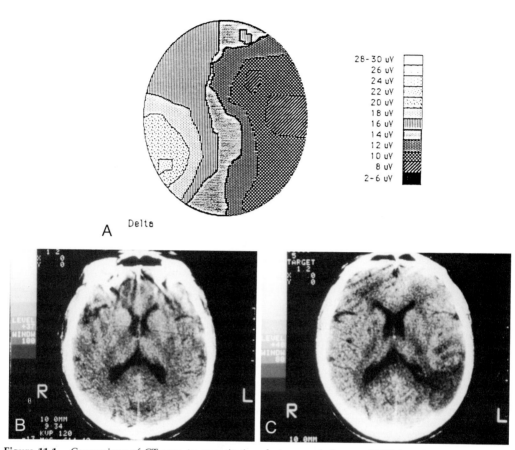

Figure 11.1. Comparison of CT scan to quantitative electroencephalogram (EEG) in a 57-year-old patient who had the sudden onset of fluent aphasia from an errant balloon while undergoing angioplasty. The EEG was being monitored during the procedure, using real-time frequency analysis and topographic mapping. *A*, the embolic ischemic change was seen immediately on EEG and indicated the anatomic localization of the errant balloon (μV = microvolts). *B*, a CT scan made later that day showed no abnormalities. *C*, a follow-up CT scan made several days later showed a wedge-shaped infarction in a location very similar to that already indicated by the changes on the quantitative EEG recording. Note that CT uses a left–right convention opposite that of EEG topographic maps. (Case and pictures courtesy of S. Jordan, M.D.)

farction. These patients showed EEG changes reflecting abnormal physiology but their neuroimaging studies revealed no signs of infarction.

Overall, these several studies suggest that quantitative EEG may provide information that is different from the information available in routine neuroimaging studies and from that available by routine EEG alone. Reasonably good sensitivity and specificity rates were achieved by these different investigators using widely differing techniques.

Comparison of Types of Quantitative Electroencephalography Tests

Hundreds of EEG parameters are available and have been studied in settings relevant to cerebral vascular disease. Investigators in this field have differed quite widely in their choices of parameters to be examined. Various ratios, absolute and relative amplitudes within set frequency bands, changes with eye opening or hand movement, peak frequencies, and mean frequencies have all been shown to change with ischemia. Review of the literature in the field gives a distinct impression that there is no clear consensus about the most accurate variables for use in assessing ischemia, but overall, across the various studies, the alpha frequency band seems to afford the best discrimination, followed by the delta frequency band activity. However, the optimal variables for detecting and localizing ischemia may vary depending on the nature of the ischemia, including its severity, location, and acuteness.

Comparison of Quantitative Electroencephalography to Other Types of Tests

The utility of quantitative EEG tests in evaluating stroke has been compared to that of other types of medical tests, including CT, MR imaging, regional cerebral blood flow (rCBF) studies, and positron emission tomography (PET) of regional cerebral glucose metabolism and regional oxygen utilization. In patients with cerebral vascular disease, quantitative EEG measurements correlate quite well with rCBF. Correlations reported are highest for percent delta power ($r = -0.76$), percent alpha power ($r = 0.76$), and mean frequency ($r = 0.67$) compared to mean rCBF (27, 39). Correlation of EEGs measured with these frequencies for mean rCBF was better than for peak flow rCBF. The correlation of mean rCBF for theta activity was much poorer, probably because theta may change in parallel with either increasing delta or decreasing alpha power. Buchsbaum et al (9) reported that quantitative EEG testing correlates well with mean rCBF and the regional metabolic rate for gray matter, but not for white matter, as measured by PET. Mean EEG frequency in the posterior scalp regions showed the best correlation (18).

Rosén et al (36) studied postischemic impairment in a rat model following a variety of changes in quantitative EEG, somatosensory evoked potential (SSEP), and measurements of brain energy metabolism. In that study, the quantitative neurophysiologic recovery in the postischemic period provided more detailed prognostic information than did brain energy metabolism for indicating the extent of brain cell damage and death.

To date, most studies comparing quantitative EEG with neuroimaging devices have focused on CT rather than MR imaging. A normal CT scan or MR image was found in nine of 19 patients with mild stroke whom we studied (33), including eight of 16 patients (50%) in whom the quantitative EEG test showed focal electrical abnormalities. These normal CT scans occurred in several clinical settings, including marginal ischemia with fluctuating symptoms and in CT testing within 2 to 3 days of the onset of symptoms. Van Huffelen et al (40), using a set of five quantitative EEG variables, were able to detect an abnormality in 72% of patients with transient ischemia whereas the CT scan showed the abnormality in only 10% of these patients. The anecdotal reports now available, however, do not indicate sufficiently what the relative sensitivities will be when comparing the MR image with the quantitative EEG examination. It is, of course, likely that detection rates will be higher with MR imaging than with other modalities in patients with mild or transient ischemia, thereby narrowing the discrepancies between neuroimaging and quantitative EEG testing. However, there remain the problematic cases in which ischemia is sufficient to cause dysfunction but insufficient to cause frank anatomic changes, such as edema or infarction. In such cases of mild ischemia, the physiologic tests may well outperform tests of anatomy.

Other Clinical Observations

Quantitative EEG tests appear to be a good means for detecting an ischemia-related abnormality and a moderately good technique for assessing its lateralization, but they are less accurate in determining the exact location of a lesion within the affected hemisphere. Although Jonkman et al (20) were able to obtain a very high rate of detection with EEG testing, they were able to indicate the side of the lesion in only 53% of their patients who had completed stroke or partial nonprogressive stroke. One difficulty was that the abnormalities were often found by using asymmetry parameters, which by definition do not test the two hemispheres separately. Another difficulty was caused by EEG diaschisis, in which physiologic changes occur in the contralateral nonischemic hemisphere. Other studies of quantitative EEG in stroke patients have also emphasized the use of asymmetry as a criterion for determining abnormality (33). Abnormalities often were detected because of localized increases in delta band activity or decreases in alpha band activity. Unfortunately, in severe ischemia the delta activity may actually be decreased locally. Alpha activity can also be increased at the site of a lesion, particularly when pseudoperiodic lateralized epileptiform discharges or other transients occur at or near the ischemic lesion.

A comparison of various cerebral abnormalities was undertaken by Mies et al (26), including studies of patients with ischemic stroke, hemorrhagic stroke, head trauma, and intracranial tumors. Asymmetry criteria were based on relative power and on frequency band ratios. These investigators were unable to differentiate the type of pathology by looking at the types of changes in the quantitative EEG tests. Such findings suggest that these EEG tests may be more useful for detecting an abnormality than for categorizing the type of pathology.

Specific subcategories of cerebral vascular disease, especially TIAs, were discriminated by quantitative EEG in several studies. Nagata et al (28) studied 25 patients with TIAs, looking for asymmetry in EEG activity within the major frequency bands. Appropriately located unilateral abnormalities were seen in 68% of the TIA patients, even long after the symptoms had completely resolved. Among those patients who were examined within 2 weeks of the most recent onset of symptoms, 88% showed corresponding abnormalities documented by quantitative EEG. Kőpruner and Pfurtscheller (22), using their multiparametric asymmetry score, studied eight

patients who had TIA. Although that score differentiated normal control subjects from patients with unequivocal stroke, it did not reveal any abnormality in some TIA patients.

Pfurtscheller et al (35) were able to distinguish superficial from deep lesions in many patients, primarily by evaluating the mu rhythm. Its desynchronization upon brief hand movements and increase in the mu amplitude predicted in 87% of cases that a lesion on that side was located deep in the brain. In contrast, mu amplitude and asymmetrical desynchronization predicted in 81% of cases that the lesion was superficial.

Intraoperative monitoring during carotid endarterectomy was done by Ahn et al (1) using 28-channel color-coded topographic maps of EEG amplitude spectra. The frequency analysis maps showed changes more often than did the simultaneously recorded routine EEG. The use of on-line frequency analysis was considered to improve communication to the surgical team, affording quick localization of changes and quantitative assessment of the degree of changes over time. Further studies may be warranted to assess whether this extra degree of sensitivity is of practical value during intraoperative monitoring.

ICU monitoring may also be carried out with quantitative EEG (3). Techniques used in the past for this purpose have included the compressed spectral array, which prints frequency analysis data without the use of topographic maps. Equipment is now sufficiently evolved, however, to permit topographic mapping in multiple frequency bands on line. Such techniques may facilitate communication of EEG features to nonspecialists, such as ICU nurses and general medical or surgical physicians. In the ICU and the operating room, artifacts are still a substantial technical problem. No organized studies have yet assessed the effectiveness of quantitative EEG, compared to other monitoring methods, in the ICU.

Traditional EEG has proved of value in intraoperative monitoring, especially during carotid endarterectomy. Minor EEG changes during the operation consist of a 25% to 50% reduction in fast-frequency EEG components together with an increase in amplitude and a decrease in the main frequency of slower EEG components. As blood flow is more severely reduced, to within the range of 16 ml/100 g/minute or less, EEG changes are more pronounced, showing an even greater reduction in fast EEG components and a decrease in amplitude of the slower components; the overall EEG amplitude decreases, leaving a relatively featureless EEG on the side the clamp is placed. Although as many as 25% of EEGs may show some changes, only about 1% to 3% of EEGs show the latter, severe, degree of change.

EEG complements other forms of monitoring during endarterectomy. Measurement of the back pressure in the distal stump of the carotid artery or the intracarotid xenon-133 (^{133}Xe) injection technique for measuring CBF are techniques that are usually employed only intermittently. The ^{133}Xe injection technique requires injection of the radionuclide into the internal carotid while the external carotid artery is clamped. Low blood flow, as measured by the ^{133}Xe injection technique, is always accompanied by EEG changes, but with measurement of the back pressure in the distal carotid stump an unexpected persistent EEG change associated with a normal blood flow or a normal stump pressure is usually caused by an embolus. EEG monitoring during endarterectomy has been encouraged by those specialists who point out that it may allow selective shunting, identify poorly functioning shunts, and permit assessment of the effects of a changing clinical status resulting from hypotension or other factors complicating the operation. By identifying the intraoperative time at which an irreversible complication has occurred, monitoring can also enable a surgeon to alter his or her technique in treating future patients. In identifying potentially reversible complications, intraoperative monitoring can help prevent some postoperative neurologic sequelae. The role of SSEPs in intraoperative monitoring is reviewed in the following section (*see also* Chapter 12, this volume).

SOMATOSENSORY EVOKED POTENTIALS

Methods and Nomenclature

SSEPs are measurements of the electrical potentials, or the voltage, evoked by the application of brief electrical stimuli to peripheral nerves, as recorded from electrodes placed on the shoulder, back, neck, and scalp (Fig. 11.2). The SSEPs reflect conduction within large fiber pathways continuing rostrally in the posterior column, medial lemniscus, internal capsule, and primary somatosensory cortex. The stimulus is usually delivered to the median nerve at the wrist. The resulting cortical potentials arise from the hand region of postcentral cortex, along with components from thalamocortical radiations and some other adjacent cortical structures. Measurements made during several hundred to several thousand individual applications of the stimulus, or trials, must be averaged to distinguish the EP activity from the ongoing EEG and from contaminating artifacts, such as muscle activity; the averaging process requires from 1 to several minutes. Equipment and technologists for EP testing are now available in most modern hospitals. Clinical applications include helping confirm a diagnosis when signs and symptoms are equivocal, identifying subclinical lesions in patients at risk for conditions such as multiple sclerosis, classifying the pathology according to the types of EP abnormality found, and monitoring neural pathways for changes over time.

The earliest peak recorded in a typical SSEP is the N9 or Erb's point peak, recorded from the proximal anterior shoulder. This is generated by a portion of the brachial plexus. The subsequent peaks N11 and N13 are recorded from the skin over the seventh spinous process. These are generated by the cervical spinal cord. Several other peaks are seen as the axon volleys ascend the neuraxis, culminating with the major negative peak N20. The latter is recorded best over the central scalp region contralateral to the wrist that was stimulated (Fig. 11.2). The N20 is followed by a

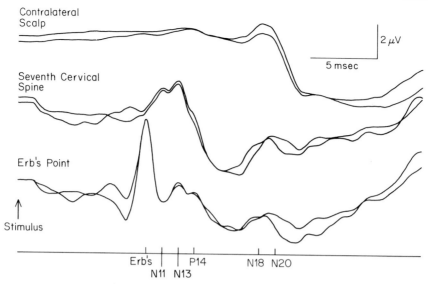

Figure 11.2. Typical median nerve SSEP's recorded from the shoulder (Erb's point), the neck over the seventh cervical spinous process, and the contralateral central scalp. Electrical stimulation of the median nerve occurred at the beginning of the traces. A series of peaks are identified and labeled with their common names. (From Nuwer MR: *Evoked Potential Monitoring in the Operating Room.* New York, Raven Press, 1986.)

positive electrical polarity peak in the same scalp region, the P22.

The early peaks are often referred to as the *subcortical* peaks, including Erb's peak and the N11–N13–P14 peaks. The later peaks N20 and P22 are referred to as the *cortical* peaks. The sources, or *generators,* of various somatosensory peaks have been studied but there is still some debate regarding the exact site of origin of some peaks. In the study of ischemia, the principal somatosensory peaks of interest are those from thalamocortical generators rather than from more rostral sources. The N18 peak may be generated from a source as deep as the thalamus. The N20 peak may be generated at the primary somatosensory cortex tucked into the central fissure. A succeeding P22–P25 peak or complex of peaks seems to arise from somatosensory cortex and adjacent structures.

Ischemia of the hemispheres can substantially attenuate or abolish the thalamocortical peaks without attenuating the peaks from more caudal structures. Ischemia of the hemisphere or brain stem may also prolong the conduction time between the N18 or N20 peak and the preceding N13 peak generated around the cuneate nucleus at the level of the foramen mag-

num. This latter interpeak conduction time has been referred to as the central conduction time (CCT).

Models of Cerebral Ischemia

SSEPs have been studied in several animal models of systemic ischemia or specific cerebral ischemia. Hargadine et al (17) produced ischemia by transorbital occlusion of the right middle cerebral artery (MCA) in nine baboons. The rCBF was recorded in both hemispheres using hydrogen clearance technique. The median nerve SSEP CCT was unaltered with flows above 15 ml/100 g/minute. Below that level, reductions in rCBF correlated well with progressively larger CCT changes. At a flow below 8 ml/100 g/minute the cortical SSEPs were lost. These results agree with earlier CCT studies by Branston et al (5), who found that there was a narrow range of cortical flow, from about 12 to 18 ml/100 g/minute, over which cortical SSEP peaks are reduced from normal amplitude to absent.

Global ischemia causes changes in cortical SSEPs more quickly than does specific occlusion of the MCA. Lesnick et al (23) produced global ischemia by the graded induction of systemic hemorrhagic hypotension following bilateral carotid artery ligation in cats. Reductions in the amplitude of the cortical SSEP began as CBF dropped below 45% of its control value, that is, below about 18 ml/100 g/minute for white matter and about 25 ml/100 g/minute for cortex. There was also an early CCT delay that correlated well with mild white matter ischemia. This study, too, showed that the cortical EP was abolished when rCBF fell to even lower levels. Brain stem ischemia might be the reason that changes in SSEP caused by systemic hypotension occur at blood flow values slightly higher than those associated with unilateral MCA occlusion.

A study by Meyer et al (25) indicated that unfavorable intraoperative EP changes correlate with unfavorable postoperative outcomes. After occluding the right MCA in 17 cats, these investigators observed a significant slowing of the cortical positive peak ipsilaterally. Maximal slowing of the positive peak was seen in the cats sustaining an infarction extending into the thalamus. Greater slowing of the first negative peak corresponded to more severe infarction of midsuprasylvian and posterior ectosylvian gyri, including the somatosensory cortex. They concluded that the SSEP central latencies and cortical amplitudes are sensitive tools not only for indicating onset of ischemia, but also for measurement of the extent of a cerebral ischemia insult.

Subcortical SSEP generators may be much more resistant to effects of ischemia than cortical SSEP generators are, as suggested by the findings of Kobrine et al (21) in five monkeys monitored through hydrogen clearance technique while systemic arterial pressure was progressively lowered. Both the cervical and the cortical SSEP peaks began to decrease in amplitude when mean arterial blood pressure (MABP) was lowered to 50 mm Hg. At half that MABP, the spinal cord blood flow became immeasurably low or absent but the spinal SSEPs disappeared only after 8 to 18 minutes of no spinal cord blood flow. In contrast, cortical SSEPs had always disappeared by the time the cortical blood flow reached 15 ml/100 g/minute or less. Indeed in one animal who died during monitoring, the cortical SSEP disappeared immediately, whereas the cervical SSEP did not disappear until an additional 6 minutes had elapsed.

Direct comparisons of animal models during systemic hypotension and hypoxia showed that SSEP changes are better than EEG changes at predicting subsequent brain tissue damage (6, 12). This difference in predictive value is probably accounted for by the greater resistance of SSEPs to ischemia change: SSEP changes occur at blood flow levels about 20% lower than the blood flow levels evoking EEG changes; therefore, the level at which SSEP change occurs lies closer to the critical point at which irreversible damage to the central nervous system (CNS) develops.

Overall, ischemia causes a loss of cortical SSEPs when cortical blood flow falls below approximately 15 ml/100 g/minute, a rate that is near but not quite at critical levels for hypoxic damage. Subcortical and cervical SSEP recordings are more resistant to ischemia and may continue to show some measurable activity even after blood flow to their generators has completely stopped for several minutes. Cortical peak latency delays often occur together with a loss in the SSEP peak amplitude during ischemia. The more severe the change in the SSEP, the more severe is the postoperative deficit. These findings seem to be consistent independent of the particular model of ischemia tested. Many investigators agree that cortical SSEPs are relatively safe, sensitive, reproducible tools for detecting systemic or carotid distribution, hypotension, and probably also hypoxia. The EPs change at just about the point in time when moderately severe nervous system ischemia is occurring but before the impairment has crossed the critical threshold for permanent damage to the CNS. (29).

Carotid Endarterectomy

SSEPs provide an alternative to EEG in monitoring the patient during carotid endarterectomy procedures. Cortical SSEP peaks become progressively smaller as hemispheric blood flow decreases below 18 ml/100 g/minute and disappear at about 15 ml/100 g/minute. In studies of SSEP during clinical endarterectomy, various investigators have noted the frequent occurrence of mild to moderate SSEP peak attenuations upon clamping of the carotid artery. Ipsilateral peaks showed attenuations of up to 50% and remained stable during the clamping interval. Contralateral changes have also been reported. Delays in latency may accompany the amplitude attenuation. Exact criteria for critical SSEP change have not been set. Loss of EPs for as short a period as 8 minutes has been associated with postoperative stroke. Even the return of SSEPs after the release of clamping is not a guarantee that the patient will awaken free of new neurologic deficits, especially if the SSEPs upon returning show a lack of late components, a reduction in peak amplitude, or an increase in CCT.

SSEP changes can alert the surgical team to significant ischemia even in circumstances when ischemia is unanticipated. Among 40 patients monitored by Gigli et al (15) during carotid endarterectomy, 30 had no SSEP changes and none of those 30 patients had postoperative neurologic sequelae. Loss of SSEP cortical amplitude or prolongation of the CCT was seen in the other 10 cases: No neurologic sequelae occurred in the five patients in whom the SSEP changes were transient; the five with persistent SSEP changes all had new neurologic deficits postoperatively. In several of these patients, carotid back pressure exceeded 50 mm Hg, suggesting that there was adequate collateral circulation, whereas SSEP monitoring revealed ischemia-related impairment of cortical function and correctly predicted postoperative impairment. The surgical team responded to these SSEP changes (Fig. 11.3), preventing permanent deficits in all but one case.

Postoperative neuropsychologic deficits have been correlated with intraoperative SSEP changes. Patients whose cortical amplitudes decreased by more than 50% performed significantly more poorly on postoperative neuropsychologic testing than those patients who had either lesser degrees of or no EP attenuation (7, 11). Such

neuropsychologic deterioration was unrelated to other factors, including age, education, or presence of a stroke preoperatively.

Overall, median nerve SSEPs appear to be a safe and effective tool for monitoring the intraoperative status of several portions of the nervous system (29). The EP changes occur in parallel with rCBF decreases. When blood flow falls to a nearly critical level, the EPs change. If blood flow impairment reaches or exceeds a critical level, the EPs disappear. Substantial attenuation of the EPs correlates with neuropsychologic impairment, even in patients who have not suffered a more classic intraoperative stroke.

Coma

In cases of coma or brain death, SSEPs can be helpful in establishing the patient's prognosis. The EPs are relatively unchanged by sedative drugs such as pentobarbital and by the relative hypothermia often found in ICU patients. Most studies in this area have been in series of patients who have suffered cardiac arrest or head trauma. Among patients who meet criteria for brain death, SSEPs usually showed relatively normal peripheral and cervical peaks but no thalamocortical activity whatever. Such a change corresponds to cessation of conduction at a low brain stem level and also provides reassurance that the stimulus was technically applied correctly. The absence of the thalamocortical peaks after a cardiac arrest is considered to be a grave prognostic sign with no likelihood of meaningful recovery.

SSEP tests are not medically necessary in simple cases of coma from hypoxia, but because the EPs are relatively unaffected by drugs they may be of great value in helping to distinguish drug effects from true CNS damage. It has been estimated that the rates of prognostic error, whether falsely optimistic or falsely pessimistic, could be cut in half through the judicious use of SSEPs concomitantly with other prognostic indicators—intracranial pressure monitoring, CT scans, and clinical data including age, Glasgow Coma Scale,

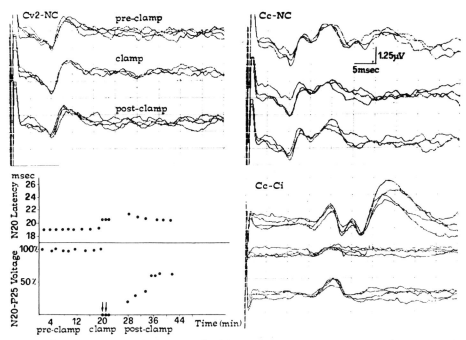

Figure 11.3. Somatosensory evoked potentials (SSEPs) during a carotid endarterectomy in a 71-year-old male patient. The N20–P25 complex and the following cortical waves entirely disappeared after a brief interval when the carotid artery was clamped, although a 90-mm Hg stump pressure was found. For this reason, the carotid artery was unclamped immediately and the procedure interrupted. Despite this action and barbiturate administration, the SSEPs did not return to baseline values. Ten minutes after the carotid artery was reopened, a delayed and prolonged N20 of depressed amplitude reappeared. Postoperative neurologic examination displayed a moderate right-sided hemiparesis and a mixed aphasia. Neurologic deficits gradually and almost completely recovered, but 3 days later the patient died from intercurrent complications. Cv2 = skin over the second cervical vertebra; Cc = contralateral central region scalp; Ci = ipsilateral central region scalp; Cv2-NC = recording made over Cv2, with a noncephalic (NC) reference; Cc-NC = recording made over the scalp contralateral to the wrist stimulated, with a noncephalic (NC) reference; Cc-Ci = recording made over the contralateral scalp, with an ipsilateral scalp reference; μV = microvolt. (From Gigli GL, Caramia M, Marciani MG, et al: Monitoring of subcortical and cortical SSEPs during carotid endarterectomy: Comparison with stump pressure levels. *Electroencephalogr Clin Neurophysiol* 68:424–432, 1987.)

and physical findings such as posturing and eye movements (8, 14, 16). The clinical setting in which SSEP testing seems most often to be worthwhile involves cases that are complex, are open to dispute, or involve organ transplantation, children under 3 years of age, or patients in whom the usual examinations are difficult to perform or interpret. The utility of SSEPs in these and other clinical settings has been discussed by Chiappa (10).

The comparison between clinical monitoring of ischemic patients with traditional EEG tests and with SSEPs also requires further study. From blood flow studies of the two techniques done separately, it appears that the SSEP becomes abnormal and attenuated and disappears at slightly lower blood flow rates than does the EEG. This lower flow rate for SSEP changes may be closer to the critical flow rate at which permanent damage will occur if flow is not soon improved.

MAGNETOENCEPHALOGRAPHY

Measurements of the brain's ongoing electromagnetic signals provide a potential methodologic alternative to measurements of the brain's electrical activity (4, 38). The magnetic fields of the brain are much smaller than the electrical fields and their measurement is much more difficult. The past 20 years have seen substantial improvements in the technology of electromagnetic measurement and an evolution in the concepts regarding the meaning of these magnetic signals.

Tools for magnetic measurement now involve Josephson junction devices, miniscule cousins of integrated circuit technology that employ principles of quantum mechanics. Because superconductivity is essential to the proper functioning of these devices, the measuring device must be kept in a thermal flask surrounded by liquid helium at near absolute zero temperatures (Fig. 11.4). The device is often referred to as a SQUID, or superconducting quantum interference device. Several separate recording devices can be packaged into this same thermal flask, allowing convenient multichannel recordings. Other magnetic fields in the environment are partially cancelled out by differential recording techniques, and especially by shielding using mu-metal, a special substance that is a particularly strong barrier to magnetic fields. The magnetic fields measured by these magenetoencephalography (MEG) techniques are 15 orders of magnitude less powerful than the fields used for MR imagers.

MEG recordings differ from EEG recordings in several important ways. Whereas MEG is particularly sensitive to intracellular electrical currents, the EEG is sensitive to extracellular currents. MEG is also particularly sensitive in recording currents tangential to the scalp. whereas the special sensitivity of routine EEG is in recording potentials whose dipole lies perpendicular to the scalp. It should be noted that the skull is transparent to magnetic fields whereas electrically it offers substantial resistance; the smearing effect of an interposed high-resistance structure is avoided with MEG.

Although little is known about the effects of ischemia on the brain's electromagnetic activity, there are several theoretical reasons to believe that MEG may not be the best technique to elucidate the effects of ischemia. Ischemia often pro-

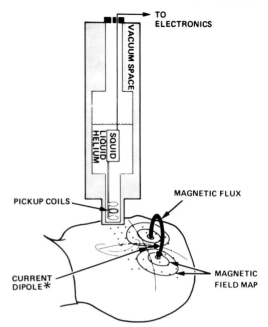

Figure 11.4. Magnetoencephalography generation and measurement with a single channel sensor. Distribution of magnetic field from the simplified model of a single equivalent current dipole* tangential to the scalp with intracellular current flowing toward the top of the head. A current dipole creates a scalp pattern with exiting and entering magnetic field "maxima," as shown. The underlying cortical source is modeled as an equivalent current dipole. The sensor is sequentially placed over each point in a rectangular matrix encompassing the field pattern and the perpendicular component of magnetic flux is measured. From these measurements, averaged traces and isocontour maps are constructed to image the instantaneous magnetic field for equivalent source localization. (From Barth DS, Sutherling W, Engel J, et al: Neuromagnetic localization of single and multiple sources underlying epileptiform spikes in the human brain. *Adv Epileptology* 15:379–384, 1984.)

duces dysfunction over broad regions of the CNS, resulting in broad magnetic fields from the impaired tissue which are much more difficult to interpret than are the localized electrical fields of dipoles. Moreover, ischemia produces slowly progressive changes, whereas MEG is more suited to the study of repeated, brief, transient activity or regular rhythmical activity. Overall, MEG provides a recording method that differs from and complements traditional EEG, but innovative use of the technique or new approaches to the application of this technology may be necessary before any substantial, new information about ischemia can be found using these elegant, new, sensitive magnetic recording devices.

References

1. Ahn SS, Jordan SE, Nuwer MR: Computerized EEG topographic brain mapping. In Moore W (ed): *Surgery for Cerebrovascular Disease.* New York, Churchill Livingstone, 1987, pp 275–280.

2. American Electroencephalographic Society: Statement on the clinical use of quantitative EEG. *J Clin Neurophysiol* 4:197, 1987.

3. Archibald JE, Drazkowski JF: Clinical applications of compressed spectral analysis (CSA) in OR/ICU settings. *Am J EEG Technol* 25:13–36, 1985.

4. Barth DS, Sutherling W, Engel J, et al: Neuromagnetic localization of single and multiple sources underlying epileptiform spikes in the human brain. *Adv Epileptology* 15:379–384, 1984.

5. Branston NM, Symon L, Crockard HA, et al: Relationships between the cortical evoked potential and local cortical blood flow following acute middle cerebral artery occlusion in the baboon. *Exp Neurol* 45:195–208, 1974.

6. Brierley JB, Brown AW, Excell BJ, et al: Brain damage in the rhesus monkey resulting from profound arterial hypotension. I. Its nature, distribution and general physiological correlates. *Brain Res* 13:68–100, 1969.

7. Brinkman SD, Braun P, Ganji S, et al: Neuropsychological performance one week after carotid endarterectomy reflects intraoperative ischemia. *Stroke* 15:497–503, 1984.

8. Brunko E, Zegers de Beyl D: Prognostic value of early cortical somatosensory evoked potentials after resuscitation from cardiac arrest. *Electroencephalogr Clin Neurophysiol* 66:15–24, 1987.

9. Buchsbaum MS, Kessler R, King A, et al: Simultaneous cerebral glucography with positron emission tomography and topographic electroencephalography. In Pfurtscheller G, Jonkman EJ, Lopes da Silva FM (eds): *Brain Ischemia: Quantitative EEG and Imaging Techniques.* Vol. 62 (Prog Brain Res). Amsterdam, Elsevier, 1984, pp 263–269.

10. Chiappa KH: *Evoked Potentials in Clinical Medicine.* New York, Raven Press, 1983.

11. Cushman L, Brinkman SD, Ganji S, et al: Neuropsychological impairment after carotid endarterectomy correlates with intraoperative ischemia. *Cortex* 20:403–412, 1984.

12. Dong WK, Bledsoe SW, Chadwick HS, et al: Electrical correlates of brain injury resulting from severe hypotension and hemodilution in monkeys. *Anesthesiology* 65:617–625, 1986.

13. Duffy FH (ed): *Topographic Mapping of Brain Electrical Activity.* Boston, Butterworths, 1986.

14. Frank LM, Furgiuele TL, Etheridge JE Jr: Prediction of chronic vegetative state in children using evoked potentials. *Neurology* 35:931–934, 1985.

15. Gigli GL, Caramia M, Marciani MG, et al: Monitoring of subcortical and cortical somatosensory evoked potentials during cartoid endarterectomy: Comparison with stump pressure levels. *Electroencephalogr Clin Neurophysiol* 68:424–432, 1987.

16. Greenberg RP, Newlong PG, Hyatt MS, et al: Prognostic implications of early multimodality evoked potentials in severely head-injured patients. *J Neurosurg* 55:227–236, 1981.

17. Hargadine JR, Branston NM, Symon L: Central conduction time in primate brain ischemia—a study in baboons. *Stroke* 11:637–642, 1980.

18. Ingvar DH, Rosén I, Johannesson G: EEG related to cerebral metabolism and blood flow. *Pharmakopsychiatr Neuropsychopharmakol* 12:200–209, 1979.

19. John ER, Prichep L, Easton P: Normative data banks and neurometrics. Basic concepts, methods and results of norm constructions. In Gevins AS, Rémond A (eds): *Handbook of Electroencephalography and Clinical Neurophysiology. Revised Series, Vol. 1. Methods of Analysis of Brain Electrical and Magnetic Signals.* Amsterdam, Elsevier, 1987, pp 449–495.

20. Jonkman EJ, Poortvliet DCJ, Veering MM, et al: The use of neurometrics in the study of patients with cerebral ischemia. *Electroencephalogr Clin Neurophysiol* 61:333–341, 1985.

21. Kobrine AI, Evans DE, Rizzoli HV: Relative vulnerability of the brain and spinal cord to ischemia. *J Neurol Sci* 45:65–72, 1980.

22. Köpruner V, Pfurtscheller G: Multiparametric asymmetry score (MAS)—distinction between normal and ischemic brains. *Electroencephalogr Clin Neurophysiol* 57:343–346, 1984.

23. Lesnick JE, Michele JJ, Simeone FA, et al: Alteration of somatosensory evoked potentials in response to global ischemia. *J Neurosurg* 60:490–494, 1984.

24. Lopes da Silva FH, van Leeuwen WS, Rémond A: *Handbook of Electroencephalography and Clinical Neurophysiology. Revised Series, Vol. 2. Clinical Applications of Computer Analysis of EEG and Other Neurophysiological Signals.* Amsterdam, Elsevier, 1986.

25. Meyer KL, Dempsey RJ, Roy MW, et al: Somatosensory evoked potentials as a measure of experimental cerebral ischemia. *J Neurosurg* 62:269–275, 1985.

26. Mies G, Hoppe G, Hossmann K-A: Limitations of EEG frequency analysis in the diagnosis of intracerebral diseases. In Pfurtscheller G, Jonkman EJ, Lopes da Silva FM (eds): *Brain Ischemia: Quantitative EEG and Imaging Techniques.* Vol. 62 (Prog Brain Res). Amsterdam, Elsevier, 1984, pp 85–103.

27. Nagata K, Tagawa K, Shishido F, et al: Topographic EEG correlates of cerebral blood flow and oxygen consumption in patients with neuropsychological disorders. In Duffy FH (ed): *Topographic Mapping of Brain Electrical Activity.* Boston, Butterworths, 1986, pp 357–370.

28. Nagata K, Yunoki K, Araki G, et al: Topographic electroencephalographic study of transient ischemic attacks. *Electroencephalogr Clin Neurophysiol* 58:291–301, 1984.

29. Nuwer MR: *Evoked Potential Monitoring in the Operating Room.* New York, Raven Press, 1986.
30. Nuwer MR: Recording electrode site nomenclature. *J Clin Neurophysiol* 4:121–133, 1987.
31. Nuwer MR: Quantitative EEG: I. Techniques and problems of frequency analysis and topographic mapping. *J Clin Neurophysiol* 5:1–43, 1988.
32. Nuwer MR: Quantitative EEG: II. Frequency analysis and topographic mapping in clinical settings. *J Clin Neurophysiol* 5:45–85, 1988.
33. Nuwer MR, Jordan SE, Ahn SS: Evaluation of stroke using EEG frequency analysis and topographic mapping. *Neurology* 37:1153–1159, 1987.
34. Pfurtscheller G, Jonkman EJ, Lopes da Silva FM (eds): *Brain Ischemia: Quantitative EEG and Imaging Techniques.* Vol. 62 (Prog Brain Res). Amsterdam, Elsevier, 1984.
35. Pfurtscheller G, Sager W, Wege W: Correlations between CT scan and sensorimotor EEG rhythms in patients with cerebrovascular disorders. *Electroencephalogr Clin Neurophysiol* 52:473–485, 1981.
36. Rosén I, Smith ML, Rehncrona S: Quantitative EEG and evoked potentials after experimental brain ischemia in the rat: Correlation with cerebral metabolism and blood flow. In Pfurtscheller G, Jonkman EJ, Lopes da Silva FM (eds): *Brain Ischemia: Quantitative EEG and Imaging Techniques.* Vol. 62 (Prog Brain Res). Amsterdam, Elsevier, 1984, pp 175–183.
37. Sainio K, Stenberg D, Keskimaki I, et al: Visual and spectral EEG analysis in the evaluation of the outcome in patients with ischemic brain infarction. *Electroencephalogr Clin Neurophysiol* 56:117–124, 1983.
38. Sutherling WW, Barth DS, Beatty J: Magnetic fields of epileptic spike foci: Equivalent localization and propagation. In Weinberg H, Stroink G, Katila T (eds): *Biomagnetism: Applications Theory.* New York, Pergamon Press, 1985, pp 249–260.
39. Tolonen U, Sulg IA: Comparison of quantitative EEG parameters from four different analysis techniques in evaluation of relationships between EEG and CBF in brain infarction. *Electroencephalogr Clin Neurophysiol* 64:274–277, 1986.
40. Van Huffelen AC, Poortvliet DCJ, van der Wulp CJM: Quantitative electroencephalography in cerebral ischemia: Detection of abnormalities in "normal" EEGs. In Pfurtscheller G, Jonkman EJ, Lopes da Silva FM (eds): *Brain Ischemia: Quantitative EEG and Imaging Techniques.* Vol. 62 (Prog Brain Res). Amsterdam, Elsevier, 1984, pp 29–50.

CHAPTER TWELVE

Intraoperative Monitoring of Cerebral Perfusion During Carotid Endarterectomy

Thoralf M. Sundt, Jr., M.D.

From January 1972 to June 1987, we performed 2,361 carotid endarterectomies for primary carotid stenosis and 62 procedures for recurrent stenosis, monitoring the cerebral blood flow (CBF) and cerebral metabolic activity intraoperatively through the intraarterial injection of xenon-133 (^{133}Xe) and continuous electroencephalography (EEG). There has been an excellent correlation between these two types of monitoring techniques which has made this operation, at least in our hands, safer and more dependable (12, 17). Because the results and complications of the operative procedures (19) and the methodology of intraoperative CBF measurements have been described elsewhere, they are reviewed only briefly as they relate to intraoperative brain protection.

CEREBRAL BLOOD FLOW MEASUREMENT

CBF is measured with a technique involving the rapid injection of 300 μCi of ^{133}Xe in 0.4 ml of isotonic saline through a 27-gauge needle into the common carotid artery with the external carotid artery occluded (20). The rate of radionuclide uptake by tissue is measured by a single scintillation detector with a sodium iodide crystal $1\frac{1}{4}$ inches in diameter and $\frac{1}{4}$-inch thick. The crystal is recessed 1 inch behind a tapered lead collimator with a $\frac{7}{8}$-inch opening widening to $1\frac{1}{8}$ inches at the surface of the crystal. The detector is mounted on a Zeiss operating microscope stand (Carl Zeiss, Oberkochen, FRG; Zeiss Inc., Thornwood, NY) and placed adjacent and perpendicular to the scalp overlying the hand and face area of the motor strip.

It is possible, after completion of the carotid endarterectomy, to compute CBF values by the kinetic ("stochastic" or "H/A") method or by exponential analysis (3, 4). During the early years of our series, this computation was done to determine a correlation with CBF values obtained at surgery which were calculated by the initial slope technique of Waltz et al (24). The calculation is made using a formula derived from the work of Waltz et al (24) comparing analytical methods for the derivation of CBF. Our confidence in the initial slope technique is now so great that we seldom use the other methods of measurement. The use of this formula is illustrated in Figure 12.1.

$$\text{CBF (ml/100 g/minute)} = \frac{3600}{T\frac{1}{2} \text{ (second)},}$$

in which $T\frac{1}{2}$ is the time required in seconds for the curve to reach a value one-half its original maximum or peak.

Flows are calculated on a computer or with a slide rule and are available to the surgeon within several minutes after the ^{133}Xe injection. Examples of typical clearance curves obtained before, during, and after carotid occlusion are depicted in Figure 12.2.

ELECTRO-ENCEPHALOGRAPHIC MONITORING

Technique

Forty-five minutes before the patient is taken to the operating room, two ear elec-

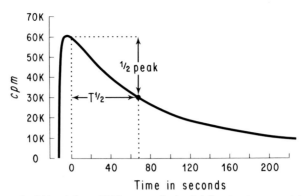

Figure 12.1. Typical cerebral blood flow (CBF) curve obtained following intraarterial injection of xenon-133 into the internal carotid artery. CBF is determined by dividing 3,600 by the time in seconds that it takes for the curve to fall to one-half its peak value. CBF here equals $3,600 \div 65 = 55.5$ ml/100 g/minute. K = kilocounts (1,000 counts), cpm = counts per minute.

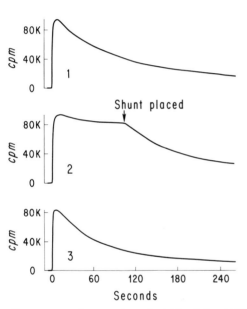

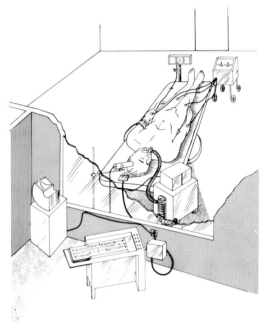

Figure 12.2. Sequential cerebral blood flow (CBF) curves in a patient during carotid endarterectomy. CBF values in ml/100 g/minute were as follows: 46, baseline; <5, with occlusion (washout slope too flat to measure accurately rapidly); 44, with placement of a shunt; and 67, following restoration of flow. K = kilocounts (1,000 counts), cpm = counts per minute.

Figure 12.3. Arrangement of equipment for simultaneous cerebral blood flow measurements and electroencephalography during carotid endarterectomy. All cumbersome equipment is housed in an adjacent monitoring room so that it does not encroach upon the work space for the surgical or anesthesia teams.

trodes and 21 scalp electrodes are applied with colloidin (18). The 10–20 international system of electrode placement is employed. A 16-channel EEG recording is obtained with a Grass Model 6 polygraph (Grass Instrument Co., Quincy, MA). A baseline trace is obtained before induction of anesthesia. The EEG is then recorded continuously throughout the operation. Both routine (30 mm/second) and slow (5 mm/second) paper speeds are employed. The EEG and CBF recording equipment are positioned in a monitoring room adjacent to the operating room or in a corner of the operating room well away from the surgical field (Fig. 12.3).

Results

Background Electroencephalographic Pattern Under Anesthesia

There are two basic patterns seen during a surgical level of anesthesia: a symmetric pattern and a grossly asymmetric pattern with a persistent delta focus (18).

The symmetric pattern is observed in most cases in which the patient has no significant preoperative neurologic deficits or persistent focal findings in his or her awake EEG. The records are usually dominated by symmetric, sustained, rhythmic activity of 10 to 14 Hz that ranges between 25 and 100 μV. Some EEG records show faster activity, 15 to 24 Hz, but the activity is usually of lesser amplitude and duration. In addition, especially with deeper levels of anesthesia, slower activity in the delta frequency range with amplitudes ranging between 50 and 150 μV becomes apparent. All of these patterns tend to show a midline maximum in either the frontal or the central cerebral regions. In Figure 12.4, these normal anesthetic patterns are demonstrated in the first eight channels, all of which record activity from a normal hemisphere.

A persistent delta focus and asymmetry of the background EEG patterns throughout anesthesia are observed in most patients who have a persistent delta focus in

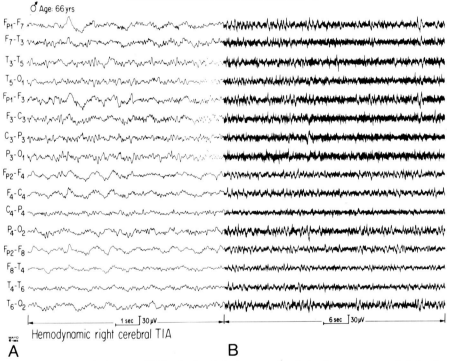

Figure 12.4. Electroencephalogram (EEG) obtained during anesthesia is shown as recorded A, at regular (30 mm/second) paper speed and B, at slow (5 mm/second) paper speed. The first eight channels record the usual anesthetic pattern from a normal left hemisphere, showing the sustained rhythmic pattern under anesthesia in the 10- to 14-Hz frequency range. In addition, there are triangular slow waves of briefer duration, maximal in the anterior frontal region, as well as lower voltage, more widespread, and irregular slow waves predominantly seen more posteriorly. The lower eight channels record from the right hemisphere where residual EEG changes seen are related to previous right hemodynamic transient ischemic attacks (TIAs). In these channels, the rhythmic anesthetic pattern is reduced (compare the lower four channels to the upper four channels), and there is an increased amount of irregular slowing. This effect can be appreciated both at the regular and slow paper speed.

their waking EEG taken before surgery. In addition, some patients show a persistent delta focus during anesthesia even though their awake tracing showed no such delta focus. Figure 12.4 illustrates the baseline anesthetic EEG in a patient with previous right cerebral hemodynamic transient ischemic attacks (TIAs) and a residual EEG abnormality on the right side which consists of reduction in the normal, faster background activity associated with persistent irregular delta slowing (last eight channels).

Major Focal Electroencephalographic Changes Occurring with Carotid Clamping

Approximately 24% of the patients in our series have shown a major focal EEG change when the carotid artery is clamped. The severity of these changes has closely paralleled the related reduction of CBF. In general, the onset of change is less rapid

and less severe with reduction of CBF to levels between 10 ml and 18 ml/100 g/minute than it is when flow is reduced to levels below 10 ml/100 g/minute. It is rare for CBF to drop to levels below 10 ml/100 g/minute without EEG evidence of ischemia, although the correlation between CBF and EEG may vary depending on the anesthetic agent used. In some cases in which the internal carotid artery opposite the side of operation is occluded, the EEG changes are bilateral but only rarely are they more severe on the contralateral side.

The EEG changes that occur with clamping almost always include attenuation of the faster background frequencies. In patients with moderate ischemia, this is associated with slow waves of higher amplitude and longer wavelength than before clamping, but in those with more severe ischemia even the slow waves are attenuated (Fig. 12.5). In most cases the EEG returns to normal within 1 to 2 minutes after the shunt is in place, but in patients who have severe changes and undergo

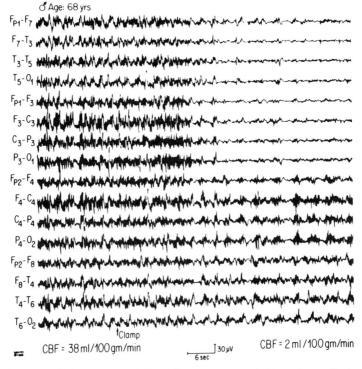

LEFT CAROTID ENDARTERECTOMY

♂ Age: 68 yrs

Fp1-F7
F7-T3
T3-T5
T5-O1
Fp1-F3
F3-C3
C3-P3
P3-O1
Fp2-F4
F4-C4
C4-P4
P4-O2
Fp2-F8
F8-T4
T4-T6
T6-O2

↑Clamp

CBF = 38 ml/100 gm/min   ⌐30 μV   CBF = 2 ml/100 gm/min
                                 6 sec

Figure 12.5. Electroencephalogram recorded at slow paper speed (5 mm/second) shows the dramatic attenuation of the faster as well as the slower components that had occurred with carotid clamping which reduced cerebral blood flow (CBF) from 38 to 2 ml/100 g/minute.

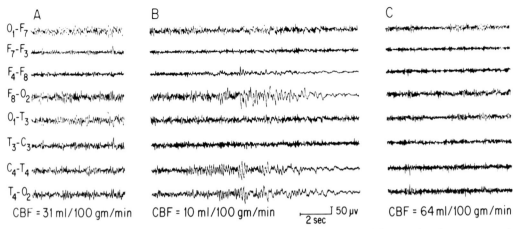

Figure 12.6. Electroencephalogram (EEG) in a 59-year-old man undergoing left carotid endarterectomy. *A*, EEG recording before clamping of the left carotid artery shows a symmetrical pattern. *B*, EEG recording 40 seconds after clamping shows left-sided delta slowing and reduced background activity when the blood flow is reduced to 10 ml/100 g/minute. *C*, EEG recorded 4 minutes after internal shunting has returned to baseline levels. CBF = cerebral blood flow.

prolonged clamping, it takes longer. In our series, the EEG returned to normal after placement of a shunt in almost every case; the focal EEG changes resolved within 2 to 7 minutes after shunting. After the shunt was in place, however, four patients sustained an EEG change that was angiographically proved to be related to small emboli arising from the patent shunt.

Major Focal Electroencephalographic Changes Not Immediately Associated with Carotid Clamping

Several patients in our series have had major transient focal or generalized slowing of the EEG not immediately associated with or caused by carotid clamping. These changes usually persisted for a few minutes and in most cases appeared in both hemispheres. Early in our experience it was our impression that, when these changes were seen predominantly on the side of surgery, they were related to the presence of small emboli to peripheral vessels. This indeed can be the case, but fortunately such changes in the EEG are more often related to subtle alterations in the level of anesthesia. When the changes develop more slowly and are seen in both hemispheres, they invariably are related

to an increase in the depth of anesthesia and quite often can be attributed to the effects of nitrous oxide rather than of the primary anesthetic agent. Lightening the level of anesthesia usually results in prompt improvement in the EEG.

In patients with a preexisting neurologic deficit and an asymmetrical baseline EEG, an increase or decrease in the level of anesthesia may be preferentially reflected in the hemisphere with the abnormal EEG. Thus, a lateralized EEG change in these patients is not necessarily attributable to intraoperative embolization.

Intraoperative embolization can usually be identified on the EEG by its focal distribution, as well as by the lack of an EEG response to altering the level of anesthesia. However, the embolic changes usually are not as dramatic as those associated with total hemispheric ischemia following occlusion of the internal carotid artery (ICA) in patients with inadequate collateral flow (Fig. 12.6).

CEREBRAL BLOOD FLOW EFFECTS OF ANESTHETIC AGENT AND PATIENT CATEGORY

Our evaluations of patients operated under anesthesia with halothane, ethrane, or

Table 12.1. Cerebral Blood Flow According to Anesthetic Used and Grade of Risk: January 1, 1972, to June 30, 1987[a]

Time of measurement	Grade 1			Grade 2			Grade 3			Grade 4		
	n[b]	CBF[c]	±SD[d]	n	CBF	±SD	n	CBF	±SD	n	CBF	±SD
Halothane ($n=478$)												
Baseline	155	62	26	91	58	28	143	51	21	82	48	21
Occlusion	153	35	18	89	30	18	145	26	16	78	24	13
Shunt	43	44	15	44	52	17	66	43	17	48	42	12
Postocclusion	156	69	27	92	69	26	145	61	23	85	60	22
Ethrane ($n=868$)												
Baseline	306	50	18	197	44	18	198	42	18	142	37	21
Occlusion	303	28	13	195	23	13	194	21	11	139	18	11
Shunt	102	39	15	102	35	11	105	36	13	89	35	14
Postocclusion	312	51	18	200	50	19	205	48	19	151	51	22
Forane[e] ($n=919$)												
Baseline	247	35	15	207	33	18	287	30	14	133	26	14
Occlusion	245	23	11	202	18	11	279	18	9	128	15	9
Shunt	66	27	9	87	29	9	121	27	10	85	28	10
Postocclusion	251	40	16	213	42	16	302	35	15	153	45	41

[a]Patients receiving an anesthetic agent other than halothane, ethrane, or a combination of forane and fentanyl were excluded from analysis.
[b]Number of cases.
[c]Cerebral blood flow.
[d]Standard deviation from the mean.
[e]Forane was supplemented in many cases with fentanyl.

a combination of forane and fentanyl show that CBF measurements obtained intraoperatively are correlated with the anesthetic agent used during the operation and with the patient's preoperative risk category (Table 12.1). In these patients, the discrepancy between the number who had a postocclusion flow and the number who had a baseline flow was related to technical problems after injection of the isotope solution in delivering the indicator to the brain in those patients with a very high-grade carotid stenosis (99.9%), causing almost complete obstruction of distal flow. There was a statistically significant difference among the baseline flow measurements in comparable risk categories (Grades 1 to 4 [19]) for the patients operated on under these three agents. Within each group of patients receiving the same anesthetic agent, there was a significant difference ($p<0.05$) in the baseline and occlusion flows between the patients considered to be in the poor risk category (Grade 4) and those in the better risk categories (Grades 1 and 2).

CORRELATION OF ELECTRO-ENCEPHALOGRAPHIC AND CEREBRAL BLOOD FLOW MEASUREMENTS

The severity of EEG changes observed in patients with varying degrees of ischemia who are operated on under halothane anesthesia is illustrated in Figure 12.7. Table 12.2 summarizes the frequency of changes seen in the EEG with carotid occlusion according to the anesthetic agent used. However, in patients who had a low CBF value, a shunt often was placed before the development of an EEG change.

CEREBRAL BLOOD FLOW AND STUMP PRESSURES

Stump pressures (23) were measured consecutively in 100 patients in order to correlate these measurements with the CBF values after carotid occlusion. These data,

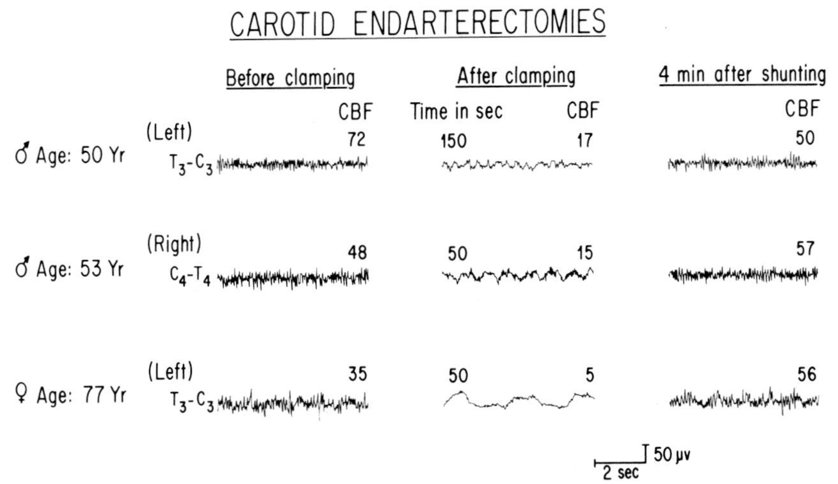

Figure 12.7. Correlation between the electroencephalogram (EEG) and cerebral blood flow (CBF) measurements obtained under halothane anesthesia. The severity of the EEG change parallels the reduction in CBF. (From McKay RD, Sundt TM Jr, Michenfelder JD, et al: Internal carotid artery stump pressure and cerebral blood flow during carotid endarterectomy: Modification by halothane, enflurane, and innovar. *Anesthesiology* 45:390–399, 1976.)

which have been reported elsewhere (14), are summarized in Figure 12.8. On the basis of our findings, we no longer use stump pressure measurements as a monitoring technique. However, other experienced groups report excellent results using this technique (8, 9, 15).

EMBOLIC COMPLICATIONS

Embolic complications during the operation are identified by focal change in the EEG. In our series, a total of 15 embolic complications that led to a major or minor neurologic deficit occurred intraoperatively in patients undergoing surgery for primary stenosis, for an incidence of about 1%. Embolic complications were more common in patients with recurrent stenosis.

There were four cases of emboli through a functioning shunt during the operation in this series. These were major events related to proximal atherosclerosis and, in retrospect, might possibly have been avoided if we had been more experienced in treating such patients. There were two

Table 12.2. Cerebral Blood Flow During Carotid Occlusion Using Halothane ($n = 469$), Ethrane ($n = 841$), and Forane ($n = 876$) Anesthesia: January 1, 1978, to June 30, 1987

Flow (ml/100 g/minute)	Electroencephalographic status within 3 minutes of occlusion											
	Cases with no change						Cases with change					
	Halothane		Ethrane		Forane		Halothane		Ethrane		Forane	
	n	Percent	n	Percent	n	Percent	n	Percent	n	Percent	n	Percent
0–4	0	0	2	0.2	14	1.5	12	2.5	23	2.7	39	4.4
5–9	1	0.2	2	0.2	55	6.2	21	4.4	76	9.0	55	6.2
10–14	8	1.7	52	6.1	122	13.9	42	8.9	74	8.7	40	4.5
15–19	25	5.3	91	10.8	149	17.0	41	8.7	46	5.4	18	2.0
20–24	49	10.4	122	14.5	148	16.8	0	0	0	0	4	0.4
25–29	56	11.9	104	12.3	94	10.7	0	0	0	0	0	0
30+	214	45.6	249	29.6	138	15.7	0	0	0	0	0	0
Total	353	75.2	622	73.9	720	82.1	116	24.7	219	26.0	156	17.8

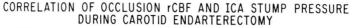

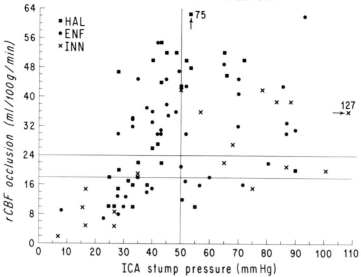

Figure 12.8. Scattergram of regional cerebral blood flow (rCBF) during occlusion plotted against stump pressure measurements in the internal carotid artery (ICA). The *vertical line* represents a stump pressure of 50 torr (considered the critical level for ischemia). The *two horizontal lines* represent the critical flow level (rCBF ≤ 18 ml/100 g/minute) and the marginal zone (rCBF 18 to 24 ml/100 g/minute). Regression lines for each anesthetic agent were calculated. Expressed for halothane (HAL), $rCBF_{occl} = 0.51$ (stump pressure) ± 9.94, $r = 0.43$. Expressed for enflurane (ENF), $rCBF_{occl} = 0.26$ (stump pressure) ± 16.51, $r = 0.39$. Expressed for Innovar (INN), $rCBF_{occl} = 0.27$ (stump pressure) ± 0.93, $r = 0.68$. (From McKay RD, Sundt TM Jr, Michenfelder JD, et al: Internal carotid artery stump pressure and cerebral blood flow during carotid endarterectomy: Modification by halothane, enflurane, and innovar. *Anesthesiology* 45:390–399, 1976.)

additional cases in which the shunt became transiently occluded from a platelet thrombus or fragment of atherosclerosis. The occlusion was identified because of an EEG change and was actually visualized through the shunt wall. Removal of the shunt with extraction of the thrombus resulted in normalization of the EEG. Both patients had normal neurologic function when they awoke after surgery.

There were 11 cases of embolic complications not related to shunt usage. Nine of these occurred during the exposure of the vessel, one with induction of anesthesia and one as the patient was awakening from surgery.

VALUE OF MONITORING AND SHUNTING DURING ENDARTERECTOMY

The correlation of CBF measurements with EEG patterns in our series has been excellent, as indicated by data from 2,186 cases operated on under halothane, ethrane, or forane anesthesia (Table 12.2). We have had 90 patients with occlusion flows between 0 and 4 ml/100 g/minute, 210 with flows between 5 and 9 ml/100 g/minute, and 338 with flows between 10 and 14 ml/100 g/minute. Using the ^{133}Xe washout technique, flows below 5 ml/100 g/minute are difficult to quantitate and can be equated essentially to zero flow. On this basis, we believe that, without placement of a shunt, 3% of the patients in our series would definitely have sustained a cerebral infarction because of inadequate collateral flow, and another 8% to 9%—those patients with CBF between 5 and 9 ml/100 g/minute—probably would have sustained an infarction with any prolonged period of occlusion.

Patients with flows between 10 and 14 ml/100 g/minute, representing 15% of the group, may or may not have withstood the period of ischemia, as we shall discuss shortly. Shunts were also used in a large number of patients with CBF between 15 and 20 ml/100 g/minute. This was done because we feared that the EEG would not reveal regions of focal ischemia in the deep white matter and basal ganglia or because the presence of borderline flow levels and a preoperative region of infarction or ischemia represented an increased risk factor for intraoperative ischemic complications. Occasionally patients with CBF above 20 ml/100 g/minute were also shunted if they had a preexisting EEG abnormality related to preoperative infarct because we have found, as have others, that these patients are particularly vulnerable to marginal flow (5–7, 10, 11, 16, 22). Shunts usually are not inserted until the plaque has been removed from the distal ICA, except in cases in which CBF is below 5 ml/100 g/minute or in which there has been a dramatic and catastrophic change in the EEG—usually these are simultaneous events and one does not occur without the other.

A total of 958 of the 2,186 patients who had endarterectomies performed while under these three anesthetic agents were successfully protected with indwelling shunts during the operation. However, there was a significant difference in the frequency of shunt usage according to both the grade of the patient and the anesthetic agent used ($p < 0.05$). Thus, 41% and 45% of patients operated under halothane and ethrane, respectively, received a shunt, whereas only 28% of patients operated on under forane (often supplemented with fentanyl) were shunted.

There was also a significant difference in CBF among patients categorized according to the anesthetic agent used. The highest flows were in patients anesthetized with halothane and the lowest, in those administered forane. A data analysis of Table 12.1 shows significant differences in baseline and postocclusion CBF in patients operated under the three agents studied ($p < 0.001$). Halothane anesthesia was associated with higher CBF than ethrane, which in turn had higher flows than forane. Halothane occlusion and shunt flows were also significantly higher compared to ethrane and forane, but the difference between the ethrane and forane flows were less striking.

A comparison of CBF according to the patients's grade, or preoperative risk cat-

egory, shows that baseline and occlusion CBF for patients in Grade 4 were significantly lower than those for patients in Grade 1 ($p < 0.001$). There were no differences in the postocclusion flow values.

Shunts were required in only 30% of Grade 1 candidates for surgery, but were required in 56% of patients who were Grade 4 candidates for surgery. Moreover, both the baseline and occlusion flows were lower in the higher risk category of patients. This leads to the conclusion that the microembolic and hemodynamic theories for TIAs and infarctions are not mutually exclusive and that areas of brain functioning on a marginal flow of 40% to 50% of normal are particularly vulnerable to the effects of emboli (20, 21, 26). In contrast, however, Whisnant et al (25) found, from a detailed multivariant analysis of a group of patients with TIAs undergoing surgery in the period of 1970 to 1974, that no patients with a high occlusion flow had an intraoperative or postoperative stroke. Furthermore, this group had no stroke in 4.5 years of follow-up evaluation, indicating that individuals with high collateral flow have a good prognosis.

CRITICAL FLOW AND ISCHEMIC TOLERANCE

There is good correlation between results observed in laboratory studies in primates and the clinical studies in humans related to the ability of the brain to tolerate ischemia (1–4). It appears that the critical flow required to maintain normal electrical activity in the brain varies somewhere between 15 and 20 ml/100 g/minute and that the critical flow required to maintain basic cell metabolism is somewhere between 10 and 15 ml/100 g/minute. There is now general agreement about the protective effects of barbiturate anesthesia for cerebral ischemia but there is less information concerning the possible beneficial effects of inhalation general anesthesia agents (13). Our data suggest that there is a difference in these critical flows related to the anesthetic agent used; for example, the critical flow is higher for halothane than it is for forane. The best available data at present suggest that flows below 10 ml/100 g/minute, regardless of the anesthetic agent in use, result in ionic shifts that may be irreversible if allowed to persist. However, the true level of tolerance for ischemia in patients who have flows between 5 and 10 ml/100 g/minute or between 10 and 15 ml/100 g/minute is unknown. Furthermore, in areas of marginal flow, brain blood flow is not homogenous, and there may be considerable focal variability among regions of incomplete focal ischemia.

We prefer not to speculate about how long a particular patient can retain a physiologic paralysis without developing neuronal damage. Therefore, we routinely place a shunt whenever there is a doubt regarding the adequacy of CBF and when placement of the shunt is safe and does not jeopardize the arterial repair. A number of other groups with considerable experience in this field have adopted intraoperative EEG monitoring as a means of increasing the safety of the procedure (5, 7, 11, 12, 16, 17, 23).

References

1. Astrup J. Siesjö BK, Symon L: Thresholds in cerebral ischemia: The ischemic penumbra. *Stroke* 12:723–725, 1981.
2. Astrup J, Symon L, Branston NM, et al: Cortical evoked potential and extracellular K^+ and H^+ at critical levels of brain ischemia. *Stroke* 8:51–57, 1977.
3. Boysen G: Cerebral blood flow measurement as a safeguard during carotid endarterectomy. *Stroke* 2:1–10, 1971.
4. Boysen G, Ladegaard-Pedersen HJ, Henriksen H, et al: The effects of $PaCO_2$ on regional cerebral blood flow and internal carotid arterial pressure during carotid clamping. *Anesthesiology* 35:286–300, 1971.
5. Callow AD, Matsumoto G, Baker D, et al: Protection of the high risk carotid endarterectomy patient by continuous electroencephalography. *J Cardiovasc Surg (Torino)* 19:55–64, 1978.
6. Callow AD, O'Donnell TF: Electroencephalogram monitoring in cerebrovascular surgery. In Bergan JJ, Yao JS (eds): *Cerebral Vascular Insufficiency.* New York, Grune & Stratton, 1983, pp 327–341.
7. Gianotta SL, Dicks RE, Kindt GW: Carotid endarterectomy: Technical improvements. *Neurosurgery* 7:309–312, 1980.
8. Hays RF, Levinson SA, Wylie EJ: Intraoperative measurement of carotid back pressure as a guide to operative management of carotid endarterectomy. *Surgery* 72:953–960, 1972.
9. Hunter GC, Sieffert G, Malone JM, et al: The accuracy of carotid back pressure as an index for shunt requirements. *Stroke* 13:319–326, 1982.
10. Imparato AM, Ramirez A, Rile T, et al: Cerebral protection in carotid surgery. *Arch Surg* 117:1073–1078, 1982.
11. Leech PJ, Miller JD, Fitch W, et al: Cerebral blood flow, internal carotid artery pressure, and the EEG as a guide to the safety of carotid ligation. *J Neurol Neurosurg Psychiatry* 37:854–862, 1974.
12. Matsumoto GH, Baker JD, Watson CW, et al: EEG surveillance as a means of extending operability in high risk carotid endarterectomy. *Stroke* 7:554–559, 1976.
13. McDowall DG: The effects of general anaesthetics on cerebral blood flow and cerebral metabolism. *Br J Anaesth* 37:236–245, 1965.
14. McKay RD, Sundt TM Jr, Michenfelder JD, et al: Internal carotid artery stump pressure and cerebral blood flow during carotid endarterectomy: Modification by halothane, enflurane, and innovar. *Anesthesiology* 45:390–399, 1976.
15. Moore WS, Hall AD: Carotid artery back pressure. A test of cerebral tolerance to temporary carotid occlusion. *Arch Surg* 99:702–710, 1969.
16. Ojemann RG, Crowell RM, Roberson GH, et al: Surgical treatment of extracranial carotid occlusive disease. *Clin Neurosurg* 22:214–263, 1975.
17. Phillips MR, Johnson WC, Scott RM, et al: Carotid endarterectomy in the presence of contralateral carotid occlusion: The role of EEG and intraluminal shunting. *Arch Surg* 114:1232–1239, 1979.
18. Sharbrough FW, Messick JM Jr, Sundt TM Jr: Correlation of continuous electroencephalograms with cerebral blood flow measurements during carotid endarterectomy. *Stroke* 4:674–683, 1973.
19. Sundt TM Jr, Sandok BA, Whisnant JP: Carotid endarterectomy: Complications and preoperative assessment of risk. *Mayo Clin Proc* 50:301–306, 1975.
20. Sundt TM Jr, Sharbrough FW, Anderson RE, et al: Cerebral blood flow measurements and electroencephalograms during carotid endarterectomy. *J Neurosurg* 41:310–320, 1974.
21. Sundt TM Jr, Sharbrough FW, Piepgras DG, et al: Correlation of cerebral blood flow and electroencephalographic changes during carotid endarterectomy. *Mayo Clin Proc* 56:533–543, 1981.
22. Thompson JE: Complications of carotid endarterectomy and their prevention. *World J Surg* 3:155–165, 1979.
23. Trojaborg W, Boysen G: Relation between EEG, regional cerebral blood flow and internal carotid artery pressure during carotid endarterectomy. *Electroencephalogr Clin Neurophysiol* 34:61–69, 1973.
24. Waltz AG, Wanek AR, Anderson RE: Comparison of analytic methods for calculation of cerebral flow after intracarotid injection of ^{133}Xe. *J Nucl Med* 13:66–72, 1972.
25. Whisnant JP, Sandok BA, Sundt TM Jr: Carotid endarterectomy for unilateral carotid system transient cerebral ischemia. *Mayo Clin Proc* 58:171–175, 1983.
26. Wylie EJ, Ehrenfeld WK: *Extracranial Occlusive Cerebrovascular Disease: Diagnosis and Management.* Philadelphia, WB Saunders, 1970.

CHAPTER THIRTEEN

Diagnosis, Prevention, and Treatment of Postoperative Ischemic Complications

Lawrence F. Marshall, M.D.

The prevention of focal or diffuse cerebral ischemia resulting from sustained intracranial hypertension following surgical intervention is imperative. Postoperative elevated intracranial pressure (ICP) often can be avoided by using a systematic preoperative plan, as well as a meticulous intraoperative approach. Prophylactic intervention may be undertaken, particularly in patients who are at risk for ischemic brain damage or brain swelling in the perioperative period. In most instances, care during the recovery from surgery is directed toward minimizing those factors which might adversely affect cerebral perfusion pressure (CPP).

In theory, all operations on the brain place it at risk of ischemic injury. Although most operations generally proceed without incident because of the advantages afforded by modern microsurgical techniques, enhanced lighting, and improved neuroanesthesia, there are three major types of surgical procedures that merit discussion in the context of postoperative ischemia: procedures for brain tumors, for trauma, and for cerebral vascular disease. In each of these, circumstances determined by the surgical findings may predispose the patient to edema or ischemic postoperative complications from which the brain requires protection. The role of ICP measurement in order to monitor CPP is discussed with respect to prevention and treatment of postoperative ischemic complications.

POSTOPERATIVE BRAIN EDEMA

Brain edema, an increase in the water content or a change in its distribution in

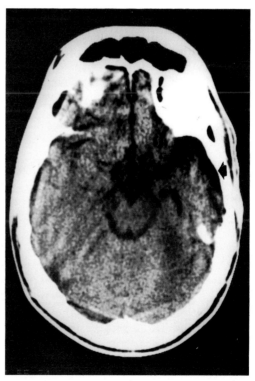

Figure 13.1. CT scan of the brain shows edema *(arrow)* often observed postoperatively as a result of brain retraction. It is usually not symptomatic.

145

the tissue, usually occurs wherever the brain is retracted. Edema is distinguished from reactive hyperemia or the increase in the volume of brain caused by vascular engorgement and an increase in blood volume, either in the arterial or venous compartment or both. The edema often seen on computerized tomography (CT) postoperatively (Fig. 13.1) is usually of little consequence in affecting neurologic function and resolves spontaneously, reaching its maximum level within 48 hours and then diminishing over the next several days. However, if the surgical exposure is extended to the base of the brain, if the operation is prolonged, and if several draining veins are sacrificed, ischemia may develop in the retracted lobe, resulting in rather severe edema which can compress vital structures. For example, approaching perimesencephalic lesions from under the temporal lobe can result in severe temporal lobe edema, uncal herniation, and brain stem compression even if the procedure is done carefully. Severe focal or diffuse postoperative edema ultimately produces or aggravates ischemia that may progress to infarction if impairment of microcirculatory, venous, or ultimately arterial blood flow is not relieved by reduction of ICP and an increase in CPP. During the postoperative period, such edema can be extremely difficult to treat and in severe cases temporal lobectomy may be required. Thus, for specific indications, surgical decompression, in addition to the usual medical methods of brain protection, is an approach by which postoperative intracranial hypertension, especially of the focal type, can be reduced.

POSTOPERATIVE BRAIN ISCHEMIA

Occlusion or vasospasm of cerebral vessels may occur in cases of aneurysm or tumor when the surgical dissection is carried into the Sylvian fissure or is at the base of the brain, such as occurs often in cerebral vascular surgery. Much of the attention directed toward brain protection has been targeted at focal brain damage produced by postoperative ischemia or stroke. Although there are analogies between atherosclerotic thrombotic occlusion and direct iatrogenic vascular occlusion, there are also important differences. Laboratory models of middle cerebral artery occlusion more commonly simulate the situation occurring in the operating room—acute and complete obstruction of blood flow through an otherwise intact major artery. Under such circumstances, two issues arise. First, what is the possibility of revascularization of the focally ischemic region? Second, what can be done to mitigate the brain damage when revascularization is done in a delayed fashion, or is not possible?

A number of approaches to these issues has been suggested over the past 15 years (see Chapters 17 and 24, this volume). Only a few have been tested in patients, even though there are several reports of successful experimental treatment. Our interests in the treatment of focal ischemic brain damage during the postoperative period have ranged from use of high-dose barbiturate therapy, which has not been successful (3); to the administration of large doses of phenytoin; to the recent experimental use of glutamate receptor antagonists (5, 7) (see Chapter 20, this volume).

TUMORS

The indications for continuous monitoring of ICP to prevent ischemic brain injury caused by intracranial hypertension during or after removal of a brain tumor have declined substantially over the past decade. This decline reflects five major improvements in neurosurgical management: (a) preoperative preparation of patients has improved with regard to hydration and the administration of glucocorticoids; (b) patients with intracranial neoplasms are recognized when their tumor is in an earlier stage because of improvements in neurodiagnostic procedures (CT, magnetic resonance imaging); (c) with intraoperative imaging methods such as ultrasound, lesions are more accurately localized or identified during surgery; (d) improved neuroanesthesia techniques afford less perioperative brain swelling because of the elimination of agents that produce vasodilation; and (e) improvements have been made in microneurosurgery techniques and lighting. Thus, postoperative neurologic deterioration is less common in the patient with a very bulky tumor who presents with signs of brain stem compression and the associated risk of acute catastrophic decompensation from herniation of brain during the induction of anesthesia. Nevertheless, in patients with large hemispheric tumors that are not amenable to extensive internal decompression, the risks of anesthesia and postoperative brain edema remain. Although in most instances ICP monitoring is not essential, it may add to the attending neurosurgeon's accuracy and efficiency in selecting and monitoring appropriate therapy for postoperative intracranial hypertension. Considering its benign nature, ICP monitoring can be done with very little risk to the patient.

In a recent report, Constantini and colleagues* described their experiences in 514 consecutive patients who underwent craniotomy and were monitored postoperatively with a subdural device. Sustained elevations of ICP (>20 mm Hg for 2 or more hours) occurred in 76 of 412 patients (18.4%) with supratentorial tumors and in 13 of 102 patients (12.7%) with infratentorial tumors. Clinical deterioration occurred in 47 patients, and in 19 the deterioration was clearly preceded by an increase in ICP. Because such monitoring is almost risk free and in some patients will forewarn of impending deterioration, its use in selected high-risk patients should be considered.

The patients potentially at highest risk for intracranial hypertension during the intraoperative and postoperative period include those requiring craniotomy whose CT scans show extensive mass effect and a midline shift preoperatively. It is impor-

tant to stress the need for a coordinated neuroanesthetic approach to these patients. If the shift is substantial and the surgeon envisions the possibility that the tumor may not be entirely removed during the procedure, then postoperative ICP monitoring for 48 hours may permit early detection of a treatable increase in ICP before clinical deterioration occurs. In this situation, a small fiberoptic monitor placed either on the surface or just into the parenchyma of the brain provides accurate detection of changes in ICP yet does not require ventricular penetration and the attendant risks of infection. In most instances, however, excision of the tumor, either complete or partial, usually reduces the brain volume sufficiently to obviate the need for ICP monitoring.

Finally, in patients in whom a prolonged deep dissection with substantial retraction of the brain is required, ICP monitoring during the postoperative period may give early evidence of brain edema before it causes compression of the deep structures. It is also important to emphasize that, in these patients, serial CT scanning may also be extremely useful, particularly if the neurologic status is somewhat depressed as a result of the operation and if ICP monitoring has not been established. CT scanning should be considered a form of discontinuous monitoring of the structural integrity and volume status of the brain. By paying particular attention to the perimesencephalic subarachnoid spaces and the position of the midline structures, much can be learned regarding abnormalities of brain volume and the risk that the patient may develop ischemia from compression and shift of the intracranial contents.

TRAUMA

Systematic recording of ICP in all patients with severe head injuries had demonstrated that a substantial number of patients who sustain diffuse brain injury for which no surgical treatment is possible or who are treated with evacuation of large intraparenchymal or intracranial mass lesions develop a significant rise in ICP (>30 mm Hg) that causes diffuse brain ischemia

*S Constantini, S Cotev, ZH Rappaport, et al: ICP monitoring after elective intracranial surgery. A study of 514 consecutive patients. In *Proceedings of the 7th International Symposium on Intracranial Pressure and Brain Injury.* Ann Arbor, MI, 1988, p 81.

Highest ICP Following Surgery

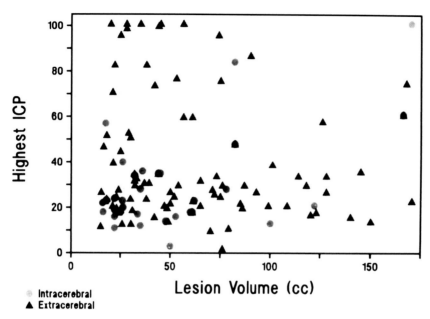

Lesion volume by CT scan before surgery related to highest ICP after surgery, during the first 72 hrs.

Figure 13.2. Occurrence of intracranial hypertension following evacuation of traumatic mass lesions. Note the prevalence of elevated intracranial pressure (ICP) and its lack of correlation with the volume of the mass. (Courtesy of Howard Eisenberg, M.D., University of Texas Medical Center, Galveston, TX.)

during the postoperative period. Estimates vary as to the frequency of postoperative ICP elevations in this setting, but it appears that approximately 50% of all patients undergoing craniotomy for a traumatic lesion will have such increases in ICP (Fig. 13.2).

In general, ICP monitoring after surgery for trauma should be restricted to: (a) patients in coma with a mass lesion (hematoma or contusion) or hemispheric swelling producing a substantial amount of shift (>5 to 6 mm); (b) patients in whom there has been a delay in hematoma removal; and (c) patients in whom neurologic deterioration has been relatively abrupt because of a hematoma, but who are not in coma at the time of operation. In such cases, there is a high incidence of postoperative intracranial hypertension and ischemia, caused in part by vasomotor paralysis and edema. It is recommended that a ventricular cannula be placed in all patients in these three categories because ICP control is often more difficult in such cases

and ventricular drainage is usually very effective, at least initially.

It is appropriate to point out here that dural closure and replacement of the bone flap can be accomplished in almost every instance after trauma surgery. Systemic medical therapy including hyperventilation and mannitol treatment usually lowers the ICP and prevents further postoperative ischemic brain injury. Leaving the dura open without replacing the bone flap often exacerbates the problem by causing extracranial herniation of the exposed brain which then becomes infarcted because of venous obstruction.

CEREBRAL VASCULAR DISEASE

In general, most operations for intracranial aneurysm are uncomplicated and postoperative ICP monitoring is not warranted. Occasionally, if the subtemporal approach is used for basilar artery aneurysms and several draining veins are sacrificed, swelling of the temporal lobe may result. Usually, a partial temporal lobectomy is the best treatment if the swelling is recognized during surgery. If, however, lobectomy has not been done and the patient's condition deteriorates, a decision must be made regarding use of medical management or further surgical intervention to decompress the brain stem. Surgical decompression appears to be more appropriate under such circumstances because the proximity of the temporal lobes to the brain stem makes ischemic edema more dangerous than when swelling occurs in more peripheral regions. Postoperative vasospasm may also result in focal, hemispheric, or diffuse brain ischemia and edema aggravated by increases in ICP. In patients at high risk, ICP monitoring may be useful.

Operations for large, high-flow, usually deeply situated arteriovenous malformations (AVMs) may also be associated with postoperative ischemia. It is not entirely clear why such lesions can be followed by malignant brain swelling and with what Spetzler et al (6) have termed "normal perfusion pressure breakthrough bleeding." It appears that in patients who have such lesions, regions of the brain contiguous to the AVMs suffer from ischemia due to low blood flow because of shunting of blood into the AVM (1). It has been proposed that these maximally dilated vessels lose their ability to autoregulate in response to changes in arterial pressure. When there is a sudden increase in arterial pressure in such regions, because of either embolization or resection of the AVM, the resulting hyperperfusion can produce edema and hemorrhage.

For such operations, which are often prolonged and thus involve sustained periods of brain retraction, ICP monitoring during the immediate postoperative period seems warranted. Those surgeons expert in the excision of such lesions (2, 4, 6) have suggested that deep barbiturate anesthesia may permit the brain to adjust more appropriately to the changes in hemodynamics which occur when the brain surrounding such lesions undergoes a sudden reduction in blood flow. Barbiturates reduce the metabolic rate and, therefore, the overall brain blood flow in such patients. Several authors have suggested that when this syndrome develops, barbiturate therapy can produce a successful outcome if administered in large enough doses (*see* Chapter 24, this volume). It appears logical to monitor the ICP continually during the period of greatest risk for patients. These patients are also at some risk for intraoperative or postoperative intracerebral hemorrhage, which may go undetected because it occasionally occurs at some distance from the site of resection. Thus, particularly if deep anesthetic techniques are used and clinical examination parameters are lost, a serial assessment of ICP seems warranted. Periodic reassessment with CT is also essential whether or not ICP monitoring is done. Knowing the structural state of the brain and its cerebral spinal fluid spaces gives the surgeon invaluable information regarding the occurrence of brain swelling and its response to therapeutic intervention.

A final indication for ICP monitoring is the presence of significant intraventricular hemorrhage. In such circumstances after a patient has undergone a craniotomy—usually for an AVM but occasionally for an aneurysm, often in the posterior circulation—ventricular drainage is necessary. The availability of combined drainage and monitoring systems within the ventricular cannula permits monitoring of the ICP concurrent with drainage. Thus, the surgeon and anesthesiologist have the advantage of being able to monitor the ICP continuously without the risks associated with the insertion of a second device. We have prevented herniation in several instances with such a system by detecting a sudden change from an incomplete to a complete obstruction of the ventricular system due to enlargement of a hematoma during intermittent ventricular drainage.

PERSPECTIVE

After craniotomy in those patients with tumor, trauma, or cerebral vascular disease who are at high risk for postoperative edema, hemorrhage, ventricular obstruction and ischemia, ICP monitoring and ventricular drainage may be useful to identify and monitor treatment of these complications. Reoperation or aggressive medical therapy for protection of the brain from delayed postoperative damage may be instituted more promptly and effectively using information provided by continuous monitoring of CPP.

References

1. Batjer HH, Devous MD, Meyer YJ, et al: Cerebrovascular hemodynamics in arteriovenous malformation complicated by normal perfusion pressure breakthrough. *Neurosurgery* 22:503–509, 1988.
2. Marshall LF, U HS: Treatment of massive intra-operative brain swelling. *Neurosurgery* 13:412–414, 1983.
3. Rockoff MA, Marshall LF, Shapiro HM: High-dose barbiturate therapy in humans: A clinical review of 60 patients. *Ann Neurol* 6:194–199, 1979.
4. Selman W, Spetzler RF, Zabramski JM: Induced barbiturate coma. In Wilkins RH, Rengachary SS (eds): *Neurosurgery.* New York, McGraw-Hill, 1985, pp 343–349.
5. Simon R, Swan J, Griffiths T, et al: Blockade of N-methyl-D-aspartate receptors may protect against ischemic damage in the brain. *Science* 226:850–852, 1984.
6. Spetzler RF, Martin NA, Carter LP, et al: Surgical management of large AVMs by staged embolization and operative excision. *J Neurosurg* 67:17–28, 1987.
7. Westerberg E, Monaghan D, Cotman C, et al: Excitatory amino acid receptors and ischemic brain damage in the rat. *Neurosci Lett* 73:119–124, 1987.

CHAPTER FOURTEEN

Management of Acute Cerebral Infarction

Harold P. Adams, Jr., M.D.

Cerebral infarction is the leading cause of acute focal neurologic deficits and the leading neurologic cause of death or disability among adults in the United States. However, no medical or surgical therapy has been proved to be effective at improving the outcome after stroke. The management of acute stroke is controversial and remains a major challenge. Its immediate goals are to stabilize the neurologic deficits, limit irreversible brain damage, and avoid neurologic or medical complications. The ultimate aim is to reduce the mortality rate and improve the likelihood of a favorable neurologic outcome. The treatment of concomitant medical problems and aggressive rehabilitation are also crucial elements in the care of stroke patients. This chapter, however, focuses on medical therapies for acute or progressing cerebral infarction (Table 14.1).

Research in animals is essential in developing new therapies for acute stroke. For a variety of reasons, however, treatments that show great promise in animals often prove to be clinically disappointing. Animal models may not be clinically relevant. The anatomy of the cerebral circulation in some species often differs markedly from that in humans; as a result, experimental models of stroke often include combinations of hypoxia, hypotension, and multiple vessel ligations. Subtle neurologic signs are hard to detect in animals. Therefore, the therapeutic response to an intervention is often determined by infarct size on pathologic examination or by changes in cerebral blood flow (CBF). In addition, experimental studies are carefully planned and controlled, whereas patients with acute cerebral infarctions have confounding clinical variables that are not found in animals.

In humans, stroke may result from sev-

Table 14.1. Medical Therapies for Treatment of Acute Cerebral Infarction

Aminophylline	GM-1 gangliosides
Ancrod	Heparin
Anticerebral edema drugs	Hyperbaric oxygen
Corticosteroids	Hypervolemic
Glycerol	hemodilution
Mannitol	Low-molecular-weight
Nonosmotic diuretics	dextran
Anticonvulsants	Low-molecular-weight
Barbiturates	heparinoids
Calcium ion entry blockers	Naloxone
Nicardipine	Pentoxifylline
Nimodipine	Phenothiazines
Dimethyl sulfoxide	Streptokinase
Drug-induced hypertension	Supportive care
Fluosol™	Tissue plasminogen
Free-radical antagonists	activators
Glutamate antagonists	Urokinase

eral types of cerebral vascular abnormalities in vessels ranging from arterioles to large arteries. Unlike experimental animals, patients with cerebral infarction often have other serious illnesses, such as heart disease, chronic pulmonary disease, or diabetes mellitus, that complicate the management of cerebral infarction. Moreover, these patients may be taking medications that can alter the response to therapy. For all these reasons, promising treatments for acute cerebral infarction must be carefully evaluated in clinical studies to determine their efficacy in humans.

NATURAL HISTORY AND PROGNOSIS OF CEREBRAL INFARCTION

The response to any therapy must be evaluated against the natural history of the disease. The complexity of the variables that influence the course of cerebral infarction makes it difficult to interpret the results of therapeutic intervention. The onset of cerebral infarction is marked by the sudden occurrence or rapid evolution of focal neurologic signs. The deficits usually reach maximal intensity within a few minutes or hours but may progress over several days or a week (11). Approximately 10% to 15% of patients die within 1 week, primarily of neurologic causes such as cerebral edema; 15% to 20% die within 1 month, primarily of nonneurologic causes, including pneumonia, sepsis, pulmonary embolism, and myocardial infarction (MI) (19, 26, 65, 67, 71).

Virtually all patients show some neurologic improvement after cerebral infarction. No factors have been identified that predict the speed of recovery or the degree of improvement. Approximately 50% of survivors recover with minimal or no disability. A large number of patients, however, have severe deficits and are often institutionalized. Several variables influence the prognosis of patients with acute cerebral infarction. The 30-day mortality rate is highest among patients with cardiogenic cerebral embolism (65). The poor prognosis reflects the underlying heart disease as well as the possibility of multiple or recurrent cerebral vascular events, which may lead to larger brain injuries. Conversely, the 30-day mortality rate among patients with lacunar infarction due to small-vessel occlusion is quite low. Therefore, it would be more difficult to prove the value of any treatment in that group of patients. The prognosis of patients with atherothrombotic occlusions of large arteries is similar to that of patients with cardiogenic cerebral embolism. Strokes caused by nonatherosclerotic vasculopathies, such as fibromuscular dysplasia or arterial dissection, have a more benign course than those related to underlying atherosclerosis.

The location of the vascular event influences the outcome of therapy. The mortality rate is higher among patients with events in the posterior circulation than in those with hemispheric lesions (71). Residual neurologic deficits from a right hemi-spheric stroke are different from those caused by stroke in the left hemisphere. Depression occurs more frequently and may be more severe in patients with left hemispheric lesions (63). Isolated subcortical infarctions carry a much lower mortality rate than larger, lobar infarctions.

The type and severity of neurologic deficits provide certain prognostic information. The level of consciousness is the most important neurologic variable (23). Patients who are comatose after cerebral infarction have an extremely poor prognosis. Coma results from large brain stem infarctions, brain stem compression, elevated intracranial pressure (ICP), or compartmental shifts associated with cerebral edema. Coma due to a hemispheric stroke reflects a large injury that may contraindicate several types of therapy, such as anticoagulation. Demonstrating a therapeutic effect may be difficult in a comatose patient.

Motor deficits are the basis of several stroke assessment scales (Tables 14.2 to 14.6) (2, 12, 20, 23, 56). Several scales that are based on components of the neurologic examination have been developed. None of these scales is universally accepted, and many have not had extensive validation.

Complicating medical conditions also influence recovery. Heart disease, for example, may hamper rehabilitation and is

Table 14.2. West Haven Veterans Administration Hospital Scale for Stroke Evaluation[a]

	Evaluation scale	
Assessed variables	Grade	Neurologic status
Mental status	I	Transient ischemic attack
Aphasia	II	Mild mental status
Comprehension		symptoms; mild to
Expression		moderate focal
Motor function		symptoms
Sensory function	III	Mental status changes;
Pin stick		mild aphasia/motor
Position sense		signs
Double	IV	Depressed
simultaneous		consciousness;
stimulation		moderate aphasia/
Visual fields		motor signs; severe
		motor symptoms

[a]Adapted from Dove HG, Schneider KC, Wallace JD: Evaluating and predicting outcome of acute cerebral vascular accident. Stroke 15:858–864, 1984.

Table 14.3. Allen Scale: Calculation for Stroke Evaluation[a]

Clinical feature	Score
Starting score	40
Complete limb paralysis	subtract 12
Higher cortical deficits, hemiparesis, hemiplegia	subtract 10
Multiply age in years × 0.4	subtract product
Loss of consciousness at onset	subtract 9
Uncomplicated hemiparesis	add 8

Total above 0 = better prognosis
Total below 0 = worse prognosis

[a]Adapted from Allen CMC: Predicting the outcome of acute stroke. A prognostic scale. *J Neurol Neurosurg Psychiatry* 47:475–480, 1984.

the leading long-term cause of death among patients with stroke. Another variable that may affect the prognosis is the interval between the onset of symptoms and the initiation of therapy. Like acute MI, acute cerebral infarction requires urgent treatment; the first few hours are critical. Treatment initiated more than 24 hours after the onset of symptoms is unlikely to affect the evolution of stroke.

TREATMENT OF ACUTE CEREBRAL INFARCTION

Supportive Care

Supportive care is the foundation for any other medical therapy. Most supportive measures have not been scientifically tested but remain part of medical tradition. The components of supportive care are bed rest, oxygenation, hydration, nutrition, treatment of associated medical conditions, prevention or treatment of neurologic or medical complications, and rehabilitation. Bed rest is an established part of the acute care of a patient with cerebral infarction. Although bed rest for up to 1 week has been advocated, this seems excessive because it increases the risk of atelectasis, pneumonia, deep vein thrombosis, and pulmonary embolism. The amount of bed rest should be determined by the condition of the patient; many do not require any restriction in activity. Early ambulation can lower the risk of deep vein thrombosis (14); pneumatic stockings may also lower the risk of deep vein thrombosis in paretic limbs. Administration of low doses of heparin or heparinoids may further lower the risk of venous thromboembolism (14, 72).

The position of the patient in bed should be decided case by case. Keeping the head flat may help maintain adequate cerebral perfusion; elevating the head by no more than 30° may improve venous drainage. If increased ICP is a concern, the head of the bed should be elevated; otherwise, the bed should be kept horizontal. Patients with acute occlusions of the basilar or internal carotid artery should be kept horizontal.

Lack of tissue oxygen is the critical metabolic problem in acute cerebral infarction. Hypoxemia may potentiate the ischemic effects of the arterial occlusion. Although there is no proof that supplemental oxygen is beneficial, correction of hypoxemia appears to be a reasonable component of supportive care during the first 24 hours after a cerebral infarction. The airway of

Table 14.4. Oxbury Scale for Stroke Evaluation[a]

Assessed variables	Number of grades	Neurologic status	Grade
Consciousness	6	Alert	0
		Deep coma	5
Visual field defects	2	Absent	1
		Present	2
External ocular movements	2	Normal	0
		Abnormal	2
Limb movements	5	Normal	0
		Plegia	5

[a]Data from Oxbury JM, Greenhall RCD, Grainger KMR: Predicting outcome of stroke. Acute state after cerebral infarction. *Br Med J* 3:125–127, 1975.

Table 14.5. Canadian Neurological Scale for Stroke Evaluation[a]

Assessed variables	Evaluation scale	
	Neurologic status	Grade
Level of alertness[b]	Alert	3
	Drowsy	1.5
Orientation	Oriented	1
	Disoriented	0
Speech	Normal	1
	Expressive deficit	0.5
	Receptive	0
Facial weakness	None	0.5
	Present	0
If no comprehension deficit		
Proximal arm weakness	None	1.5
	Mild	1
	Significant	0.5
	Total	0
Distal arm weakness	None	1.5
	Mild	1
	Significant	0.5
	Total	0
Leg weakness	None	1.5
	Mild	1
	Significant	0.5
	Total	0
If comprehension impaired		
Face	Symmetrical	0.5
	Asymmetrical	0
Arms	Equal	1.5
	Unequal	0
Legs	Equal	1.5
	Unequal	0
		—Total score added—

[a] Adapted from Cote R, Hachinski VC, Shurvell BL, et al: The Canadian Neurological Scale. A preliminary study in acute stroke. *Stroke* 17:731–737, 1986.
[b] If the patient is comatose, the Glasgow Coma Scale is used.

an obtunded patient should be protected. Some critically ill patients require ventilatory assistance. Hyperventilation can help patients with signs of transtentorial herniation due to acute intracranial hypertension. Hyperbaric oxygen therapy has been proposed as an effective treatment for acute or progressing cerebral infarction (37, 52) (*see* Chapter 19, this volume), but its potential has not been carefully evaluated in a controlled trial.

Fluid and electrolyte balance must be carefully managed in patients with acute stroke. Although there is no proof that fluid restriction limits the development of cerebral edema, it is a traditional component of the management of patients with large cerebral infarctions. If fluids are re-stricted, the limitation should be modest (approximately 1,500 to 2,000 ml/day); severe restrictions should be avoided. Patients who are not at risk for intracranial hypertension should not have fluids limited. Most patients with severe strokes receive intravenous fluids during the first few days. Hypo-osmolar agents, such as 5% dextrose in water, may exacerbate cerebral edema and should be avoided. If normal saline is used, the patient should be observed for the development of congestive heart failure.

Maintaining nutrition is an essential component of long-term care but is less important during the acute phase of stroke. Patients in whom aspiration is a concern should not be fed during the first few

Table 14.6. National Institutes of Health Scale for Stroke Evaluation[a]

Assessed variables	Number of grades	Evaluation scale	
		Neurologic status	Grade
LOC[b]	4	Alert	0
		Coma	3
LOC questions	3	Normal	0
		Incorrect	2
LOC commands	3	Obeys	0
		Incorrect	2
Best gaze	3	Normal	0
		Forced deviation	2
Best visual	4	Normal	0
		Bilateral field cuts	3
Facial palsy	4	Normal	0
		Complete facial paresis	3
Best motor arm	5	Normal	0
		No movement	4
Best motor leg	5	Normal	0
		No movement	4
Limb ataxia	3	Absent	0
		Present bilaterally	2
Sensory	3	Normal	0
		Dense loss	2
Neglect	3	None	0
		Complete	2
Dysarthria	3	None	0
		Nearly unintelligible	2
Best language	4	Normal	0
		Mute	3

[a]From Brott T, Adams HP Jr, Olinger CP, et al: Developing measurements of acute cerebral infarction I. A reliable, valid, and brief clinical examination scale. *Stroke* 20:864–870, 1989.
[b]LOC = level of consciousness.

hours after cerebral infarction. In some animal models, hyperglycemia exacerbates ischemia (21, 60); combined with hypoxia, hyperglycemia may enhance anaerobic metabolism and lactic acidosis, which may result in more extensive brain injury (13). Cerebral infarction may be more severe in diabetic or hyperglycemic patients (7, 59), although an elevated blood glucose is also a stress response to stroke (15). Some clinical reports have not found a strong correlation between the blood glucose concentration or glycosylated hemoglobin and either the severity or the outcome of cerebral infarction (1, 34). It has been suggested that the blood sugar be vigorously lowered to low normal values (less than 100 mg/dl or 5.6 mmol/liter) in all patients with cerebral infarction, but this advice appears premature (59, 62). As with other acutely ill patients, the best approach is not to lower the blood glucose to hypoglycemic values.

TREATMENT OF CEREBRAL EDEMA

How to treat cerebral edema complicating acute cerebral infarction remains a subject of debate. Dexamethasone has been evaluated in several small series, with mixed results (6, 53). There is no evidence that larger doses of steroids are better than lower doses in ischemic brain edema (54). Osmotherapy acts only in areas where the blood–brain barrier is intact; therefore, any reduction in tissue water will occur primarily in areas of normal brain. Glycerol has been reported to be effective, but side effects (vomiting with oral doses and hemolysis with intravenous doses) limit its applicability (16, 49, 70). Urea is contraindicated because of the potential for postinfusion rebound.

Mannitol appears to be the best medical agent to control increased ICP complicating cerebral infarction. It has not been extensively evaluated in clinical trials and often is given only when a patient is deteriorating neurologically. Not surprisingly, it is difficult to prove the efficacy of mannitol in this setting. Mannitol should be given as a life-saving measure when a patient's level of consciousness becomes impaired. Mannitol should be combined with hyperventilation in patients with signs of transtentorial herniation. The usual regimen is a rapid intravenous infusion of 20% mannitol, followed by maintenance therapy of 0.25 g/kg intravenously every 4 to 6 hours (46, 48). The daily dose should not exceed 2 g/kg (46). The effects of mannitol begin within 20 minutes and persist for 4 to 6 hours. Measures to avoid a hyperosmolar state should be included if recurrent doses of mannitol are given; ICP monitoring may be useful (64).

Patients with massive cerebral edema after cerebral infarction might not respond to mannitol. Other options include barbiturate-induced coma or craniectomy (22). There is no proof that either therapy will be effective. Resection of necrotic tissue may be a life-saving procedure in cases of massive cerebellar infarction.

ANTICOAGULANTS

Anticoagulants have been prescribed to prevent neurologic deterioration in patients with acute cerebral infarction. Anticoagulation may help stop propagation of the intraarterial clot, lyse the clot, and avoid distal embolization, as well as maintain the patency of collateral vessels. The most widely used anticoagulant is heparin, a mixture of polysaccharides of various molecular weights (4,000 to 40,000 daltons) derived from animal tissues. Heparin increases the rate at which antithrombin III inhibits thrombin, activated clotting Factor X, and other serine proteases and also alters platelet function (73). Heparin

is believed to act by inhibiting conversion of prothombin to thrombin, and thus fibrinogen to fibrin; it also prevents platelet aggregation and thus prevents thrombus formation. The response to an intravenous bolus of heparin is almost immediate, and its effects can be reversed by protamine sulfate. Despite these attributes, which make it an ideal agent for treating progressing cerebral infarctions, heparin has substantial side effects (61).

The risk of intracranial hemorrage is the major limitation of heparin therapy for recent cerebral infarction. Infarcted brain tissue is susceptible to spontaneous hemorrhagic transformation; sequential computerized tomography (CT) studies have shown that bleeding can occur in 40% of cases (3, 39). The use of anticoagulants may increase the risk of hemorrhage. Advanced age, hypertension, or an extensive brain injury also increases the risk of bleeding during heparin therapy. High doses of heparin may cause intraspinal, adrenal, renal, or gastrointestinal hemorrhage (61). Treatment with heparin can also cause thrombocytopenia or the "white-clot" syndrome (61). Many of the side effects of heparin appear to be related to the antiplatelet aggregating effects of its components.

Heparin has been evaluated in several clinical trials but with conflicting results. Two trials in the 1960s indicated a beneficial effect for heparin (5, 17). In a more recent randomized study of patients with acute, stable, noncardiogenic strokes, Duke et al (24) found no benefit from the use of heparin. Similarly, in a small, uncontrolled study of patients with evolving stroke, Haley et al (31) could show no benefit from heparin. The therapeutic value of intravenous heparin for acute noncardiogenic or worsening cerebral infarction has not been established.

Anticoagulants may also have a role in preventing recurrent embolism in a patient with a recent, nonseptic, cardiogenic cerebral infarction (18, 25, 78); the risk of recurrent events nears 10% within 10 days of cerebral infarction (44). The Cerebral Embolism Study Group reported that heparin can be given safely and might lower the risk of recurrent stroke when given within a few days of cerebral infarction (18); however, this was a small study. Recently, Yatsu and Zivin (79) recommended that early anticoagulation be reserved for patients with mild neurologic deficits in whom CT scans do not show a hemorrhagic lesion. In patients with more severe deficits, heparin should be withheld for 3 to 5 days and then be given only if CT scans continue to demonstrate the absence of hemorrhage. Heparin should be given as a continuous intravenous infusion after a loading bolus dose; the usual regimen is 5,000 U, followed by 800 to 1,000 U/hour. The dose should be adjusted to maintain a partial thromboplastin time of 1.5 to 2 times control.

Fractionation of heparin leads to dissociation of its antithrombotic and anticoagulant actions. Low-molecular-weight heparins and heparinoids inhibit activated clotting Factor X (38, 73) but do not significantly affect platelets or thrombin. Heparinoids cause fewer bleeding complications than heparin and therefore appear to be safer. Several disorders that predispose patients to thrombosis have been treated successfully with heparinoids (33, 36). One study of heparinoids in patients with intracerebral hemorrhage and evidence of deep vein thrombosis or an intracardiac clot showed that these compounds could be given safely (69). Turpie et al (72) found that the heparinoid ORG 10172 is useful in preventing deep vein thrombosis in patients with recent stroke. Biller et al (8) reported that large-dose infusions of ORG 10172 appear safe in patients with acute or evolving cerebral infarction. The efficacy of heparinoids in reversing the evolution of cerebral infarction is under investigation.

The therapeutic response to oral anticoagulants may be delayed for more than 48 hours. Therefore, these drugs cannot be used to treat acute cerebral infarction. Their use is limited to patients at risk of recurrent cardiogenic embolism. The utility of long-term oral anticoagulant therapy to prevent second strokes in patients with atherosclerosis has not been established.

The role of antiplatelet aggregating agents and thrombolytic agents in treating acute cerebral infarction is discussed elsewhere in this volume (see Chapters 21 and 22, this volume).

THERAPIES THAT ALTER BLOOD VISCOSITY/RHEOLOGY

Cerebral blood flow is influenced by the viscosity of blood. Blood is a non-Newtonian fluid, so its viscosity increases rapidly as the rate of flow decreases. Viscosity is also affected by the hematocrit level, fibrinogen level, erythrocyte deformability, and platelet aggregation. In most patients with cerebral infarction, hematocrit is the major influence on blood viscosity. Indeed, Harrison et al (32) reported that the severity of cerebral infarction parallels the hematocrit levels. Lowering the hematocrit to low normal values (approximately 30% to 35%), can greatly reduce blood viscosity without affecting oxygen delivery to the brain (77). Lowering viscosity may increase blood flow, particularly in small-caliber vessels.

Hemodilution reduces viscosity and increases blood flow. It can be achieved by hypervolemic or isovolemic methods. Several regimens have been proposed, but the most elaborately developed is that outlined by Wood and Kee (77). Hemodilution with low-molecular-weight dextran has been evaluated in several clinical stroke trials; in some, venesection or vasopressors were included in the study protocol, but the results have been negative or inconclusive (28, 29, 41, 43, 47, 66, 68, 76). The efficacy of hemodilution with low-molecular-weight dextran is not yet proved.

Hydroxyethyl starch, albumin, human plasma protein fraction, and other intravenous colloid replacement fluids also can be used to accomplish hemodilution (35). Studies of hypervolemic hemodilution to treat ischemic symptoms caused by vasospasm in patients with aneurysmal subarachnoid hemorrhage suggest that such treatment may be useful (4, 42). However, hypervolemic hemodilution may be dangerous because congestive heart failure, MI, or increased cerebral edema can occur. Pentoxifylline, a drug that improves blood rheology and is effective in treating intermittent claudication, has not been found to be effective in patients with acute cerebral infarction (58). Perfluorohydrocarbons, especially Fluosol™ (Alpha Therapeutics, Los Angeles, CA), are blood substitutes that have the oxygen characteristics of hemoglobin and have been reported to improve outcome after experimental cerebral ischemia (57). Fluosol, however, has major side effects, in particular anaphylaxis, that limit its clinical usefulness.

THERAPIES THAT AFFECT CEREBRAL PERFUSION PRESSURE

Normal cerebral vascular autoregulation is lost in acute cerebral infarction. As a result, blood flows becomes directly dependent upon blood pressure (79). Lowering ICP improves cerebral perfusion pressure. Increasing mean arterial pressure (MAP) also increases cerebral perfusion pressure in areas where blood flow is critically low.

In the past, acute cerebral infarction was an indication for vigorous lowering of hypertensive blood pressures. An elevation of blood pressure can be a physiologic compensation to improve cerebral perfusion pressure and impaired blood flow (74). Institution of aggressive antihypertensive therapy may worsen the vascular event (9). Conversely, markedly elevated systemic blood pressures after an acute cerebral infarction are probably very dangerous and should be treated; high pressures may predispose to hemorrhagic transformation and increase the risk of cerebral edema. The most prudent approach appears to be restriction of antihypertensive drugs to those patients with severe hypertension (MAP greater than 130 torr) (9). Antihypertensive therapy should be used to control the blood pressure before administering anticoagulants or thrombolytic drugs. MAP should be lowered to 110 to 120 torr. Antihypertensive drugs that may be useful in this situation are nifedipine, labetalol, minoxidil, hydralazine, or angiotensin-converting enzyme inhibitors. If the patient's neurologic condition worsens

as the blood pressure drops, the dosage of the antihypertensive drug should be adjusted or discontinued (9). As the patient stabilizes or as ICP drops, the blood pressure usually returns toward normal. If not, antihypertensive therapy can be started later. Antihypertensive drugs, particularly those with a vasodilatory action, should be used with caution in a patient who has evidence of intracranial hypertension.

Because CBF becomes dependent on systemic blood pressure after acute cerebral infarction, inducing hypertension in a hypotensive or normotensive patient may improve collateral flow (75). To elicit a clinical response, MAP may need to be raised by at least 40 to 50 torr. Dopamine is the most common vasopressor given to patients with acute cerebral infarction. Although drug-induced hypertension has many potential benefits, it has not been extensively studied in cerebral infarction. The most frequent clinical use is for treating vasospasm after subarachnoid hemorrhage; it is usually combined with hypervolemic hemodilution (4, 42). Drug-induced hypertension may be dangerous in patients receiving anticoagulants or thrombolytic drugs. The potential complications of drug-induced hypertension are MI, cardiac arrhythmias, aggravation of cerebral edema, or hemorrhagic transformation of the cerebral infarction (42).

VASODILATORS AND VASOCONSTRICTORS

Evidence that vasodilators, such as papaverine, are of any value in acute cerebral infarction is lacking (50, 55). In one study (51), prostacyclin, a potent vasodilator and antiplatelet aggregating agent produced from endoperoxides by endothelial cells, showed potential efficacy in acute cerebral infarction. However, a randomized, controlled clinical trial failed to demonstrate any efficacy (40).

Aminophylline causes vasoconstriction of normal cerebral arteries (27, 30, 45). Constriction of normal arteries in patients with cerebral infarction might divert flow from normal areas of the brain to the already dilated vessels in the ischemic area. Anecdotal reports that aminophylline had a therapeutic effect led Britton et al (10) to conduct a small controlled trial of the drug in patients with acute cerebral infarction. No therapeutic effect could be demonstrated. This trial has been criticized for the long delay (average 40 to 46 hours) between the onset of symptoms and therapy. Seizures and cardiac arrhythmia are potential side effects.

OTHER THERAPIES

A variety of other experimental therapies have been examined in animal and clinical studies. Many of these therapies are discussed in detail in other chapters in this volume, including opiate antagonists (*see* Chapter 26), calcium channel blockers (*see* Chapter 25), excitotoxic antagonists (*see* Chapter 20), thrombolytic agents (*see* Chapter 22), anesthetics (*see* Chapter 24), free-radical scavengers (*see* Chapter 5), arachidonic acid cascade antagonists (*see* Chapter 27), and antiplatelet aggregating agents (*see* Chapter 21). Controlled clinical studies will be required to further assess the potential benefits of these therapies.

References

1. Adams HP Jr, Olinger CP, Marler JR, et al: Comparison of admission serum glucose concentration to neurological outcome in acute cerebral infarction. A study in patients given naloxone. *Stroke* 19:455–458, 1988.
2. Allen CMC: Predicting the outcome of acute stroke. A prognostic scale. *J Neurol Neurosurg Psychiatry* 47:475–480, 1984.
3. Allen GS, Ahn HS, Preziosi TJ, et al: Cerebral arterial spasm. A controlled trial of nimodipine in patients with subarachnoid hemorrhage. *N Engl J Med* 308:619–624, 1983.
4. Awad IA, Carter LP, Spetzler RF, et al: Clinical vasospasm after subarachnoid hemorrhage. Response to hypervolemic hemodilution and arterial hypertension. *Stroke* 18:365–372, 1987.
5. Baker RN: An evaluation of anticoagulant therapy in the treatment of cerebrovascular disease. Report of the Veterans Administration Cooperative Study of Atherosclerosis (Neurology Section). *Neurology* 11:132–138, 1961.
6. Bauer RB, Tellez H: Dexamethasone as treatment in cerebrovascular disease. 2. A controlled study in acute cerebral infarction. *Stroke* 4:547–555, 1973.
7. Berger L, Hakim AM: The association of hyperglycemia with cerebral edema in stroke. *Stroke* 17:865–871, 1986.
8. Biller J, Massey EW, Marler JR, et al: A dose escalation study of ORG 10172 (low-molecular-weight heparinoid) in stroke. *Neurology* 39:262–265, 1989.
9. Britton M, deFaire V, Helmers C: Hazards of therapy for excessive hypertension in acute stroke. *Acta Med Scand* 207:253–257, 1980.
10. Britton M, deFaire, V, Helmers C, et al: Lack of effect of theophylline on the outcome of acute cerebral infarction. *Acta Neurol Scand* 62:116–123, 1980.
11. Britton M, Roden A: Progression of stroke after arrival at hospital. *Stroke* 16:629–635, 1985.
12. Brott T, Adams HP Jr, Olinger CP, et al: Developing measurements of acute cerebral infarction. I. A reliable, valid, and brief clinical examination scale. *Stroke* 20:864–870, 1989.
13. Brott T, Haley EC, Levy DE, et al: Very early therapy for cerebral infarction with tissue plasminogen activator (tPA) (abstract). *Stroke* 19:133, 1988.
14. Buonanno F, Toole JF: Management of patients with established cerebral infarction. *Stroke* 12:7–16, 1981.
15. Candelise L, Landi G, Orazio EN, et al: Prognostic significance of hyperglycemia in acute stroke. *Arch Neurol* 432:661–663, 1985.
16. Cantore G, Guidetti B, Virno M: Oral glycerol for the reduction of intracranial pressure. *J Neurosurg* 21:278–283, 1964.
17. Carter AB: Anticoagulant treatment in progressing stroke. *Br Med J* 2:70–73, 1961.
18. Cerebral Embolism Study Group: Cardioembolic stroke, early anticoagulation and brain hemorrhage. *Arch Intern Med* 147:636–640, 1987.
19. Chambers BR, Norris JW, Shurvell BL, et al: Prognosis of acute stroke. *Neurology* 37:221–225, 1987.
20. Cote R, Hachinski VC, Shurvell BL, et al: The Canadian neurological scale. A preliminary study in acute stroke. *Stroke* 17:731–737, 1986.
21. de Courten-Myers GM, Schoolfield L, Myers RE: Effect of glucose pretreatment on experimental stroke outcome (abstract). *Stroke* 16:143, 1985.
22. Delashaw JB, Kassell NF, Vollmer DG, et al: Treatment of hemispheric cerebral infarction by hemicraniectomy (abstract). *Stroke* 19:130, 1988.
23. Dove HG, Schneider KC, Wallace JD: Evaluating and predicting outcome of acute cerebral vascular accident. *Stroke* 15:858–864, 1984.
24. Duke RJ, Bloch RF, Turpie AGG, et al: Intravenous heparin for the prevention of stroke progression in acute partial stable stroke. A randomized controlled trial. *Ann Intern Med* 105:825–828, 1986.
25. Furlan AJ, Cavalier SJ, Hobbs RE, et al: Hemorrhage and anticoagulation after non-septic embolic brain infarction. *Neurology* 32:280–282, 1982.
26. Garraway WM, Whisnant JP, Furlan AJ, et al: The declining incidence of stroke. *N Engl J Med* 300:449–452, 1979.
27. Geismar P Marquardsen J, Sylvest J: Controlled trial of intravenous aminophylline in acute cerebral infarction. *Acta Neurol Scand* 54:173–180, 1976.

28. Gilroy J, Barnhart MI, Meyers JS: Treatment of acute stroke with dextran 40. *JAMA* 210:293–298, 1969.

29. Gottstein U, Sedlmeyer I, Heuss A: Treatment of acute cerebral ischemia with low molecular dextran. Results of a retrospective study. *Dtsch Med Wochenschr* 101:223–227, 1976.

30. Gottstein U, Paulson OB: The effect of intracarotid aminophylline infusion on the cerebral circulation. *Stroke* 3:560–565, 1972.

31. Haley EC Jr, Kassell NF, Torner JC: Failure of heparin to prevent progression in progressing cerebral infarction. *Stroke* 19:10–14, 1988.

32. Harrison MJ, Pollock S, Kendall BE, et al: Effect of haematocrit on carotid stenosis and cerebral infarction. *Lancet* 2:114–115, 1981.

33. Harteberg J, Zimmermann R, Schwarz F, et al: Treatment of heparin-induced thrombocytopenia with thrombosis by a new heparinoid. *Lancet* 1:986–987, 1983.

34. Helgason CM, Kuhmen D: The significance of glycosylated hemoglobin for stroke outcome (abstract). *Stroke* 18:296, 1987.

35. Hemodilution in Stroke Study Group: Effect of hypervolemic hemodilution treatment of acute stroke (abstract). *Stroke* 19:150, 1988.

36. Henny CP, TenCate H, TenCate JW, et al: Use of a new heparinoid as anticoagulant during acute hemodialysis of patients with bleeding complications. *Lancet* 1:890–893, 1983.

37. Heyman A, Saltzman H, Whalen RE: Use of hyperbaric oxygen in the treatment of cerebral ischemia and infarction. *Circulation* 33(Suppl II):2–20, 1966.

38. Holmer E, Lindahl U, Bäckström G, et al: Anticoagulant activities and effects on platelets of a heparin fragment with high affinity for antithrombin. *Thromb Res* 18:861–869, 1980.

39. Hornig CR, Dorndorf W, Agnoli AL: Hemorrhagic cerebral infarction—a prospective study. *Stroke* 17:179–185, 1986.

40. Hsu CY, Faught RE, Furlan AJ, et al: Intravenous prostacyclin in acute nonhemorrhagic stroke: A placebo-controlled, double-blind trial. *Stroke* 18:352–358, 1987.

41. Italian Acute Stroke Study Group: Hemodilution in acute stroke. Results of the Italian hemodilution trial. *Lancet* 1:318–321, 1988.

42. Kassell NF, Peerless SJ, Durward QJ, et al: Treatment of ischemic deficits from vasospasm with intravascular volume expansion and induced arterial hypertension. *Neurosurgery* 11:337–343, 1982.

43. Kaste M, Fogelholm R, Waltimo O: Combined dexamethasone and low-molecular-weight dextran in acute brain infarction. Double-blind study. *Br Med J* 2:1409–1410, 1976.

44. Koller RL: Recurrent embolic cerebral infarction and anticoagulation. *Neurology* 32:283–285, 1982.

45. Magnussen I, Hoedt-Rasmussen K: The effect of intraarterial administered aminophylline on cerebral hemodynamics in man. *Acta Neurol Scand* 55:131–136, 1977.

46. Marshall LF, Smith RW, Rauscher LA, et al: Mannitol dose requirements in brain-injured patients. *J Neurosurg* 48:169–172, 1978.

47. Matthews WB, Oxbury JM, Grainger KMR, et al: A blind controlled trial of dextran 40 in the treatment of ischaemic stroke. *Brain* 99:193–206, 1976.

48. McGraw CP, Howard G: Effect of mannitol on increased intracranial pressure. *Neurosurgery* 13:269–271, 1983.

49. Meyer JS, Fukuuchi Y, Shimazu K, et al: Effect of intravenous infusion of glycerol on hemispheric blood flow and metabolism in patients with acute cerebral infarction. *Stroke* 3:168–180, 1972.

50. Meyer JS, Gotoh F, Gilroy J, et al: Improvement in brain oxygenation and clinical improvements in patients with strokes treated with papaverine hydrochloride. *JAMA* 194:957–961, 1965.

51. Miller VT, Coull BM, Yatsu FM, et al: Prostacyclin infusion in acute cerebral infarction. *Neurology* 34:1431–1435, 1984.

52. Neubauer RA: Hyperbaric oxygen treatment and stroke. *JAMA* 246:2574, 1981.

53. Norris JW: Steroid therapy in acute cerebral infarction. *Arch Neurol* 33:69–71, 1976.

54. Norris JW, Hachinski V: High dose steroid treatment in cerebral infarction. *Br Med J* 292:21–23, 1986.

55. Olesen J, Paulson OB: The effect of intra-arterial papaverine on the regional cerebral blood flow in patients with stroke or intracranial tumor. *Stroke* 2:148–159, 1971.

56. Oxbury JM, Greenhall RCD, Grainger KMR: Predicting outcome of stroke. Acute stage after cerebral infarction. *Br Med J* 3:125–127, 1975.

57. Peerless SJ, Ishikawa R, Hunter IG, et al: Protective effect of Fluosol-DA in acute cerebral ischemia. *Stroke* 12:558–563, 1981.

58. Pentoxifylline Study Group: Pentoxifylline (PTX) in acute ischemic stroke (abstract). *Stroke* 18:298, 1987.

59. Pulsinelli WA, Levy DE, Sigsbee B, et al: Decreased damage after ischemic stroke in patients with hyperglycemia with or without established diabetes mellitus. *Am J Med* 74:540–544, 1983.

60. Pulsinelli WA, Weldman S, Rawlinson D, et al: Moderate hyperglycemia augments ischemic brain damage. A neuropathologic study in the rat. *Neurology* 32:1239–1246, 1982.

61. Ramirez-Lassepas M, Quinnones MR: Heparin for stroke: Hemorrhagic complications and risk factors for intracerebral hemorrhage. *Neurology* 34:114–117, 1984.

62. Rehncrona S: Brain acidosis. *Ann Emerg Med* 14:770–776, 1985.

63. Robinson RG, Price TR: Post-stroke depressive disorders. A follow-up study of 103 patients. *Stroke* 13:635–641, 1982.

64. Ropper AH, Kennedy SK, Zervas NT: *Neurological and Neurosurgical Intensive Care*. Baltimore, University Park Press, 1983.

65. Sacco RL, Wolf PA, Kannell WB, et al: Survival and recurrence following stroke. The Framingham Study. *Stroke* 13:290–295, 1982.

66. Scandinavian Stroke Study Group: Multicenter trial of hemodilution in acute ischemic stroke. I. Results in the total patient population. *Stroke* 18:691–699, 1987.

67. Silver FL, Norris JW, Lewis AJ, et al: Early mortality following stroke. A prospective review. *Stroke* 15:492–496, 1984.
68. Strand T, Asplund K, Eriksson S, et al: A randomized controlled trial of hemodilution therapy in acute ischemic stroke. *Stroke* 15:980–989, 1984.
69. TenCate H, Henny CP, Buller HR, et al: Use of a heparinoid in patients with hemorrhagic stroke and thromboembolic disease. *Ann Neurol* 15:268–270, 1984.
70. Tourtellotte WW, Reinglass JL, Newkirk TA: Cerebral dehydration action of glycerol. I. Historical aspects with emphasis on the toxicity and intravenous administration. *Clin Pharmacol Ther* 13:159–171, 1972.
71. Turney TM, Garraway WM, Whisnant JP, et al: The natural history of hemispheric and brainstem infarction in Rochester, Minnesota. *Stroke* 15:790–794, 1984.
72. Turpie AG, Levine MN, Hirsh J, et al: Double-blind randomised trial of ORG 10172 low-molecular-weight heparinoid in prevention of deep-vein thrombosis in thrombotic stroke. *Lancet* 1:523–529, 1987.
73. Verstraete M, Vermylen J: *Thrombosis.* Oxford, Pergamon Press, 1984.
74. Wallace JD, Levy LL: Blood pressure after stroke. *JAMA* 246:2177–2180, 1981.
75. Wise G, Sutter R, Burkholder J: The treatment of brain ischemia with vasopressor drugs. *Stroke* 3:135–140, 1972.
76. Wood JH, Fleischer AS: Observations during hypervolemic hemodilution of patients with acute focal cerebral ischemia. *JAMA* 248:2999–3004, 1982.
77. Wood JH, Kee DB Jr: Hemorheology of the cerebral circulation in stroke. *Stroke* 16:765–772, 1985.
78. Yatsu FM, Hart RG, Mohr JP, et al: Anticoagulation of embolic strokes of cardiac origin. An update. *Neurology* 38:314–316, 1988.
79. Yatsu FM, Zivin J: Hypertension in acute ischemic strokes. Not to treat. *Arch Neurol* 42:999–1000, 1985.

CHAPTER FIFTEEN

Cardiac Causes of Stroke

Antonio V. Salgado, M.D.
Anthony J. Furlan, M.D.

Cardiogenic embolism is a major cause of brain infarction. In the Harvard Stroke Registry, 20% of brain infarcts occurred in patients with an identified cardiac source of emboli (57). Traditionally, the diagnosis of cardiogenic embolic stroke has been considered in any patient with a cardiac source of emboli who has a focal neurologic deficit that occurs suddenly and is maximal at or near its onset. Additional clues include age below 45 years; absence of risk factors for atherosclerosis; rapid resolution of the neurologic deficit; certain localized deficits, such as Wernicke's aphasia, monoparesis, or isolated hemianopsia; and a history of stroke in a different vascular distribution.

Unfortunately, the cause of stroke cannot be determined from the clinical presentation alone (9, 45, 65, 70). Even the demonstration of a cardiac source of emboli does not necessarily establish a diagnosis of cardiogenic embolic stroke. Many patients, especially the elderly, have coexistent carotid artery disease (8). Diagnostic tests such as computerized tomography (CT), cerebral angiography, and two-dimensional echocardiography may clarify the etiology of the symptoms, particularly when evaluated in the context of the clinical history (Table 15.1).

CARDIAC CAUSES OF EMBOLISM

Cardiogenic cerebral vascular embolism may be caused by disorders affecting the myocardium, heart valves, or heart rhythm; or it may occur during or after invasive procedures, such as coronary artery bypass grafting, percutaneous transluminal coronary angioplasty, and cardiac catheterization (Table 15.2).

Table 15.1. Predictive Value of Clinical and Diagnostic Findings in the Diagnosis of Cardiogenic Embolism[a]

Findings	Likelihood of embolism	
	Present (percent)	Absent (percent)
Potential cardiac source	56	1
Prior transient ischemic attack	5	21
Maximal deficit	20	7
Onset while awake	19	10
Hemorrhagic infarct on computerized tomographic scan	50	15

[a]Data from Hart RG: Prevention and treatment of cardioembolic stroke. In Furlan AJ (ed): *The Heart and Stroke*. New York, Springer-Verlag, 1987, pp 117–138.

Myocardial Disorders

About 3% of patients who have a myocardial infarction (MI) subsequently have a stroke (4, 77). In 85% of those patients, the stroke occurs in the first month after the MI (52, 77). Up to 70% of patients who have a stroke after MI die within 1 year (19, 52). Large anterior wall infarcts, septal involvement, and congestive heart failure increase the risk of cerebral embolism after acute MI (4, 77). There is some evidence that treatment with anticoagulants may lower the risk of embolism in selected patients with acute MI (25, 82, 84).

Ventricular dyskinesia or aneurysm after MI predisposes to local thrombus formation. The long-term risk of embolism from ventricular mural thrombus appears to be low (5%) and is not reduced by treatment with anticoagulants (66, 73).

Disorders of the Myocardium
  Acute myocardial infarction
  Ventricular dyskinesia
  Cardiomyopathies
  Atrial myxoma
  Paradoxical embolism
Disorders of the Heart Valves
  Rheumatic valvular disease
  Mitral valve prolapse
  Mitral annulus calcification
  Infective endocarditis
  Nonbacterial thrombotic endocarditis
  Prosthetic heart valves
Disorders of Heart Rhythm
  Atrial fibrillation
  Sick sinus syndrome
Diagnostic and Therapeutic Cardiac Procedures
  Cardiac catheterization
  Percutaneous transluminal coronary angioplasty
  Coronary artery bypass graft surgery

Disorders Affecting the Heart Valves

Rheumatic heart disease usually affects the mitral valve, causing it to become deformed, fibrotic, and, finally, calcified. Mitral stenosis and mitral insufficiency combined with atrial dilatation and atrial fibrillation are associated with a 20% risk of embolism, usually to the brain (1). The incidence of cerebral embolism in patients with rheumatic mitral stenosis is 3% to 4% per year (21). The risk of stroke is 17-fold greater in patients with atrial fibrillation and mitral stenosis than in matched control subjects (83).

Prosthetic heart valves are likely sources of cerebral emboli (33). Even when anticoagulants are taken, there is a 4% per year risk of embolism from mitral valves and a 2% per year risk from aortic valves (12, 27, 64). Patients with mitral bioprostheses, regardless of whether they take anticoagulants, have a 1% to 2% per year risk of cerebral embolic complications (39, 58).

Mitral valve prolapse is present in 6% of the normal population. Although it is a major cause of stroke in patients under age 45, the overall incidence of stroke from mitral valve prolapse is low (estimated 1/5,000 per year) (3, 46). Therefore, other causes of stroke should be sought in patients with mitral valve prolapse who are older than 45 years of age (70).

It is difficult to establish a cause-and-effect relationship between calcification of the mitral annulus and embolic stroke. In one study of 63 patients with mitral annular calcification, two patients had transient ischemic attacks (TIAs) and three had strokes during a mean follow-up of 3 years (36). Since atherosclerosis and atrial fibrillation are common in patients with mitral annular calcification, it is often difficult to unequivocally implicate mitral annulus calcification as the cause of stroke (36).

Infective endocarditis causes neurologic complications in 30% to 40% of patients. Strokes and TIAs account for more than 50% and mycotic aneurysms for approximately 5% of the neurologic complications (51, 63), regardless of whether the valve is native (34%) or prosthetic (36%) (69).

Cardiomyopathies are associated with stroke in 15% of patients due either to thrombus formation or to associated arrythmias such as atrial fibrillation (35, 40). The risk of stroke is higher in patients with dilated rather than restrictive cardiomyopathies (5, 35, 37, 42).

Atrial myxoma is a rare pedunculated, gelatinous, and friable tumor that usually causes symptoms of polymyalgia rheumatica or cardiac outflow obstruction. In 20% of patients, however, a fragment of tumor or local thrombus causes an embolic stroke (71, 72). Tumor emboli may invade the vascular wall or the brain, resulting in aneurysm, parenchymal metastases, or hematoma (24, 32, 62).

Paradoxical embolism is being recognized with increased frequency as a cause of cerebral embolism (17, 50, 55). Paradoxical cerebral emboli occur as a result of a patent foramen ovale, an atrial septal defect, or, rarely, a pulmonary arteriovenous fistula (68, 74). The diagnosis should be considered in any stroke patient who has evidence of (a) venous thrombosis; (b) pulmonary embolism; or (c) right-to-left cardiac shunt and systemic arterial embolism. A history of focal neurologic deficit after Valsalva's maneuver also suggests a paradoxical embolus.

Staphylococcus endocarditis carries a greater risk of neurologic complications and a higher mortality rate than endocarditis caused by other infective organisms (69).

Nonbacterial thrombotic endocarditis is a rare condition seen most often in patients with cancer (particularly adenocarcinoma of the lung and gastrointestinal tract), debilitating diseases such as uremia and lupus (6, 11, 53), or acquired immunodeficiency syndrome (54, 76). In these patients, stroke is caused by the breakdown and embolization of sterile vegetations, which are usually too small to be detected by two-dimensional echocardiography. These patients may also have disseminated intravascular coagulation, which may cause brain hemorrhage or vascular occlusion (43, 67).

Disorders of Heart Rhythm

Nonvalvular atrial fibrillation is the most common cause of cardiogenic embolic stroke. The risk of stroke is six times greater in patients with nonvalvular atrial fibrillation than in normal control subjects and 17 times greater in patients with rheumatic atrial fibrillation (83). Nonvalvular atrial fibrillation increases in prevalence with age; therefore, atherosclerosis is often present as well. Embolism occurs most frequently at the onset of fibrillation.

There appears to be a relationship between sick sinus syndrome and the development of global cerebral ischemia (30). However, strokes in patients with sick sinus syndrome are rare and are probably related to other types of cardiac dysrhythmias or atherosclerosis.

Invasive Intracardiac Procedures

Stroke occurs in 5% of patients undergoing coronary artery bypass graft surgery (CABG), although only 2% of postoperative strokes are severe (10). In most cases, the stroke is caused by embolism; however, atherosclerosis, hypotension, and other factors need to be excluded. Most patients with asymptomatic carotid stenosis or occlusion are not at increased risk during CABG (34).

Embolic stroke occurs in less than 1% of patients who undergo cardiac catheterization (23) or percutaneous transluminal coronary angioplasty (38).

DIAGNOSIS OF CARDIOGENIC EMBOLIC STROKE

Occasionally, the history, physical examination, and routine laboratory workup can identify a cardiac source of emboli in stroke patients. In most cases, however, additional studies are required.

CT scans of the brain may show one or more hypodense lesions, usually in the distribution of the middle cerebral artery (MCA). In 3% to 5% of patients with embolic brain infarcts, CT brain scans obtained within 48 hours after the stroke show hemorrhage, but this finding is not specific (14) (Fig. 15.1).

Cerebral angiography may show occlusion or delayed perfusion, usually in one of the branches of the MCA. In many patients with embolic occlusions, the occluded vessel recanalizes; thus, the likelihood of finding an angiographic abnormality is greater if the study is done within the first hours after the stroke (Fig. 15.2).

Holter electrocardiographic monitoring may show a variety of dysrhythmias in patients with cerebral ischemia. Occasionally an unsuspected dysrhythmia that pre-

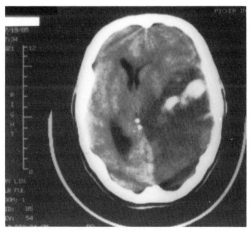

Figure 15.1. Noncontrast CT scan shows a large hemorrhagic brain infarct caused by cardiogenic embolism of the middle cerebral artery.

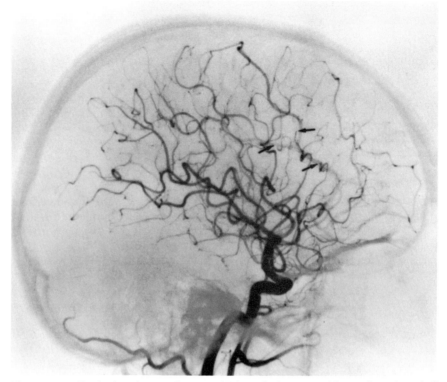

Figure 15.2.   Cerebral angiogram shows multiple occlusions caused by cardiogenic emboli.

disposes to stroke, such as paroxysmal atrial fibrillation, will be found. It might be difficult to determine if the findings on prolonged monitoring are the cause or the result of the stroke (56). Two-dimensional echocardiography should be performed in patients with unexplained strokes, especially in patients under 45 years of age and in those with signs or symptoms of heart disease. Echocardiography may be helpful in identifying mural or valvular thrombi or vegetations, mitral valve prolapse, and mitral annulus calcification.

Newer techniques, such as contrast echocardiography, transesophageal echocardiography, and magnetic resonance (MR) imaging of the heart, may also help to diagnose a cardiac cause of stroke. Contrast echocardiography seems to be as sensitive as cardiac catheterization in identifying a right-to-left shunt (40, 80). MR imaging of the heart can demonstrate left ventricular thrombus, aneurysms (47), and intracardiac neoplasms (41).

TREATMENT OF CARDIOGENIC EMBOLIC INFARCTION

Acute Anticoagulation and Thrombolysis

Since embolic strokes are often hemorrhagic (14) (Fig. 15.3), the risk of producing a clinically significant brain hematoma by early treatment with anticoagulants should be weighed against the risk of recurrent embolization. About 10% to 13% of patients have a recurrent embolism within 2 weeks after cardiogenic embolic stroke (14, 26). However, 20% of patients with large embolic infarcts who receive immediate treatment with anticoagulants will experience clinical worsening associated with brain hemorrhage; this risk exceeds the risk of early recurrent embolism (15, 16). The Cerebral Embolism Study

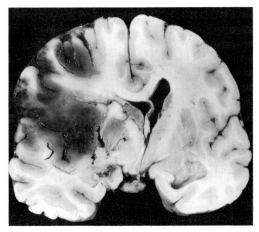

Figure 15.3. Gross brain specimen from a patient with a hemorrhagic infarct. Multiple petechiae are seen throughout the infarcted area.

Group and the Cerebral Embolism Task Force recommend anticoagulation for small- to moderate-sized infarcts if CT scans performed 24 to 48 hours after the onset of stroke show no blood. Patients with large infarcts should not receive anticoagulants for at least 7 days (15, 16). In rare circumstances, treatment with heparin has been safely continued despite CT evidence of hemorrhagic infarction (58, 60).

The optimal level of anticoagulation with heparin has not been defined. Heparin should be given by constant intravenous infusion at a rate of 300 to 400 U/kg/24 hours or to maintain the activated partial thromboplastin time at 1.5 to 2 times control. An initial intravenous bolus injection should not be given.

A new thrombolytic agent, tissue plasminogen activator, has the ability to dissolve blood clots and therefore recanalize obstructed vessels (20, 44, 78, 81). Its use in patients with cerebral ischemia, including those with cardiogenic embolic strokes, is under clinical investigation. Also under investigation are heparinoids—small fragments of the heparin molecule that retain antithrombotic effect and may be associated with lower bleeding risks (7, 13).

Long-Term Therapy

Antiplatelet therapy with aspirin is the initial treatment in patients with mitral valve prolapse and stroke. Dipyridamole may provide an additional protective effect against embolism when combined with warfarin sodium in patients with prosthetic heart valves (18, 22). The role of antiplatelet treatment in other cardiac conditions that place patients at increased risk of embolic stroke is unclear or of no proven benefit. In patients with atrial fibrillation, warfarin is usually withheld until embolism occurs. However, a recent study found warfarin to be effective in primary stroke prevention in patients with atrial fibrillation (61). Treatment with warfarin effectively prevents embolism in patients with rheumatic valvular disease (2, 31) and mechanical valves (27, 32).

Chronic anticoagulation with warfarin sodium often has major hemorrhagic complications; among patients over age 64, the risk of brain hemorrhage is 1% per year (28, 29, 59, 75, 79) and the risk of systemic hemorrhage in patients anticoagulated for a variety of reasons is 2% to 4% per year (29, 75). The current recommendation is to use less intensive anticoagulation that maintains a prothrombin time of 1.25 to 1.5 times control levels (48, 49).

References

1. Abernathy WS, Willis PW: Thromboembolic complications of rheumatic heart disease. *Cardiovasc Clin* 5:131–135, 1973.
2. Adams GF, Merrett JD, Hutchinson WM, et al: Cerebral embolism and mitral stenosis: Survival with and without anticoagulants. *J Neurol Neurosurg Psychiatry* 37:378–383, 1974.
3. Barnett HJM: Embolism in mitral valve prolapse. *Ann Rev Med* 33:489–507, 1982.
4. Bean WB: Infarction of the heart. III. Clinical course and morphological findings. *Ann Intern Med* 12:71–94, 1938.
5. Becker BJP, Chatgidakis CB, Van Lingen B: Cardiovascular collagenosis with parietal endocardial thrombosis. *Circulation* 7:345, 1953.
6. Biller J, Challa VR, Toole JF, et al: Nonbacterial thrombotic endocarditis. *Arch Neurol* 39:95–98, 1982.
7. Biller J, Massey EW, Adams HP, et al: A dose escalation study of ORG 10172 (low-molecular-weight heparinoid) in the treatment of acute cerebral infarction (abstract). *Ann Neurol* 222:159, 1987.
8. Bogousslavsky J, Hachinski VC, Boughner DR, et al: Cardiac and arterial lesions in carotid transient ischemic attacks. *Arch Neurol* 43:223–228, 1984.
9. Bogousslavsky J, Hachinski VC, Boughner DR, et al: Clinical predictors of cardiac and arterial

lesions in carotid transient ischemic attacks. *Arch Neurol* 43:229–233, 1986.

10. Breuer AC, Furlan AJ, Hanson M, et al: Central nervous system complications of coronary artery bypass graft surgery: Prospective analysis of 421 patients. *Stroke* 14:682–687, 1983.

11. Bryan CS: Nonbacterial thrombotic endocarditis with malignant tumors. *Am J Med* 46:787–793, 1969.

12. Burckhart D, Hoffman A, Vogt S, et al: Clinical evaluation of the St. Jude mechanical heart valve prosthesis. *J Thorac Cardiovasc Surg* 88:432–438, 1984.

13. Cate HT, Henny CP, Buller HR, et al: Use of a heparinoid in patients with hemorrhagic stroke and thromboembolic disease. *Ann Neurol* 15:268–270, 1984.

14. Cerebral Embolism Study Group: Immediate anticoagulation of embolic stroke: A randomized trial. *Stroke* 14:668–676, 1983.

15. Cerebral Embolism Study Group: Immediate anticoagulation of embolic stroke. Brain hemorrhage and management options. *Stroke* 15:779–789, 1984.

16. Cerebral Embolism Task Force: Cardiogenic brain embolism. *Arch Neurol* 43:71–84, 1986.

17. Cheng TO: Paradoxical embolism: A diagnostic challenge and its detection during life. *Circulation* 53:565–569, 1976.

18. Cheseboro JH, Fuster V, Elveback LR, et al: Trial of combined warfarin plus dipyridamole or aspirin therapy in prosthetic heart valve replacement: Danger of aspirin compared with dipyridamole. *Am J Cardiol* 51:1537–1541, 1983.

19. Chin PL: Relationship between acute stroke and myocardial infarction in the elderly. *Internal Medicine* 3:45–52, 1982.

20. Collen D, Topol EJ, Tiefenbrum AJ, et al. Coronary thrombolysis with recombinant human tissue-type plasminogen activator: A prospective randomized placebo controlled trial. *Circulation* 70:1012–1017, 1984.

21. Coulshed N, Epstein EJ, McKendrick CS, et al: Systemic embolism in mitral valve disease. *Br Heart J* 32:26–34, 1970.

22. Dale J, Myhre E, Stortstein O, et al: Prevention of arterial thromboembolism with acetylsalicylic acid: A controlled clinical study in patients with aortic ball valves. *Am Heart J* 94:101–111, 1977.

23. Dawson DM, Fischer EG: Neurologic complications of cardiac catheterization. *Neurology* 27:496–497, 1977.

24. DeSousa AL, Muller J, Campbell RL, et al: Atrial myxoma: A review of neurological complications, metastases and recurrences. *J Neurol Neurosurg Psychiatry* 41:1119–1124, 1978.

25. Drapkin A, Mersky C: Anticoagulant therapy after acute myocardial infarction: Relation of therapeutic benefit to patient's age, sex and severity of infarction. *JAMA* 222:541–549, 1972.

26. Easton JD, Sherman DG: Management of cerebral embolism of cardiac origin. *Stroke* 11:433–442, 1980.

27. Edmunds LH: Thromboembolic complications of current cardiac valvular prosthesis. *Ann Thorac Surg* 34:96–106, 1982.

28. EPSIM Research Group: A controlled comparison of aspirin and oral anticoagulants in prevention of death after myocardial infarction. *N Engl J Med* 307:701–708, 1982.

29. Erickson SE, Link H: Evaluation of anticoagulants in patients with cerebral infarction with slight to moderate neurologic deficit. *Acta Neurol Scand* 68:96–106, 1983.

30. Fairfax AJ, Lambert CD, Leatham A: Systemic embolism in chronic sinoatrial disorders. *N Engl J Med* 295:190, 1983.

31. Fleming HA, Bailey SM: Mitral valve disease, systemic embolism and anticoagulants. *Postgrad Med J* 47:599–604, 1971.

32. Frank RA, Shalen PR, Harvey DG, et al: Atrial myxoma with intellectual decline and cerebral growths on CT scan. *Ann Neurol* 5:396–400, 1979.

33. Friedli B, Aerichide N, Grondi P, et al: Thromboembolic complications of heart valve prostheses. *Am Heart J* 81:702–708, 1971.

34. Furlan AJ, Craciun AR: Risk of stroke during coronary artery bypass graft surgery in patients with internal carotid artery disease documented by angiography. *Stroke* 16:797–799, 1985.

35. Furlan AJ, Craciun AR, Raju NR, et al: Cerebrovascular complications with idiopathic hypertrophic subaortic stenosis. *Stroke* 15:282–284, 1984.

36. Furlan AJ, Craciun AR, Salcedo EE, et al: Risk of stroke in patients with mitral annulus calcification. *Stroke* 15:801–803, 1984.

37. Fuster V, Gersh BJ, Guiliani ER, et al: The natural history of idiopathic dilated cardiomyopathy. *Am J Cardiol* 47:525–531, 1981.

38. Galbraith C, Salgado E, Furlan AJ, et al: Cerebrovascular complications of percutaneous transluminal coronary angioplasty. *Stroke* 17:616–619, 1986.

39. Gallo I, Ruiz B, Duran CG: Isolated mitral valve replacement with the Hancock porcine bioprosthesis in rheumatic heart disease: Analysis of 213 operative survivors followed up 4.5 to 8.5 years. *Am J Cardiol* 53:173–181, 1984.

40. Ginzton LE, French W, Mena I: Combined contrast echocardiography and radionuclide diagnosis of atrial septal defect: Accuracy of the technique and analysis of erroneous diagnosis. *Am J Cardiol* 53:1639–1642, 1984.

41. Go RT, O'Donnel JK, Underwood DA, et al: Comparison of gated cardiac MRI and 2D echocardiography of intracardiac neoplasms. *AJR* 145:21–25, 1985.

42. Gottdiener JS, Gay JA, Van Voorhees L, et al: Frequency and embolic potential of left ventricular thrombus in dilated cardiomyopathy: 2D echocardiography. *Am J Cardiol* 52:1281–1285, 1983.

43. Graus F, Rogers LR, Posner JB: Cerebrovascular complications in patients with cancer. *Medicine* 64:16–35, 1985.

44. Grossbard EB, Gold H, Tiefenbrum A, et al: Coronary thrombolysis with recombinant human tissue-type plasminogen activator. *Circulation* 70 (Suppl II):11–27, 1984.

45. Hart RG: Prevention and treatment of cardioembolic stroke. In Furlan AJ (ed): *The Heart and Stroke* New York, Springer-Verlag, 1987, pp 117–138.

46. Hart RG, Easton JD: Mitral valve prolapse and cerebral infarction. *Stroke* 18:429–430, 1982.

47. Higgins CB, Lanzer P, Stark D, et al: Imaging by

nuclear magnetic resonance in patients with chronic ischemic heart disease. *Circulation* 69:523–531, 1984.

48. Hirsh J, Levine M: Therapeutic range for the control of oral anticoagulant therapy. *Arch Neurol* 43:1162–1164, 1986.

49. Hull R, Hirsh J, Jay R, et al: Different intensities of oral anticoagulant therapy in treatment of proximal vein thrombosis. *N Engl J Med* 307:1676–1680, 1980.

50. Jones HR, Caplan LR, Come PC, et al: Cerebral emboli of paradoxical origin. *Ann Neurol* 13:314–319, 1983.

51. Jones HR, Siekert RG, Geraci JE: Neurologic manifestations of bacterial endocarditis. *Ann Intern Med* 71:21–28, 1969.

52. Komrad MS, Coffey KS, McKinnis R, et al: Myocardial infarction and stroke. *Neurology* 34:1403–1409, 1984.

53. Kosiker JC, Maclean JM, Sumi SJ: Cerebral embolism, marantic endocarditis and cancer. *Arch Neurol* 33:260–264, 1976.

54. Levy RM, Bredesen DE, Rosenblum ML: Neurologic manifestations of the acquired immunodeficiency syndrome (AIDS): Experience at UCSF and review of the literature. *J Neurosurg* 62:475–495, 1985.

55. Meister SG, Grossman W, Dexter L, et al: Paradoxical embolism. Diagnosis during life. *Am J Med* 53:292–298, 1972.

56. Meyers MG, Norris JW, Hachinsky VC, et al: Cardiac sequelae of acute stroke. *Stroke* 13:838–842, 1982.

57. Mohr JP, Caplan LR, Melski JW, et al: Stroke registry: A prospective study. *Neurology* 28:754–762, 1978.

58. Nunez L, Aguado MG, Larrea JL, et al: Prevention of thromboembolism using aspirin after mitral valve replacement with porcine bioprosthesis. *Ann Thorac Surg* 37:84–87, 1984.

59. Olson JE: Recent advances in the treatment of cerebrovascular disorders. *Acta Neurol Scand* (Suppl) 62:77–95, 1980.

60. Ott BR, Zamani A, Kleefield J, et al: The clinical spectrum of hemorrhagic infarct. *Stroke* 17:630–637, 1986.

61. Petersen P, Boysen G, Godtfredsen J, et al: Placebo-controlled randomized trial of warfarin and aspirin for prevention of thromboembolic complications in chronic atrial fibrillation. The Copenhagen AF ASAK study. *Lancet* 1:175–179, 1989.

62. Price DL, Harris JL, New PFJ, et al: Cardiac myxoma. A clinicopathologic and angiographic study. *Arch Neurol* 23:558–567, 1970.

63. Pruit AA, Rubin RH, Karchmer AW: Neurologic complications of bacterial endocarditis. *Medicine* 57:329–343, 1978.

64. Rahimtoola SH: Valvular heart disease: A perspective. *J Am Coll Cardiol* 1:199–215, 1983.

65. Ramirez-Lassepas M, Cipolle RJ, Bjok RJ, et al: Is there a neurologic profile for embolic stroke? *Arch Neurol* 44:87–89, 1987.

66. Reeder GS, Lengyel M, Tapik AJ, et al: Mural thrombus in left ventricular aneurysm. Incidence, role of angiography and relation between anticoagulation and embolization. *Mayo Clin Proc* 56:77–81, 1981.

67. Rogers LR, Graus F, Posner JB: Central nervous system vascular complications occurring in patients with cancer: Changes within the past decade. *Medicine* 64:16–35, 1985.

68. Roman G, Fisher M, Perl DP, et al: Neurological manifestations of hereditary hemorrhagic telangiectasis (Rendu-Osler-Weber disease): Report of 2 cases and review of the literature. *Ann Neurol* 4:130–144, 1978.

69. Salgado AV, Furlan AJ, Keys TF, et al: Neurologic complications of endocarditis: A 12-year experience. *Neurology* 39:173–178, 1989.

70. Sandok BA: Evaluation of patients with suspected cardioembolic brain infarctions. In Furlan AJ (ed): *The Heart and Stroke*. New York, Springer-Verlag, 1987, pp 37–45.

71. Sandok BA, Van Estorff I, Giuliana E: CNS embolism due to atrial myxoma. Clinical features and diagnosis. *Arch Neurol* 37:485–488, 1980.

72. Silverman J, Olwin JS, Graethinger JS: Cardiac myxomas with systemic embolization: Review of the literature and report of a case. *Circulation* 26:99–103, 1979.

73. Simpson MT, Oberman A, Kouchoukos NT, et al: Prevalence of mural thrombi and systemic embolization with left ventricular aneurysms. *Chest* 77:463–469, 1980.

74. Sisel RJ, Parker BM, Bahl OP: Cerebral symptoms in pulmonary arteriovenous fistula. A result of paradoxical emboli (?). *Circulation* 41:123–128, 1970.

75. Sixty Plus Reinfarction Study Research Group: Risks of long-term oral anticoagulant therapy in elderly patients after myocardial infarction. Second report. *Lancet* 1:64–68, 1982.

76. Snider WD, Simpson DM, Nielsen S, et al: Neurological complications of acquired immune deficiency syndrome: Analysis of 50 cases. *Ann Neurol* 14:403–418, 1983.

77. Thompson PL, Robinson JS: Stroke after myocardial infarctioin: Relation to infarct size. *Br Med J* 12:457–459, 1978.

78. TIMI Study Group: The thrombolysis in myocardial infarction (TIMI) trial. *N Engl J Med* 32:932–936, 1985.

79. Trent A, Andersson B: The outcome of patients with TIA and stroke treated with anticoagulants. *Acta Med Scand* 208:359–367, 1980.

80. Valdes-Cruz LM, Pieroni DR, Roland JM, et al: Echocardiographic detection of intracardiac right-to-left shunts following peripheral vein injections. *Circulation* 54:558–562, 1976.

81. Van de Werf F, Ludbrook PA, Baguaran SR, et al: Coronary thrombolysis with tissue-type plasminogen activator in patients with evolving myocardial infarction. *N Engl J Med* 310:609–613, 1984.

82. Veterans Cooperative Study: Anticoagulants in acute myocardial infarction. Results of a cooperative clinical trial. *JAMA* 225:724–729, 1973.

83. Wolf PA, Dawber TR, Thomas HE, et al: Epidemiologic assessment of chronic atrial fibrillation and risk of stroke: The Framingham study. *Neurology* 28:973–977, 1978.

84. Working Party on Anticoagulant Therapy in Coronary Thrombosis: Assessment of short-term anticoagulant administration after cardiac infarction. Report to the Medical Research Council. *Br Med J* 1:335–342, 1969.

CHAPTER SIXTEEN

Brain Trauma and Ischemia

Lawrence H. Pitts, M.D.

It is well established that either ischemia or hypoxia or both contributes significantly to a poor outcome after traumatic cerebral injuries (6, 33, 36). Major systemic trauma, whether or not the brain is involved, can produce both shock and hypoxia and such ischemic insults have been implicated in secondary injury to a variety of organs including the kidneys and gastrointestinal tract. In addition, these ischemic insults almost certainly contribute to delayed systemic pathology including adult respiratory distress syndrome and multiple organ failure. Although ischemia has a grave impact in these systems, it has its most devastating effects on the brain and, most specifically, on the already injured brain (31). This chapter focuses first on the clinical importance of hypoxic and hypotensive ischemia in terms of known clinical effects. Subsequently, experimental evidence is examined to describe the specific physiologic and biochemical consequences on the injured central nervous system (CNS).

ISCHEMIA AND HEAD INJURY IN HUMANS

Hypoxia

Breathing abnormalities frequently occur after head injury. Significant cerebral impact in humans (27) and animals is usually accompanied immediately by apnea (9, 19, 38) that lasts for varying, sometimes prolonged, periods. Brain trauma also can produce pulmonary edema acutely, and it is often associated with atelectasis, pneumonia, and oxygen diffusion abnormalities in the hours and days after injury (8). In as many as 50% of patients, arterial oxygen tension (PaO$_2$) is below 80 torr on admission to the hospital (23), and in one-

third of those patients it is below 65 torr (43). Emergency medical services now initiate ventilation and resuscitation at the scene of injury, resulting in treatment or prevention of hypoxia. However, despite these efforts, 20% to 36% of patients have PaO$_2$ below 60 torr when they arrive at the hospital (7, 29).

Hypoxia has been shown to correlate significantly with worsened outcome in a number of clinical studies. The National Coma Data Bank reported that the incidence of posttraumatic vegetative status or mortality was 20% higher among patients who were hypoxic when admitted to the study centers than among other trauma patients (7) (Fig. 16.1). Other reports have described similar adverse effects of hypoxia on outcome after head injury in humans (29, 31, 39). Although it cannot be demonstrated conclusively from clinical studies that the association be-

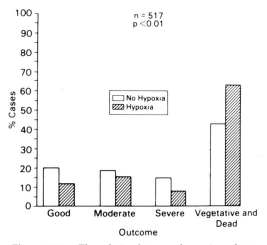

Figure 16.1. The relation between hypoxia and outcome from brain injury. (From Eisenberg HM, Cayard C, Papanicolaou AC, et al: The effects of three potentially preventable complications on outcome after severe closed head injury. In Ishii S, Nagai H, Brock M (eds): *Intracranial Pressure V.* New York, Springer-Verlag, 1983, pp 549–553.)

tween hypoxia and a poor outcome are causally related, data obtained in experimental animal studies show that hypoxia can selectively injure traumatized cells that would otherwise survive. Thus, it seems reasonable to infer that hypoxia increases tissue damage after cerebral trauma, increasing the likelihood of a poor outcome.

Shock

Systemic hypotension is one of two mechanisms that contributes directly to traumatic ischemia. The second cause of cerebral hypoperfusion or reduced cerebral perfusion pressure (CPP) is increased intracranial pressure (ICP). These parameters are defined by the equation,

$$CPP = MAP - ICP,$$

in which MAP is mean systemic arterial pressure. Many authors have reported that shock, often defined as systolic arterial pressure below 90 torr, correlates with a worsened outcome after head injury (7, 29, 35, 38, 39) (Fig. 16.2). Significant injury to other regions of the body and body systems, such as the thorax, abdominal viscera, head and neck, or extremities, frequently accompanies head injury. At least

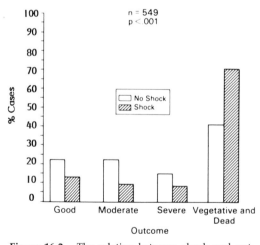

Figure 16.2. The relation between shock and outcome from brain injury. (From Eisenberg HM, Cayard C, Papanicolaou AC, et al: The effects of three potentially preventable complications on outcome after severe closed head injury. In Ishii S, Nagai H, Brock M (eds): *Intracranial Pressure V*. New York, Springer-Verlag, 1983, pp 549–553.)

one other body system in addition to the head is significantly injured in as many as 40% of patients who have severe head injury. In some cases, trauma to as many as four or five systems, including the CNS, can occur. The incidence of shock at the time of the patient's hospital admission increases with the number of organ systems injured (38). Some series (5, 38), but not all (26), have shown multiple injuries to be associated with worsened outcome after head injury. Shock has been associated with as much as a 30% increase in the incidence of death or vegetative status in patients with severe head injury (7). Again, as in cases of hypoxia, it is not possible to prove a causal relationship between systemic hypotension and worsened outcome after severe head injury based on the data accrued from studies in humans. However, experimental evidence with controlled hypotension clearly describes an adverse effect on cerebral function after head injury in experimental animals (20).

Intracranial Hypertension

Cerebral ischemia is, by definition, inadequate local or global cerebral perfusion which, if severe enough, can cause cell death. Systemic blood pressure is one major determinant of CPP, the other being ICP. If ICP rises as high as systemic arterial pressure, then all cerebral perfusion stops and brain death occurs. Lesser degrees of ICP elevation, depending on the MAP, can cause or aggravate focal cerebral injury at sites of traumatic edema, contusion, or hemorrhage. In normal brain, cerebral autoregulation maintains a relatively constant cerebral blood flow (CBF) over a wide range of CPPs (34). However, CBF begins to decline in the normal brain when CPP falls below about 50 torr. Because ICP is usually measured by intraventricular catheters or by subarachnoid or subdural catheters, the recorded ICP represents a generalized pressure that may not reflect focal tissue pressures at sites of traumatic injury. In head-injured patients, increases in ICP may result from a variety of causes which, except for the case of diffuse brain

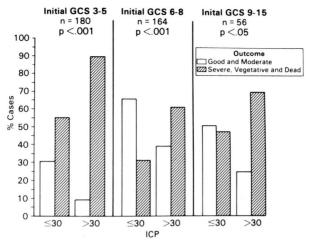

Figure 16.3. The relation between intracranial pressure (ICP) and outcome at three levels of the Glasgow Coma Scale (GCS). (From Eisenberg HM, Cayard C, Papanicolaou AC, et al: The effects of three potentially preventable complications on outcome after severe closed head injury. In Ishii S, Nagai H, Brock M (eds): *Intracranial Pressure V*. New York, Springer-Verlag, 1983, pp 549–553.)

injury, are relatively focal. These include regions of cerebral edema, brain contusion, and intracerebral or extracerebral hematomas; under these conditions, generalized ICP may be disproportionately lower than focal ICP at the injury site. The brain is viscoelastic and there can be a gradient of pressures across brain tissue (45). ICP gradients can be demonstrated in various regions of the brain, such as in supratentorial brain compartments following removal of intracerebral hematomas (44). Because of the varying degrees of tissue injury among head-injured patients and the likely differing gradients of pressure across brain tissue, it has been difficult to establish the precise level of ICP, as recorded by standard monitoring techniques, at which progressive ischemia occurs.

ICP levels have been correlated with outcome after head injury in humans. In general, when ICP remains normal in head-injured patients there is a relatively low mortality rate (14% in one series) (32), but the mortality rate is substantially higher (51% to 55%) in those patients whose ICP remains above 20 torr despite aggressive management (32, 36). A pilot study from the National Traumatic Coma Data Bank showed a significant relationship between rising ICP and poor outcome regardless of the patient's initial Glasgow coma score (7)

(Fig. 16.3). ICP levels above 40 to 60 torr are associated with exceedingly high mortality rates (24, 32). It is impossible to distinguish the dependent from the independent relationships between intracranial hypertension and head injury in humans. Although a significant correlation can be demonstrated between the two, as just indicated, whether intracranial hypertension causes secondary brain injury or is merely a measure of the severity of injury in a patient cannot be determined. Undoubtedly, in some instances increased ICP merely reflects the overall severity of injury whereas in other cases progressive intracranial hypertension actually adds an ischemic component to the other brain injuries. There is no question that extracerebral masses such as subdural hematomas can cause subjacent ischemia resulting in brain swelling from edema and hyperemia. Thus, unilateral brain swelling can be demonstrated on computerized tomography (CT) scanning after unilateral removal of an extracerebral mass. Such findings indicate that an exceedingly high probability of mortality exists (28). Posthemorrhagic edema undoubtedly contributes to increases in ICP that occur in as many as 52% of patients after surgery for traumatic hematoma (32). Thus, hematomas may be responsible for increased focal

ICP and cause adjacent ischemia, which in turn causes hyperemia and brain edema that make their own contributions to intracranial hypertension. From a therapeutic standpoint, it is best to assume that intracranial hypertension can and may lead to progressive cerebral ischemia that produces additional injury, and that controlling intracranial hypertension is probably beneficial to the patient. In those instances in which intracranial hypertension merely indicates the severity of injury, its control will not reduce the level of injury and no benefit results from controlling the ICP. At present we cannot distinguish such cases a priori without observing the neurologic effects of reduction of ICP in each patient.

Although the efficacy of ICP monitoring and control has not been definitely established, control of posttraumatic and postoperative ICP elevation is now a commonly used therapy (see Chapter 13, this volume). Moreover, because suggestive evidence of such efficacy is available, a randomized clinical trial probably cannot be justified (6).

Ischemic Pathology in Head Injury in Humans

Graham, Adams, and their colleagues (2, 12–14) have extensively evaluated neuropathologic changes after head injury in animals and humans. Brain ischemia from one or more of several possible etiologies is seen in more than 90% of patients who die from head injury. Areas of cerebral infarction often can be seen on CT scans in patients who have severe brain injuries (33). Ischemic damage can be identified in some patients in the "watershed" territory supplied in part by both the anterior cerebral and the middle cerebral arteries. This boundary-zone ischemia can be demonstrated in cases of systemic hypotension, such as cardiac arrest after myocardial infarction, and represents inadequate cerebral perfusion in these regions because of shock (16). With elevated ICP, cerebral perfusion in these regions is most severely affected, accounting for the boundary-zone infarctions in some patients. Cerebral vasospasm, found on angiograms in some

patients with head injury, can further embarrass focal cerebral perfusion and has been associated with an increased incidence of boundary-zone ischemic damage following head injury (30). Pulmonary complications that may contribute to hypoxia also seem to increase this type of cerebral ischemia (22).

Intracranial hypertension also produces brain damage, including ischemia (14). Changes include hemorrhage into the brain stem and ischemia and hemorrhage in the medial temporal lobe. In one series of 151 patients who died after head injury, 125 (83%) had evidence of elevated ICP. About 40% of patients with intracranial hypertension had ischemic damage in the posterior cerebral artery distribution owing to tentorial herniation (3). These changes were more common in patients who did not have diffuse axonal injury than in those who did (13). This perhaps suggests two major different types of fatal head injury, one with unrecoverable diffuse axonal injury and the other with a significant component of irreversible ischemic lesions, although there must be considerable overlap of these two pathologies in some patients. Brain swelling from either increased blood volume or local increases in brain water, both of which can occur in association with ischemia, can be seen adjacent to focal contusions, subjacent to extracerebral mass lesions, and occasionally bilaterally in both cerebral hemispheres. It could be hypothesized that this latter form of diffuse swelling results from hypoxia, ischemia, or both, during the early period after head injury.

Some of the neuropathologic changes seen in human head injury have been evaluated in acceleration models of experimental head injury in subhuman primates (9–11). Although the acceleration model produces a number of lesions seen in humans, such as acute subdural hematoma, diffuse axonal injury, and focal contusions, some features of human traumatic neuropathology are not reproduced. For instance, without the formation of acute subdural hematomas, intracranial hypertension is not usually seen in these models (11). In addition, ventilation is controlled in the experimental animals so that hypoxia is not a concomitant of their head injury. It is not surprising, therefore, that medial temporal ischemia and hemorrhage, generally seen with intracranial hypertension, are not present in these experimental models. Also, cortical ischemic damage was found only occasionally in the animals with acceleration injury in which hypotension or hypoxia did not occur. This finding further suggests a potential role for shock and hypoxia as major contributors to brain injury in humans. Conversely, the subhuman primates that do develop subdural hematomas in the experimental model have marked brain swelling subjacent to the hematoma (1) that is consistent with some degree of focal ischemia as the cause of the brain swelling observed. Additional causes of focal or global brain swelling could be related to unilateral or bilateral loss of cerebral autoregulation after head injury caused directly by trauma or brain compression (25) rather than indirectly by ischemia.

EXPERIMENTAL BRAIN INJURY AND ISCHEMIA

Hypoxia

To evaluate a causal relationship between brain trauma and hypoxia, Ishige and colleagues (17, 19, 20) evaluated the effect of brain impact and hypoxia, separately and together, on neurologic outcome and a variety of physiologic and metabolic variables in a lateral fluid percussion brain injury model in rats. Physiologic changes were those seen in usual head injury models, including an immediate hypertension of 30 to 70 torr which returned to baseline levels within several minutes (9, 41). With the impact used in this study, the rats became apneic for 15 to 45 seconds and then resumed spontaneous ventilation. Hypoxia was produced by placing the animals in a chamber with 13% oxygen, which lowered PaO_2 to 35 to 40 torr for 30 minutes. The rats were hypotensive (50 to 65 torr) during the period of hypoxia, after which the arterial pressure returned to normal.

Compressed spectral array (CSA) electroencephalographic (EEG) recordings were done as a continuous measure of brain function in these animals with severe concussion (19) (Fig. 16.4). This EEG technique has also been used in anesthetized human beings to monitor ischemic effects of vascular occlusion during carotid endarterectomy (40). Hypoxia had no appreciable effect on the CSA. Impact injury alone produced remarkable EEG slowing for about 10 minutes in the uninjured hemisphere and for up to 20 minutes in the injured hemisphere. The combination of head injury plus hypoxia produced a similar 10-minute electrical slowing in the noninjured hemisphere, but the combined lesions produced a marked reduction of electrical potentials in the injured hemisphere throughout the entire 30 minutes of hypoxia and for a period of 10 to 20 minutes after normoxia was reestablished.

The effect of hypoxia and impact injury on brain acidosis and high-energy phosphorus metabolites was evaluated in this same rat model (20). It was possible to measure at 3-minute intervals the brain phosphocreatine (PCr), β-adenosine triphosphate (β-ATP), inorganic phosphate (P_i), and brain pH. Hypoxia alone produced no change in brain high-energy phosphates as measured by the PCr/P_i ratio during the 30 minutes of hypoxia and the subsequent 30 minutes of recovery (20) (Fig. 16.5). A moderate impact injury produced a 10% decline in the PCr/P_i ratio within 10 minutes of injury, after which time the high-energy phosphate levels returned to within 5% of baseline values. The combined injury of hypoxia and impact produced a steady decline in brain high-energy phosphates after impact and during almost the entire period of hypoxia. When normoxia was reestablished, the PCr/P_i ratio returned toward normal, but at 1 hour after injury it was still at only 80% of control values—significantly below that of animals suffering only impact injuries. Brain pH fell to the lowest levels in animals that had both the hypoxic and impact injuries as compared with those with impact injuries only.

The effect of impact plus hypoxia in this rat model also was evaluated regarding its effect on the production of cerebral edema

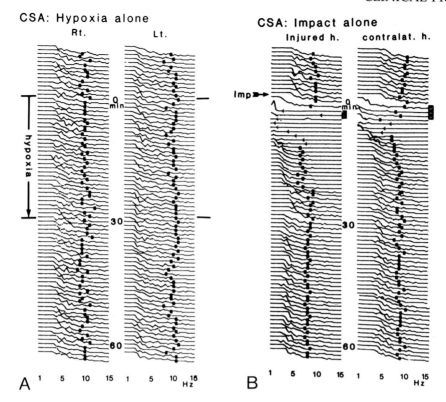

CSA: Hypoxia alone
Rt.   Lt.

CSA: Impact alone
Injured h.   contralat. h.

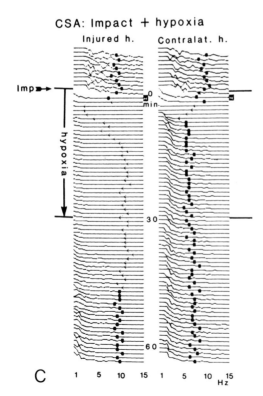

CSA: Impact + hypoxia
Injured h.   Contralat. h.

Figure 16.4. Compressed spectral array (CSA) electroencephalograms after *A,* hypoxia, *B,* impact brain injury, or *C,* both types of insults in combination. Each line represents the power spectrum for 1 minute. Rt = right; Lt = left; h = hemisphere; Imp = impact. (From Ishige N, Pitts LH, Hashimoto T, et al: The effect of hypoxia on traumatic brain injury in rats. Part 1: Changes in neurological function, electroencephalograms, and histopathology. *Neurosurgery* 20:848–853, 1987.)

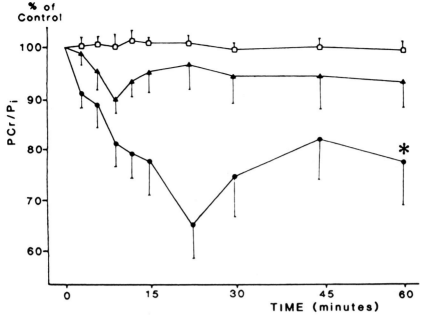

Figure 16.5. The changes over 60 minutes in the phosphocreatine/inorganic phosphate (PCr/P_i) ratio after hypoxia (□), impact (▲), or both (●). The asterisk indicates that the PCr/P_i ratio at 60 minutes after impact was significantly lower in animals subjected to both insults than after impact alone ($p<0.05$). (From Ishige N, Pitts LH, Pogliani L, et al: The effect of hypoxia on traumatic head injury in rats. Part 2: Changes in high-energy phosphate metabolism. *Neurosurgery* 20:854–858, 1987.)

and alterations in regional CBF. Cerebral edema after impact injury increased during the first 12 to 18 hours after the impact (15). At 24 hours after an hypoxic insult, rats showed no increase in brain water in either hemisphere and those with an impact injury only showed increased brain water immediately subjacent to the impact site (17) (Fig. 16.6). The combined hypoxic and impact insults, however, produced widespread increases in brain water throughout the cortex ipsilateral to the impact site.

The regions of altered regional CBF were virtually identical to the regions with altered brain water (17) (Fig. 16.7). Hypoxia alone caused no change in regional CBF at 24 hours in either hemisphere. Impact alone caused relative hypoperfusion immediately under the region of impact but blood flow was otherwise normal in both the ipsilateral and the contralateral hemispheres. The combination injury, however, caused a more substantial reduction in blood flow immediately under the impact as well as significantly lowered CBF in other regions of the hemisphere ipsilateral to the impact site (17).

Nelson et al (37) similarly found that the combination of head injury and hypoxia produced a poorer outcome in cats than either lesion alone. Anderson et al (4) also combined hypoventilation with head injury in cats and, similar to the results of the study cited above, found marked alterations in CBF and metabolic rates of oxygen and glucose in addition to reduction in the PCr/P_i ratio and decreased brain pH.

Not unexpectedly, in addition to the multiple metabolic changes caused by the addition of hypoxia to brain trauma, the outcome after a combined hypoxic–impact injury in animals is worse than after either an hypoxic or an impact injury alone. Ishige et al (19) found no neurologic abnormalities 24 hours after a 30-minute hypoxic insult in rats. Many rats subjected to impact alone were more inactive than normal rats, and some of the injured rats had a

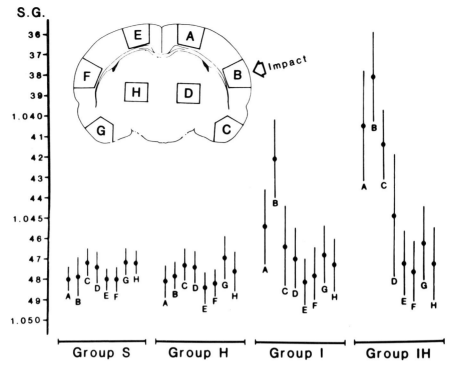

Figure 16.6. Specific gravities (S.G.) measured at eight brain areas in sham-operated rats (S) and in rats receiving hypoxic (H), impact (I), or combined impact plus hypoxic (IH) insults. The brain areas are indicated on the schematic cross-section of the rat brain. (From Ishige N, Pitts LH, Berry I, et al: The effect of hypoxia on traumatic head injury in rats: Alterations in neurologic function, brain edema, and cerebral blood flow. *J Cereb Blood Flow Metab* 7:759–767, 1987.)

hemiparesis. However, 70% of the rats with an impact–hypoxic insult had focal neurologic deficits, were unresponsive, or died—a significantly worse outcome than in animals subjected to either hypoxia or impact alone.

Hypotension

Hypotension alone, if sufficiently severe, can deplete brain high-energy metabolites (42). In one rat model of hemorrhagic hypotension, the brain PCr and P_i did not change with systemic arterial pressures of 40 torr but did change at 30 torr (18). Systemic hypotension does not immediately follow impact injury to brain (17, 18, 20) but may develop some minutes after a severe and ultimately fatal brain injury. In human head injury, shock more typically occurs either as a result of very severe brain injuries leading to medullary

failure and death or in the multiply injured patient with hypovolemic shock.

In rats, hypovolemic shock to MAP of 40 torr for 60 minutes had no effect on PCr, β-ATP, or P_i (18). MAP of 30 torr for 1 hour caused decrements of approximately 10% in PCr and 50% increases in P_i with minimal reduction in β-ATP. Impact alone produced slight and transient falls in PCr and elevations in P_i with no change in β-ATP. However, the combination of impact with hypotension to MAP of either 40 or 30 torr produced significant reductions in PCr and elevations of P_i; only the more severe degree of hypotension with impact injury caused a reduction in β-ATP. Brain pH decreased somewhat with all of the three types of insults, the smallest changes occurring after impact alone and progressively greater changes with progressive degrees of hypotension. The most dramatic and significant reductions

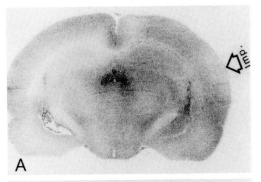

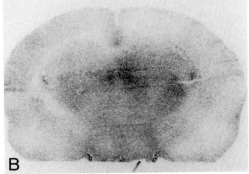

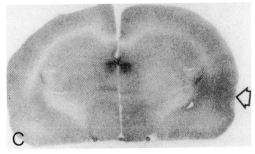

Figure 16.7. Coronal autoradiograms 24 hours after *A*, impact, or *B*, combined impact plus hypoxic (IH) insults. *C*, the region immediately beneath the impact region in the IH image shows hyperemia. Note site of impact *(arrow)*. (From Ishige N, Pitts LH, Berry I, et al: The effect of hypoxia on traumatic head injury in rats: Alterations in neurologic function, brain edema, and cerebral blood flow. *J Cereb Blood Flow Metab* 7:759–767, 1987.)

in pH were in the impact–shock groups of animals. In a rat model, relatively mild concussive impact injury and carotid occlusion with forebrain ischemia significantly reduced the animal's ability to retain learned behavior 1 week after the combined insult. This deficit was considerably worse than that observed in animals having either ischemia or impact injuries alone (21).

PERSPECTIVE

Although, in humans, it is possible to draw only a correlation between ischemia, either hypoxic or hypotensive, and outcome after head injury, it is evident from the experimental data that there is a causal relationship between ischemia and worsened outcome after a traumatic insult. It would appear, particularly from the various regional studies involving CBF and edema, that a number of brain cells are reversibly injured by impact but are at risk for subsequent failure and death when subjected to additional ischemic insults. The cellular or subcellular mechanism for this susceptibility is unknown. A variety of biochemical phenomena, such as altered lipid metabolism, the presence and activity of various neuropeptides and other neurotransmitters, and the activation of rapidly induced proteins, are all being investigated intensively. Discovering exactly how ischemia causes cell death after brain trauma very probably will allow us to treat some of the secondary brain injuries that worsen outcome in head-injured patients and to improve the outcome from this enormously important public health problem.

References

1. Adams JH, Graham DI, Gennarelli TA: Neuropathology of acceleration-induced head injury in the subhuman primate. In Grossman RG, Gildenberg PL (eds): *Headj Injury: Basic and Clinical Aspects.* New York, Raven Press, 1982, pp 141–150.
2. Adams JH, Graham DI, Gennarelli TA: Head injury in man and experimental animals: Neuropathology. *Acta Neurochir [Suppl] (Wien)* 32:15–30, 1983.
3. Adams JH, Graham DI, Scott G: Brain damage in fatal non-missile head injury. *J Clin Pathol* 33:1132–1145, 1980.
4. Anderson BJ, Unterberg AW, Clarke GD, et al: Effect of post-traumatic hypoventilation on cerebral energy metabolism. *J Neurosurg* 68:601–607, 1988.
5. Bowers SA, Marshall LF: Outcome in 200 consecutive cases of severe head injury treated in San Diego County: A prospective analysis. *Neurosurgery* 6:237–242, 1980.
6. Cooper PR: Delayed brain injury: Secondary insults. In Becker DP, Povlishock JT (eds): *Central Nervous System Trauma Status Report.* Bethesda, MD, National Institute of Neurological and Com-

municative Disorders and Stroke, National Institutes of Health, 1985, pp 217–228.

7. Eisenberg HM, Cayard C, Papanicolaou AC, et al: The effects of three potentially preventable complications on outcome after severe closed head injury. In Ishii S, Nagai H, Brock M (eds): *Intracranial Pressure V*. New York, Springer-Verlag, 1983, pp 549–553.

8. Frost EAM: The physiopathology of respiration in neurosurgical patients. *J Neurosurg* 50:699–714, 1979.

9. Gennarelli TA, Segawa H, Wald U, et al: Physiological response to angular acceleration of the head. In Grossman RG, Gildenberg PL (eds): *Head Injury: Basic and Clinical Aspects*. New York, Raven Press, 1982, pp 129–140.

10. Gennarelli TA, Thibault LE: Biomechanics of acute subdural hematoma. *J Trauma* 22:680–686, 1982.

11. Gennarelli TA, Thibault LE: Biological models of head injury. In Becker DP, Povlishock JT (eds): *Central Nervous System Trauma Status Report*. Bethesda, MD, National Institute of Neurological and Communicative Disorders and Stroke, National Institutes of Health, 1985, pp 391–404.

12. Graham DI, Adams JH, Doyle D: Ischemic brain damage in fatal non-missile head injuries. *J Neurol Sci* 139:213–234, 1978.

13. Graham DI, Adams JH, Gennarelli TA: Mechanisms of non-penetrating head injury. In Bond RF (ed): *Perspectives in Shock Research* (Proceedings of the 10th Annual Conference on Shock and the 1st International Shock Congress, Montreal, June, 1987). New York, Alan R. Liss, 1988, pp 159–168.

14. Graham DI, Lawrence AE, Adams JH, et al: Brain damage in non-missile head injury secondary to high intracranial pressure. *Neuropathol Appl Neurobiol* 13:209–217, 1987.

15. Hashimoto T, Pitts LH, Moseley M, et al: In vitro proton NMR spectroscopy and in vivo imaging in traumatic brain edema. In Inaba Y, Klatzo I, Spatz M (eds): *Brain Edema*. New York, Springer-Verlag, 1985, pp 601–605.

16. Howard R, Trend P, Russell RWR: Clinical features of ischemia in cerebral arterial border zones after periods of reduced cerebral blood flow. *Arch Neurol* 44:934–940, 1987.

17. Ishige N, Pitts LH, Berry I, et al: The effect of hypoxia on traumatic head injury in rats: Alterations in neurologic function, brain edema, and cerebral blood flow. *J Cereb Blood Flow Metab* 7:759–767, 1987.

18. Ishige N, Pitts LH, Berry I, et al: The effects of hypovolemic hypotension on high energy phosphate metabolism of traumatized brains in rats. *J Neurosurg* 68:129–136, 1988.

19. Ishige N, Pitts LH, Hashimoto T, et al: The effect of hypoxia on traumatic brain injury in rats. Part 1: Changes in neurological function, electroencephalograms, and histopathology. *Neurosurgery* 20:848–853, 1987.

20. Ishige N, Pitts LH, Pogliani L, et al: The effect of hypoxia on traumatic head injury in rats. Part 2: Changes in high-energy phosphate metabolism. *Neurosurgery* 20:854–858, 1987.

21. Jenkins LW, Lyeth BG, Hayes RL: The role of agonist-receptor interactions in the pathophysiology of mild and moderate head injury. In Hoff JT, Anderson TE, Cole TM (eds): *Mile to Moderate Head Injury*. Boston, Blackwell Scientific, 1989, pp 47–61.

22. Jennett S: Pulmonary function in the head injured patient. In Fitch W, Barker J (eds): *Head Injury and the Anesthetist*. Amsterdam, Elsevier, 1985, pp 53–82.

23. Katsurada K, Yamada R, Sugimoto T: Respiratory insufficiency in patients with severe head injury. *Surgery* 73:191–199, 1973.

24. Langfitt TW, Gennarelli TA: Can the outcome from head injury be improved? *J Neurosurg* 56:19–25, 1982.

25. Leach PJ, Miller JD: Intracranial volume/pressure relationships during experimental brain compression in primates. *J Neurol Neurosurg Psychiatry* 37:1093–1098, 1974.

26. Levati A, Farina ML, Vecchi G, et al: Prognosis of severe head injury. *J Neurosurg* 57:779–783, 1982.

27. Levine JE, Becker DP: Reversal of incipient brain death from head-injury apnea at the scene of accidents (letter). *N Engl J Med* 301:109, 1979.

28. Lobato RD, Sarabia R, Rivas JJ, et al: Normal computerized tomography in severe head injury. Prognostic and clinical management implications. *J Neurosurg* 65:784–789, 1986.

29. Lutz HA, Becker DP, Miller JD, et al: Monitoring, management, and the analysis of outcome. In Grossman RG, Gildenberg PL (eds): *Head Injury: Basic and Clinical Aspects*. New York, Raven Press, 1982, pp 221–228.

30. MacPherson P, Graham DI: Correlation between angiographic findings and the ischemia of head injury. *J Neurol Neurosurg Psychiatry* 41:122–127, 1978.

31. Miller JD: Head injury and brain ischemia—Implication for therapy. *Br J Anaesth* 57:120–129, 1985.

32. Miller JD, Becker DP, Ward JD, et al: Significance of intracranial hypertension in severe head injury. *J Neurosurg* 47:503–516, 1977.

33. Miller JD, Gudeman SK, Kishore PRS, et al: Computed tomography, brain edema and ICP in head injury. *Adv Neurol* 28:413–421, 1980.

34. Miller JD, Stanek A, Langfitt TW: Concepts of cerebral perfusion pressure and vascular compression during intracranial hypertension. *Prog Brain Res* 35:411–432, 1971.

35. Miller JD, Sweet RC, Narayan RK, et al: Early insults to the injured brain. *JAMA* 240:439–442, 1978.

36. Narayan RK, Kishore RS, Becker DP, et al: Intracranial pressure: To monitor or not to monitor? *J Neurosurg* 56:650–659, 1982.

37. Nelson LR, Auen EL, Bourke RS, et al: A comparison of animal head injury models developed for treatment modality evaluation. In Grossman RG, Gildenberg PL (eds): *Head Injury: Basic and Clinical Aspects*. New York, Raven Press, 1982, pp 117–127.

38. Newfield P, Pitts LH, Kaktis JV: The influence of shock on mortality after head trauma (abstract). *Crit Care Med* 8:254, 1980.

39. Price DJE, Murray A: The influence of hypoxia and hypotension on recovery from head injury. *Injury* 3:218–225, 1972.
40. Rampil IJ, Holzer JA, Quest DO, et al: Prognostic value of computerized EEG analysis during carotid endarterectomy. *Anesth Analg* 62:186–192, 1983.
41. Rosner MJ, Newsome HH, Becker DP: Mechanical brain injury: The sympatho-adrenal response. *J Neurosurg* 61:76–86, 1984.
42. Siesjö BK, Zwetnow NN: The effect of hypovolemic hypotension on extra- and intracellular acid–base parameters and energy metabolites in the rat brain. *Acta Physiol Scand* 79:114–124, 1970.
43. Sinha RP, Ducker TB, Perot PL Jr: Arterial oxygenation. Findings and its significance in central nervous system trauma patients. *JAMA* 224:1258–1260, 1973.
44. Suzuki A, Yasui N, Ito Z, et al: Sequential changes of the epidural, the ventricular and the surrounding tissue pressure in hypertensive intracerebral hemorrhage. In Ishii S, Nagai H, Brock M (eds): *Intracranial Pressure V*. New York, Springer-Verlag, 1983, pp 721–723.
45. Walsh EK, Schettini A: Calculation of brain elastic parameters in vivo. *Am J Physiol* 247:R693–R700, 1984.

CHAPTER SEVENTEEN

Subarachnoid and Intracerebral Hemorrhage

J. Max Findlay, M.D., Ph.D., F.R.C.S.C.
Bryce Weir, M.D., C.M., M.Sc., F.R.C.S.C., F.A.C.S

CEREBRAL ISCHEMIA AFTER SUBARACHNOID HEMORRHAGE

The most common cause of primary subarachnoid bleeding and the fourth most common cause of stroke is ruptured saccular arterial aneurysms. Approximately 50% of patients are either killed or severely disabled by the initial rupture. Those who recover are subject to a number of complications of aneurysmal subarachnoid hemorrhage (SAH), which include rebleeding from the aneurysm, obstructive hydrocephalus, and seizures. Cerebral ischemia, however, is the leading cause of morbidity and mortality in survivors of SAH. Delayed ischemia occurs in 20% to 30% of patients, and one-half of them will perish or be incapacitated as a result. The occurrence of cerebral ischemia after SAH depends on several factors, the most important of which is vasospasm.

Etiology and Pathophysiology

The onset of vasospasm and cerebral ischemia after SAH is delayed, peaking in incidence approximately 1 week after rupture of the aneurysm. Arterial narrowing occurs mostly in the larger, extraparenchymal cerebral arteries that course through the network of basal subarachnoid cisterns, the same vessels from which saccular aneurysms arise. When an aneurysm bursts, it frequently encases the parent artery and other arteries in the subarachnoid cisterns with clotted blood. The location and volume of subarachnoid hematoma are directly related to the occurrence, distribution, and severity of ensuing vasospasm (30). There is no longer any question that vasospasm is a delayed response of the vessel wall to thick periarterial blood clot, but the biochemical mechanisms of that response have not been fully explained.

The major contemporary theory of the pathogenesis of vasospasm after SAH is that the periarterial blood clot, during its degradation, releases vasoactive substances that elicit sustained spasm of vascular smooth muscle (53); also released are vasotoxins that injure the vessel wall, impairing its ability to synthesize endogenous vasodilatory substances (40) and inciting a destructive vessel wall reaction (Fig. 17.1). Histologic examination of vasospastic human and animal cerebral arteries has shown structural changes, such as intimal hypercellularity (59), corrugation and fragmentation of the internal elastic lamina (36), and medial myonecrosis and edema (15), but it is unlikely that these changes are by themselves sufficient to cause any significant degree of luminal narrowing. Often, angiography shows resolution of the vasospasm within a few weeks after SAH despite persistence of the structural abnormalities (25). The predominant physiologic and morphologic change that could account for vasospasm is smooth muscle contraction (37, 64). However, the irreversibility of the vasoconstriction during the period of vasospasm (31) suggests that the condition is more than simple physiologic smooth muscle contraction; the finding of medial myonecrosis in vasospastic vessels (15) is evidence that extreme vasoconstriction damages the structural integrity of the arterial wall.

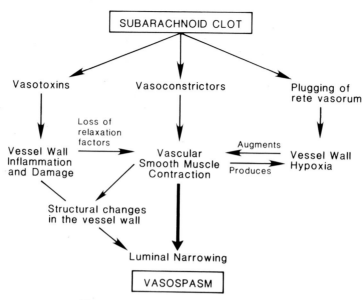

Figure 17.1.   Pathogenesis of vasospasm.

Although a number of clot-derived spasmogens have been postulated, there is accumulating evidence that products of erythrocyte breakdown, such as oxyhemoglobin, are especially important in the genesis of vasospasm (12, 37). Oxyhemoglobin is liberated during hemolysis; the time course of its release into the periarterial clot from erythrocytes appears to follow the time course of vasospasm as determined angiographically and clinically (47). It has been speculated that free radicals produced during oxidative conversion of oxyhemoglobin to methemoglobin generate vasoconstrictive and vasotoxic lipid peroxides and prostaglandins (3, 57). Finally, it has been suggested that the periarterial clot may prevent cerebral spinal fluid (CSF) from reaching the surface of the arteries and the intraadventitial rete vasorum of the vessel wall (analogous to the vasa vasorum of noncerebral vessels), thereby interfering with normal nutrition and oxygenation of the vessel wall (14, 70). Vessel wall hypoxia might also contribute to the pathogenesis of vasospasm (41, 62).

As many as two-thirds of patients have some degree of angiographic vasospasm after aneurysmal SAH, but only about one-half of them develop a delayed ischemic deficit. Several factors influence the development of ischemia in individual patients (Table 17.1). These factors determine the degree of impairment in local cerebral blood flow (CBF) and oxygen delivery and influence the ischemia thresholds, below which ischemic symptoms and brain infarction will occur. Normal cerebral tissue can tolerate CBF as low as approximately 18 ml/100 g/minute without neurologic symptoms; levels of 12 to 18 ml/100 g/minute interrupt neuronal function but maintain the viability of these neurons for a period of time, and levels below 12 ml/100 g/minute will result in cerebral infarction (4). An appreciation of factors affecting brain perfusion is important in the management of vasospasm after SAH.

Other causes of SAH are rarely associ-

Table 17.1.   Factors Determining the Development of Cerebral Ischemia Following Subarachnoid Hemorrhage

Degree and distribution of vasospasm
Cerebral perfusion pressure
Blood viscosity
Blood hemoglobin and oxygen content
Collateral cerebral blood supply
Associated direct brain or vascular injury from aneurysm rupture and/or surgery

ated with vasospasm and cerebral ischemia. Only aneurysm rupture routinely discharges enough blood into the basal cisterns to evoke vasospasm in the arteries exposed there.

Clinical Features

Vasospasm rarely occurs earlier than 4 days after SAH; the peak incidence is 7 to 10 days after rupture of the aneurysm. The occurrence of vasospasm depends on the severity of the SAH, and since there is also a positive correlation between the amount of subarachnoid blood in the basal cisterns and clinical grade of the patient, patients in poor neurologic condition are at greatest risk of developing vasospasm. The onset of vasospasm is frequently heralded by increasing headache and drowsiness, followed by focal deficits referrable to the distribution of the vasospastic vessels (19). In the anterior circulation, the middle cerebral artery (MCA) is most commonly affected, resulting in hemiparesis, hemianopsia, dysphasia (dominant hemisphere), and neglect (nondominant hemisphere). Vasospasm of the anterior cerebral arteries can result in abulia, somnolence, and lower extremity weakness. Vasospasm is commonly associated with mild pyrexia. Severe and multivessel vasospasm can lead to massive cerebral infarction, intracranial hypertension, cerebral herniation, and death.

Diagnosis

Although the diagnosis of delayed cerebral ischemia is suggested by the typical time of onset and nature of the neurologic deterioration, other complications such as aneurysmal rebleeding, hydrocephalus, seizures, increasing edema around an intracerebral hematoma, postoperative intracranial clots, electrolyte disorders (most commonly hyponatremia), hypoxemia, and sepsis must be considered. Computerized tomography (CT), useful in the diagnosis of SAH and identification of patients with a large volume of subarachnoid clot and therefore at high risk of developing vasospasm, should be done to rule out alter-

native intracranial causes for neurologic deterioration and to look for evidence of cerebral swelling or hypodensity suggestive of impending infarction (Fig. 17.2). Magnetic resonance (MR) imaging is more sensitive in detecting the presence and distribution of edema, and may become useful in detecting evolving cerebral ischemia before it is recognizable on CT scans, providing the patient has not been treated with a ferromagnetic aneurysm clip and is not too seriously ill to undergo the imaging procedure.

Transcranial Doppler sonography is very useful for detecting vasospasm (21, 24, 54). (Fig. 17.3). As the lumen of a vessel narrows, the velocity of blood flow increases (being inversely related to the square of vessel diameter). Increased blood flow in narrowed vessels at the base of the brain can be detected as an increase in Doppler frequency shifts recorded with a handheld ultrasound probe. The absolute velocity calculated from the Doppler signal is not always accurate, so that changes over time or side-to-side differences often give more important information than absolute values. The easiest vessel to record, the MCA, is usually one vessel involved in patients with clinically significant vasospasm. In one center with extensive experience with transcranial Doppler sonography, vasospasm could be diagnosed with a sensitivity of 75% and a specificity of 85% (21). The simplicity, noninvasiveness, and repeatability of this technique make it a valuable tool for evaluating patients with SAH. The detection of an early, significant increase in CBF velocity may permit early institution of measures to prevent impending symptomatic cerebral ischemia and infarction.

The CBF response to SAH and vasospasm has been evaluated both for diagnostic purposes and to provide insight into the pathophysiology of vasospasm and cerebral ischemia (22, 68). The majority of these studies have shown only a rough correlation among vasospasm, reduction in CBF, and delayed ischemic deficit. Positron emission tomography (PET) has also been used to evaluate patients with SAH (35). Xenon-enhanced CT blood flow mapping (69) promises to overcome many of

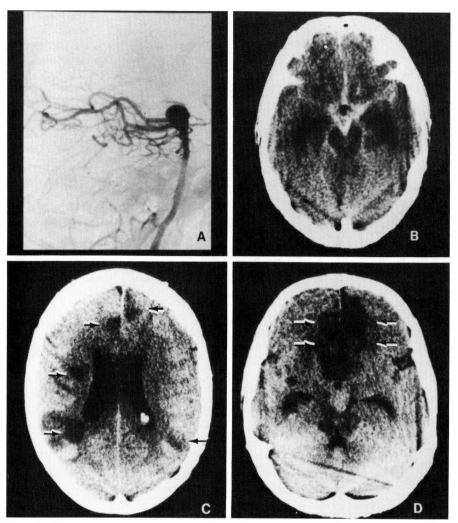

Figure 17.2. Radiologic studies from a 34-year-old man with subarachnoid hemorrhage. *A,* angiogram in the lateral projection shows a large aneurysm at the tip of the basilar artery. *B,* CT scan obtained immediately after angiography shows a large volume of blood in the basal subarachnoid cisterns, predictive of vasospasm. *C* and *D,* CT scans obtained 19 days after the hemorrhage show bilateral infarcts *(arrows)* due to severe vasospasm of the anterior and middle cerebral arteries.

the difficulties encountered in previous clinical application of CBF studies (*see* Chapter 8, this volume).

The definitive diagnosis of vasospasm still depends on cerebral angiography to demonstrate arterial narrowing. Vasospasm may appear as a tapering and smooth reduction in arterial caliber or it may be segmental (between bifurcations). It may remain localized, affecting only a single vessel, or it may be diffuse, extending from all major brain arteries to the small parenchymal vessels (Fig. 17.4). A recent review of 1,002 cerebral angiographic procedures, 33% of which were for aneurysm or related conditions, revealed a total ischemic event rate of 3.1%, and approximately one-half were permanent (11). It is possible that the use of nonionic contrast media and arterial digital subtraction angiography may reduce the risk of ischemic complications in the future. In our experience, the difficulty of diagnosing vasospasm clinically in some

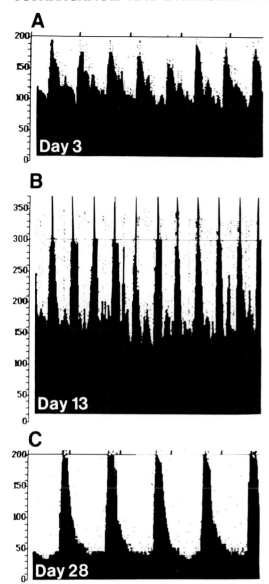

Figure 17.3. Transcranial Doppler studies of the right middle cerebral artery from the same patient as in Figure 17.2. *A,* study done 3 days after subarachnoid hemorrhage (SAH) shows marginally elevated blood flow velocity of 125 cm/second. *B,* study done 13 days after SAH shows a marked increase in blood flow velocity to 210 cm/second. Flow in the left middle cerebral artery was also elevated (280 cm/second, not shown). *C,* 28 days after SAH, the Doppler tracing shows a marked diminution in end diastolic blood flow velocity, which is characteristic of impending cerebral circulatory arrest. The patient died 2 days later.

instances necessitates cerebral angiography, particularly when surgery or an experimental or potentially dangerous treatment for vasospasm is being contemplated.

Treatment

The delayed onset of vasospasm and cerebral ischemia after aneurysm rupture, combined with the clinician's ability to predict from CT scans which patients are at greatest risk of developing these complications, appear to be ideal circumstances for effective intervention and prevention. It is discouraging to report, therefore, that despite an enormous effort to identify an agent or treatment protocol capable of preventing or reversing vasospasm, none has met with more than limited success. These treatments can be placed in five categories: vasodilator treatment to prevent or reverse arterial smooth muscle contraction; hemodynamic therapy to augment CBF despite vasospasm; cerebral protection with agents to prevent ischemic neuronal damage; antiinflammatory, antithrombotic, and miscellaneous other drugs to prevent vessel wall damage and inflammation; and methods to remove the subarachnoid periarterial blood clot and thereby prevent the occurrence of vasospasm. Wilkins has reviewed these agents and therapeutic protocols in detail (66, 67).

Vasodilators

Since it was first recognized, vasospasm has been considered largely a problem of vascular smooth-muscle contraction. Consequently many vasodilators have been tested experimentally and clinically for their effect on vasospasm. Recently, much interest has focused on the calcium antagonists, particularly the more cerebroselective agent nimodipine. Nimodipine is thought to relax smooth muscle by inhibiting the influx of extracellular calcium and by preventing the accumulation of free calcium ions, which are necessary for myofilament activation, in the myoplasm. There is evidence that cerebral vessels may be particularly susceptible to certain cal-

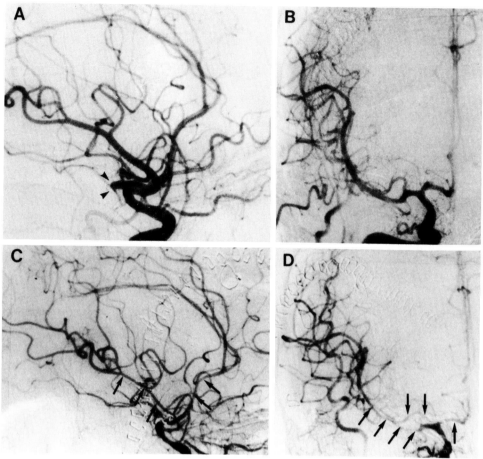

Figure 17.4. Right carotid angiograms from a patient with a ruptured aneurysm of the right posterior communicating artery. *A,* lateral and *B,* anteroposterior projections obtained on the day of subarachnoid hemorrhage (SAH) shows the aneurysm *(arrows)* with no evidence of vasospasm in the carotid artery or its branches. *C,* lateral and *D,* anteroposterior projections obtained 7 days after SAH and 6 days after aneurysm clipping show severe vasospasm in the middle and anterior cerebral arteries *(arrows).*

cium entry blockers since there is a greater dependence on extracellular pools of calcium in initiating and maintaining contraction in cerebral vascular smooth muscle than in vascular smooth muscle elsewhere in the body. Numerous in vitro investigations have shown the effectiveness of calcium antagonists in preventing and reversing cerebral vascular smooth-muscle contraction in response to various vasoactive agents, including blood.

Several controlled trials have shown that treatment with nimodipine results in a modest but significant reduction in severe neurologic deficits from vasospasm alone (2, 49, 50, 55). This effect may not be due

to any reduction in large-vessel vasospasm demonstrated angiographically and it may not reduce the mortality rate after SAH. In a randomized, prospective, double-blind, multiinstitutional trial of patients in good neurologic condition Allen et al (2) showed that oral nimodipine reduced the number of severe neurologic deficits attributed to vasospasm alone. The treatment group received nimodipine, 0.35 mg/kg, every 4 hours for 21 days; the control group received a placebo. Severe neurologic deficit occurred in 8 of 60 (13.3%) control patients but in only 1 of 56 (1.8%) nimodipine-treated patients ($p = 0.03$, Fisher's exact test). The overall outcome was not different in the two groups, presumably because of other complications. Angiography was not performed consistently, so it was not possible to determine the effect of nimodipine on the incidence or severity of vasospasm. Philippon et al (50) showed a significant reduction in poor outcomes from vasospasm in a group of patients receiving 60 mg of nimodipine every 4 hours for 21 days. Severe neurologic deficits or death from vasospasm occurred in 10 (25.6%) of 39 patients who received placebo but in only 2 (6.4%) of 31 treated with nimodipine. Again, the overall outcome did not differ significantly between the two groups.

Seiler et al (55) studied 70 consecutive patients admitted within 4 days of SAH, determining their risk of developing vasospasm from the amount of subarachnoid blood on CT scans and then evaluating them daily with transcranial Doppler sonography. The first 33 patients received no nimodipine; subsequently, 37 patients received intravenous nimodipine, 2 mg/hour, for 1 to 2 weeks followed by oral nimodipine, 60 mg every 4 hours, for an additional week. Although nimodipine did not prevent vasospasm as determined by Doppler studies, it did significantly reduce the incidence of delayed ischemic deficits and improved functional outcome in patients considered to be at high risk for the development of vasospasm. Most recently, a multicenter, randomized, placebo-controlled trial of oral nimodipine in poor-grade aneurysm patients demonstrated a significantly better outcome at 3 months in nimodipine-treated patients (49). Delayed ischemic deficits from vasospasm alone were significantly less frequent in the nimodipine group: Permanent deficits occurred in 5 (6.9%) of 72 treated patients and in 22 (26.8%) of 82 control patients ($p < 0.05$). No significant difference was seen in the incidence of moderate to severe diffuse vasospasm (64.3% vs. 66.2%). Several uncontrolled trials have been conducted to investigate the use of intravenous nimodipine after SAH (6, 33), and these also suggest that it is efficacious in preventing delayed ischemia. The apparent failure of nimodipine to affect angiographic vasospasm is in keeping with the results of a clinical study in which nimodipine lowered CBF only mildly (38), and with the results of experimental studies that failed to show any effect of nimodipine administered either orally (13, 44) or intrathecally (32) on the development of angiographic vasospasm in a primate model of SAH.

It has been suggested that the beneficial effect of nimodipine might be the dilation of smaller arterioles not seen angiographically (32, 58). Alternatively, the drug may have a direct cerebral protective effect, possibly by inhibiting calcium flux into ischemic neurons (see Chapter 25, this volume). Whatever its mode of action, nimodipine appears to help prevent cerebral ischemic damage resulting from vasospasm. Another promising calcium antagonist, nicardipine, is currently being tested in a multicenter, randomized trial (20).

Hemodynamic Therapy

Because vasospastic cerebral arteries are constricted and rigid, CBF becomes passively dependent on cerebral perfusion pressure (CPP) and blood viscosity. Realizing that it may be impossible to dilate these spastic vessels, clinicians have sought to improve CBF by increasing CPP and lowering blood viscosity. Theoretically, it might be possible through a modest improvement in blood flow to raise CPP from levels of symptomatic ischemia and impending infarction to a range of asymptomatic oligemia, which can maintain neuronal viability.

Elevation of CPP is acomplished by simultaneously decreasing elevated ICP and increasing intravascular volume, sometimes combining the latter with administration of cardiac inotropic agents to augment cardiac output and mean arterial blood pressure. Volume expansion usually reduces blood viscosity by hemodilution as well. In patients who have heart disease or require vasopressor agents, a pulmonary artery catheter must be inserted to monitor left-heart filling pressures, since aggressive hemodynamic therapy may induce congestive heart failure. Because inducing hypertension increases the risk of aneurysmal bleeding, this therapy should be reserved for postoperative patients in whom the aneurysm has already been secured. These dangers notwithstanding, hemodynamic therapy is currently the most effective treatment for symptomatic vasospasm. Several uncontrolled trials have shown some sustained neurologic improvement in 60% to 75% of patients (7, 29).

Subarachnoid Clot Removal

Because it has not been possible to dilate vasospastic cerebral vessels pharmacologically, medical therapies to date have only been able to modify the effect of the vasospasm rather than to prevent or reverse it. Consequently, some neurosurgeons have sought to prevent the onset of vasospasm by surgically removing the subarachnoid clot before it can harm the vessel wall (60). This approach of aggressive removal of clot during aneurysm clipping within 48 hours after SAH appears to reduce the risk of vasospasm and delayed ischemia. These findings have been confirmed by Nosko et al (45) and Handa et al (23) in a primate model. Clinical adoption of this practice has been hampered by the technical difficulties and dangers of extensive clot removal in the basal subarachnoid cisterns. A nonmechanical and less traumatic method of clearing subarachnoid hematoma by intrathecal administration of the thrombolytic agent tissue-type plasminogen activator (t-PA) has been investigated in primates (18). Administered into the basal cisterns beginning 24 hours after experimental SAH, t-PA completely lysed the subarachnoid clot in 11 of 12 animals. Angiographic vasospasm at 7 days was significantly less frequent than in placebo-treated animals. There was no adverse effect on coagulation and t-PA did not cause meningeal or parenchymal inflammation that could be detected histologically.

Other Treatments

On the premise that vasospasm may be due, in part, to free radicals and lipid peroxides generated by the degenerating subarachnoid clot, we administered 21-aminosteroid U74006F, a potent inhibitor of iron-dependent lipid peroxidation to monkeys after experimental SAH (57). The severity of vasospasm was modestly reduced in treated animals compared with placebo-treated controls. This study also suggested that the drug had a cerebral cytoprotective effect (57).

Recommendations

Our present policy for managing patients with SAH from aneurysms of the anterior circulation and most posterior circulation aneurysms is to operate as early as possible to clip the aneurysm and prevent catastrophic recurrent hemorrhage. At operation, as much subarachnoid clot as possible is aspirated from the exposed basal cisterns. Hypotension and temporary clips are used only if absolutely necessary. Moderate volume expansion with a mixture of crystalloid and colloid solutions is instituted to increase cardiac output, improve cerebral perfusion, and achieve a degree of hemodilution. Intracranial hypertension is treated by CSF drainage with a ventricular or cisternal catheter, hyperventilation, and osmotherapy if necessary. Delayed ischemia is treated with more aggressive hemodynamic therapy, including inotropic cardiac support with invasive hemodynamic monitoring. The left-heart filling pressure is incrementally elevated with volume expansion to the point of optimal cardiac output (a pulmonary artery capillary pressure of approximately 18 to 20 mm Hg), and systolic blood pressure is increased as high as 200 mm Hg in order to reverse the neurologic deficit. The oxygenation and acid–base status of the patient are closely monitored and supported, because cardiopulmonary complications are common.

Patients referred to us late after SAH who already have angiographic vasospasm are also treated by prompt aneurysm clipping, unless they are comatose or have severe, diffuse vasospasm. We seldom use antifibrinolytic agents, partly because of our policy of early surgery and partly because of the increased risk of delayed ischemic deficits (61, 65). Antifibrinolytic agents would be considered only for treating technically difficult posterior circulation aneurysms in patients who are not candidates for early operation and whose initial CT scans show a low-volume SAH.

Recently available for clinical use, calcium antagonists are useful in preventing delayed ischemic tissue damage. Prevention of vasospasm through thrombolytic clearance of the subarachnoid clot warrants further investigation. The development of effective pharmacologic reversal of vasospasm awaits further clarification of the pathogenesis of this disorder.

CEREBRAL ISCHEMIA AFTER INTRACEREBRAL HEMORRHAGE

Spontaneous intracerebral hematomas account for about 10% of all strokes and, like aneurysmal SAH, are associated with high morbidity and mortality rates (34). Spontaneous brain hematomas have a diverse etiology and are considered to injure the brain primarily through their destructive effect on tissue and by their volume, which increases ICP. The delayed neurologic deterioration that is not uncommon after intracerebral hemorrhage is usually ascribed to the development of cerebral edema, although rebleeding is occasionally responsible. The role of cerebral ischemia in either the acute or delayed phase of intracerebral hematoma is speculative, but recent experimental work suggests it may be important. Thus, reversal of cerebral ischemia might be useful in the management of these lesions.

Etiology and Pathophysiology

It is commonly believed that the most frequent cause of spontaneous brain hemorrhage is rupture of an arteriole weakened by chronic hypertension. The pathogenesis of intracerebral hematoma may be inferred from the location of the lesion and the age of the patient (28, 61). Hypertensive intracerebral hematomas have a pre-

dilection for the putamen or adjacent internal capsule, thalamus, cerebellum, and pons, which are served at least in part by penetrating arterioles arising from major cerebral arterial trunks. The precise natures of the underlying vascular lesion and the mechanism of rupture have been debated since the demonstration of miliary microaneurysms on the penetrating cerebral arterioles by Charcot and Bouchard in 1868 (10). A variety of degenerative changes have been described in these vessels, including hyalinization of the media sometimes accompanied by lipid-laden macrophages (lipohyalinosis) and fibrinoid necrosis. These changes are clearly associated with chronic hypertension and, to a lesser extent, diabetes mellitus (8).

A multitude of other etiologies are associated with spontaneous intracerebral hematomas: ruptured saccular aneurysms (about 20% cause intracerebral hematoma); ruptured arteriovenous malformations (AVMs) (about 80% cause intracerebral hematoma); primary or, more commonly, metastatic brain tumors, particularly renal cell carcinoma and malignant melanoma; cerebral vasculitides and angiopathies, including amyloid angiopathy; and congenital and acquired bleeding diatheses, such as those associated with hematopoietic malignancies like leukemia, and hemorrhagic cerebral infarction (19, 48). In some instances of lobar hemorrhage, no underlying cause can be identified. Multiple intracerebral hematomas are associated with bleeding diatheses, cerebral vasculitis, and amyloid angiopathy (48).

Massive intracerebral hematomas wreak havoc by their direct destructive effect and by elevating the ICP. Supratentorial hypertensive hemorrhages commonly rupture into the ventricles and cause obstructive hydrocephalus. Such large intracerebral hematomas are often fatal. Within brain parenchyma, the hemorrhage follows the path of least resistance, preferentially penetrating white matter along major tracts.

An intracerebral hematoma compresses the adjacent parenchyma and its microcirculation. This pressure may result in a decrease in local CBF, causing cerebral ischemia that could contribute to the initial neurologic deficit and, later, to the development of cerebral edema. However, in studying the effect of experimental intracerebral hematoma in rats, Nath et al (42) found that after 10 minutes of temporary reduction, hemispheral CBF ipsilateral to the hematoma began to increase within 10 minutes and reached normal levels by 3 hours. Histologic evidence of ischemia was most commonly found in the parenchyma near the hematoma injection site rather than at the site of the intracerebral lesion. Reduction in the enzyme glycogen phosphorylase, a marker of ischemia, did not closely correlate with either of these areas.

In another study from the same laboratory, Sinar et al (56) inserted a microballoon stereotactically into rat caudate nucleus. The balloon could be inflated and then deflated to simulate surgical evacuation of an intracerebral hematoma. CBF was significantly depressed 4 hours after a 10-minute balloon inflation that caused a marked transient elevation in ICP. Light microscopy showed a large area of damage in the caudate nucleus. It was concluded that evacuation of the lesion does not prevent substantial persistent ischemic brain injury. Presumably, differences in the size of the lesions accounted for the discrepancy in the CBF response in this study and that of Nath et al (42).

The dynamic changes in regional CBF (rCBF) in response to a developing intracerebral hematoma were studied in primates by Bullock et al (9). The lesions were created by allowing the animal's femoral arterial blood to flow through a needle implanted in the caudate nucleus. CBF decreased in all brain regions in the first hour, but the decrease was greatest and most persistent in the area surrounding the clot. The threshold for ischemic neuronal damage was exceeded for 90 minutes after the initiation of the intracerebral hematoma. Changes in ICP or CPP did not account for the persistent reductions in rCBF. In perfusion-fixed brains from animals sacrificed after 3 hours, the specific gravity was lower around the lesion than in other areas, which suggests that the ischemia may have been caused by progressive cytotoxic edema.

Mizukami and Tawaza used intracarotid xenon-133 injections to study rCBF in 14 hypertensive patients with intracerebral hematoma (39). CBF was reduced in 13 patients, independent of changes in CPP. In areas adjacent to the hematoma, rCBF was depressed despite a normal ICP and could be increased by hyperosmolar therapy. From these findings, the authors concluded that brain deformation and local pressure from the hematoma, rather than decreases in CPP associated with elevated ICP, reduced rCBF. They advocated hyperosmolar therapy or surgical evacuation of the intracerebral hematoma to decompress the microcirculation and avert ischemia.

Using PET to study patients with spontaneous intracerebral hematomas of various etiologies, Ackerman et al (1) demonstrated that CBF and cerebral metabolism were depressed in the area occupied by the hematoma. In the adjacent cerebral tissue, there was no evidence of anaerobic (ischemic) metabolism, which suggested that these hematomas were not producing ischemia beyond the confines of the clot. In one patient, an intact area of cortex adjacent to the mass showed an increased blood flow. There was little in this preliminary study to support the view that there is a significant area of ischemia around an intracerebral hematoma. However, these results must be interpreted with caution because the study was not performed in the first few hours or days after the intracerebral hemorrhage occurred.

Although experimental studies have not provided conclusive results, it seems likely that clinically significant intracerebral hematomas, like other mass lesions in the central nervous system, do cause a certain degree of ischemia due to local pressure. It is difficult, however, to isolate and quantify this vascular disturbance from the many other deleterious effects of intracerebral hematoma on surrounding brain. More persuasive demonstrations of a significant and reversible local microcirculatory failure due to the presence of intracerebral hematoma are needed to justify decompressive neurosurgical procedures for patients with these lesions.

Other causes for delayed clinical deterioration besides progressive cerebral ischemia have been postulated. Enlargement and extension of the hematoma should be considered. It is also possible that as it dissolves, the hematoma exerts a noxious chemical effect on the adjacent brain and its circulation that leads to a breakdown of the blood–brain barrier and development of vasogenic edema. This explanation would account for the frequent observation of ring enhancement on contrast-enhanced CT scans of patients with resorbing intracerebral hematomas.

Clinical Features

The symptom complexes of hemorrhages in typical locations such as the thalamus, lentiform nucleus, cerebellum, and brain stem have been reviewed (19). Patients may stabilize initially after intracerebral brain hemorrhage and then deteriorate some days later. Before attributing this entirely to the hematoma or its se-

quelae, a search for other possible causes, including electrolyte disorders, hypoxemia, sepsis, pulmonary emboli, and obstructive hydrocephalus, should be carried out.

Diagnosis

CT scanning establishes the diagnosis of intracerebral hematoma and is superior to MR imaging in rapidly distinguishing hematoma from infarction. A typically located hemorrhage in an older, hypertensive patient usually presents no difficulty in diagnosis (Fig. 17.5). Certain other possibilities, such as bleeding diatheses and some of the vasculitides, may be apparent after a review of the patient's history and the results of laboratory investigations. If the presence of extensive edema suggests an underlying brain tumor, then a contrast-enhanced CT scan should be per-

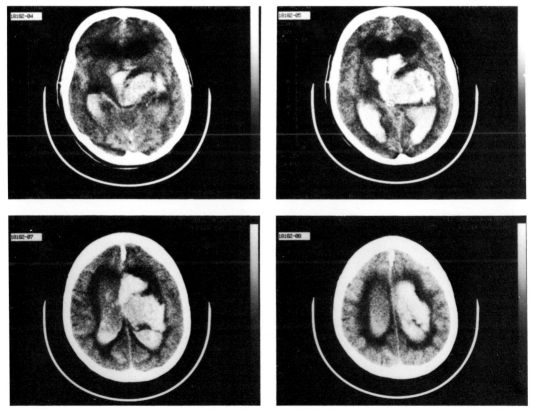

Figure 17.5. CT scans from an 81-year-old woman who collapsed at home shows a large left thalamic hemorrhage that has dissected into adjacent brain and ruptured into the lateral ventricles. Autopsy confirmed a hypertensive etiology.

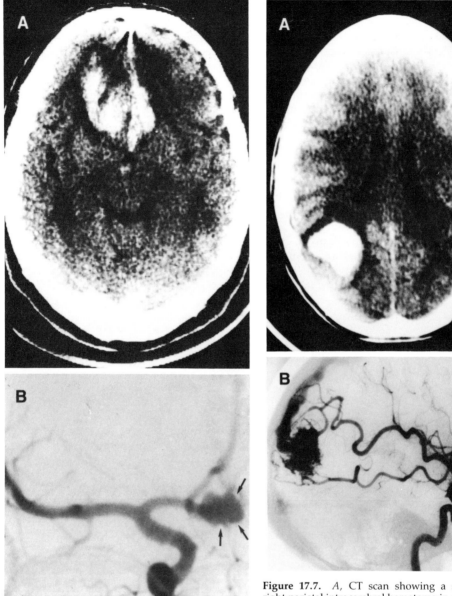

Figure 17.6. *A,* CT scan showing bilateral, medial frontal blood clots associated with blood in the inter-hemispheric fissure suggested the presence of an anterior communicating artery aneurysm. *B,* left ca-rotid angiogram demonstrates the aneurysm *(arrows).*

Figure 17.7. *A,* CT scan showing a spontaneous right parietal intracerebral hematoma in a 21-year-old woman raised the suspicion of an underlying arteri-ovenous malformation (AVM). *B,* lateral angiogram of the right carotid artery confirms the presence of the AVM.

formed to look for areas of abnormal en-hancement, although these areas may not become apparent until the hematoma has begun to be resorbed. The presence of a large Sylvian clot or bilateral midline fron-tal clots suggests an underlying ruptured aneurysm, especially if there is blood in the basal cisterns (Fig. 17.6). If there is any suspicion of an underlying aneurysm or AVM, cerebral angiography should be per-formed, particularly if surgery is being contemplated (Fig. 17.7). A small AVM may either be destroyed by the hemor-rhage or compressed by the intracerebral hematoma so that it cannot be demonstrated angiographically in the acute phase (the so-called cryptic AVM). If no cause for the intracerebral hematoma can be found and the initial angiogram is negative, MR imaging, repeat cerebral angiography, or contrast-enhanced CT scanning should be performed. The typical high density of an acute intracerebral hematoma on CT scans is lost over several weeks.

Treatment

Medical management of patients with spontaneous intracerebral hematoma is primarily supportive. Anticonvulsants are used when there is risk of seizures. Corticosteroids are also used by some doctors, although dexamethasone was not found to be useful in primary supratentorial intracerebral hematomas in a randomized trial, and we do not routinely employ them (52). Elevated blood pressure should be treated judiciously in order not to precipitate a hypotensive cerebral insult. Appropriate medical intervention should be taken to correct any underlying coagulopathy. The usual measures for controlling intracranial hypertension, including hyperventilation and osmotherapy, are undertaken for large, inoperable hematomas and in some postoperative patients. Such patients often require ICP monitoring. There may be little to gain from aggressive treatment, medical or surgical, in patients who are already neurologically devastated.

The history of surgery for hypertensive intracerebral hematoma has been reviewed by Luessenhop (34). The current surgical indications have been outlined by Ojemann and Heros (48). Generally, all but the smallest cerebellar hematomas should be evacuated, even if the patient is in a deep coma, since they are life-threatening lesions and remarkable neurologic recoveries are frequently observed postoperatively. The exceptions are those cases where there is evidence of a large extension of the hematoma into the brain stem. There is seldom any indication to operate for thalamic, deep putamenal, or brain stem hemorrhages. Surgery is reserved for those patients with lobar, lateral putamenal or capsular hematomas who continue to deteriorate from the mass effect of the lesion despite medical therapy. In some cases, the hematoma may be at least partially aspirated with a cannula under CT guidance. However, an open microsurgical procedure is often necessary. There is insufficient evidence at this time to support routine evacuation of hematomas in neurologically stable patients in the hope that this will relieve pressure on the adjacent microcirculation and prevent ischemic damage.

In fact, there is evidence that aggressive surgical treatment makes little difference in the outcome of a great many patients (16, 34). Volpin et al (63) studied 132 cases of spontaneous intracerebral hematoma, 50 of which were treated surgically; 42% of the patients were comatose at admission. The volume of the hematomas, determined from CT scans, ranged from 2 to 115 ml (average, 54 ml). All patients with a hematoma volume under 26 ml survived, while all those with a volume over 85 ml died, regardless of whether they were treated medically or surgically. Among comatose patients with hematoma volumes of 26 to 85 ml, medical treatment resulted in a mortality rate of 100% (11 of 11 cases), whereas only 7 (32%) of 22 patients treated surgically died or had a vegetative outcome; unfortunately, only 9% of comatose patients who had surgery were completely independent at hospital discharge.

If a controlled trial showed that early decompressive surgery enhanced recovery then the role for stereotactic removal of the hematoma, possibly combined with injection of thrombolytic agents into the thrombus to speed its dissolution, will need to be investigated (43). Such measures would probably need to be instituted early and combined with agents to protect the brain against ischemia and edema.

PERSPECTIVE

During the past year, several additional randomized controlled trials have confirmed the efficacy of both oral (51) and intravenous (26, 46) nimodipine in reducing secondary ischemic brain damage and improving outcome after aneurysmal subarachnoid hemorrhage. At the experimental level the 21-aminosteroid U74006F (71) and intrathecal thrombolytic therapy rt-PA (17) still appear promising as preventative therapies for vasospasm.

In a randomized controlled trial Auer et al (5) compared endoscopic evacuation of spontaneous supratentorial hematomas through a burr hole versus medical treatment in 100 patients where the interval between stroke and the start of treatment was less than 48 hours. It was found that patients with subcortical hematomas fared better with surgery, whereas the outcome of surgery for putamenal or thalamic hemorrhage was no better than with medical treatment. In a similar randomized controlled study (27) it was found that conventional surgery within 48 hours of the bleed, while prolonging the life of some semi-comatose patients, did not improve the overall mortality or morbidity rate compared to conservative therapy. It has not yet been shown, therefore, that with the exception of large subcortical hematomas urgent decompressive surgery improves overall outcome after spontaneous supratentorial intracerebral bleeding.

Acknowledgments—The authors thank Dr. Lew Disney for providing several of the radiologic studies, Dr. Ken Hutchinson for the transcranial Doppler investigations, and Arlene MacLean for preparing the manuscript.

References

1. Ackerman RH, Kelley RE, Davis SM, et al: Positron imaging of CBF and metabolism in nontraumatic intracerebral hemorrhage. In Mizukami M, Kogure K, Kanaya H, et al (eds): *Hypertensive Intracerebral Hemorrhage*. New York, Raven Press, 1983, pp 165–176.
2. Allen GS, Ahn HS, Prezosi TJ, et al: Cerebral arterial spasm—a controlled trial of nimodipine in patients with subarachnoid hemorrhage. *N Engl J Med* 308:619–624, 1983.
3. Asano T, Tanishima T, Sasaki T, et al: Possible participation of free-radical reactions initiated by clot lysis in the pathogenesis of vasospasm after subarachnoid hemorrhage. In Wilkins RH (ed): *Cerebral Arterial Spasm*. Baltimore, Williams & Wilkins, 1980, pp 190–201.
4. Astrup J, Siesjö BK, Symon L: Thresholds in cerebral ischemia—the ischemic penumbra (editorial). *Stroke* 12:723–725, 1981.
5. Auer LM, Deinsberger W, Niederkorn K, et al: Endoscopic surgery versus medical treatment for spontaneous intracerebral hematoma: A randomized study. *J Neurosurg* 70:530–535, 1989.
6. Auer LM, Ljunggren B, Brandt L, et al: Acute aneurysm surgery and nimodipine for the prevention of symptomatic vasospasm. In Auer LM (ed): *Timing of Aneurysm Surgery*. Berlin, Walter de Gryter, 1985, pp 493–502.
7. Awad IA, Carter LP, Spetzler RF, et al: Clinical vasospasm after subarachnoid hemorrhage: Response to hypervolemic hemodilution and arterial hypertension. *Stroke* 18:365–372, 1987.
8. Brott T, Thalinger K, Hertzberg VS: Hypertension as a risk factor for spontaneous intracerebral hemorrhage. *Stroke* 17:1078–1083, 1986.
9. Bullock R, Brock-Utne J, van Dellen J, et al: Intracerebral hemorrhage in a primate model: Effect of regional cerebral blood flow. *Surg Neurol* 29:101–107, 1988.
10. Charcot & Bouchard: Nouvelles recherches sur la pathogénie de l'hémorrhagie cérébrale. *Archives de Physiologie Normale et de Pathologie* 1:110–127, 643–665, 1868.
11. Dion JE, Gates PC, Fox AJ, et al: Clinical events following neuroangiography: A prospective study. *Stroke* 18:997–1004, 1987.
12. Duff TA, Louie J, Feilbach JA, et al: Erythrocytes are essential for development of cerebral vasculopathy resulting from subarachnoid hemorrhage in cats. *Stroke* 19:68–72, 1988.
13. Espinosa F, Weir B, Overton T, et al: A randomized placebo-controlled double-blind trial of nimodipine after SAH in monkeys. Part 1: Clinical and radiological findings. *J Neurosurg* 60:1167–1175, 1984.
14. Espinosa F, Weir B, Shnitka T: Electron microscopy of simian cerebral horseradish peroxidase. *Neurosurgery* 19:935–945, 1986.
15. Fein JM, Flor WJ, Cohan SL, et al: Sequential changes of vascular ultrastructure in experimental cerebral vasospasm. Myonecrosis of subarachnoid arteries. *J Neurosurg* 41:49–58, 1974.
16. Fieschi C, Carolei A, Fiorelli M, et al: Changing prognosis of primary intracerebral hemorrhage: Results of a clinical and computed tomographic follow-up study of 104 patients. *Stroke* 19:192–195, 1988.
17. Findlay JM, Weir BKA, Gordon P, et al: Safety and efficacy of intrathecal thrombolytic therapy in a primate model of cerebral vasospasm. *Neurosurgery* 24:491–498, 1989.
18. Findlay JM, Weir BK, Steinke D, et al: Effect of intrathecal thrombolytic therapy on subarachnoid clot and chronic vasospasm in a primate model of SAH. *J Neurosurg* 69:723–735, 1988.
19. Fisher CM: Clinical syndromes in cerebral thrombosis, hypertensive hemorrhage and ruptured saccular aneurysm. *Clin Neurosurg* 22:117–147, 1975.
20. Flamm ES, Adams HP Jr, Beck DW, et al: Dose-escalation study of intravenous nicardipine in patients with aneurysmal subarachnoid hemorrhage. *J Neurosurg* 68:393–400, 1988.
21. Grolimund P, Seiler RW, Aaslid R, et al: Evaluation of cerebrovascular disease by combined extracranial and transcranial Doppler sonography.

Experience in 1,039 patients. *Stroke* 18:1018–1024, 1987.

22. Grubb RJ Jr, Raichle ME, Eichling JO, et al: Effects of subarachnoid hemorrhage on cerebral blood volume, blood flow and oxygen utilization in humans. *J Neurosurg* 44:446–452, 1977.

23. Handa Y, Weir BKA, Nosko M, et al: The effect of timing of clot removal on chronic vasospasm in a primate model. *J Neurosurg* 67:558–564, 1987.

24. Hennerici M, Rautenberg W, Schwartz A: Transcranial Doppler ultrasound for the assessment of intracranial flow velocity. Part 2: Evaluation of intracranial arterial disease. *Surg Neurol* 27:523–532, 1987.

25. Hughes JT, Schianchi PM: Cerebral arterial spasm. A histological study at necroscopy of the blood vessels in cases of subarachnoid hemorrhage. *J Neurosurg* 48:515–525, 1978.

26. Jan M, Buchheit F, Tremoulet M: Therapeutic trial of intravenous nimodipine in patients with established cerebral vasospasm after rupture of intracranial aneurysms. *Neurosurgery* 23:154–157, 1988.

27. Juvela S, Heiskanen O, Poranen A, et al: The treatment of spontaneous intracerebral hemorrhage. *J Neurosurg* 70:755–758, 1989.

28. Kase CS: Intracerebral hemorrhage: Non-hypertensive causes. *Stroke* 17:590–595, 1986.

29. Kassell NF, Peerless SJ, Durward QJ, et al: Treatment of ischemic deficits from vasospasm with intravascular volume expansion and induced arterial hypertension. *Neurosurgery* 11:337–342, 1982.

30. Kistler JP, Crowell RM, Davis KR, et al: The relation of cerebral vasospasm to the extent and location of subarachnoid blood visualized by CT scan: A prospective study. *Neurology* 33:424–426, 1983.

31. Krueger C, Weir B, Nosko M, et al: Nimodipine and chronic vasospasm in monkeys. Part 2: Pharmacological studies of vessels in spasm. *Neurosurgery* 16:137–140, 1985.

32. Lewis PJ, Weir BK, Nosko MG, et al: Intrathecal nimodipine therapy in a primate model of chronic cerebral vasospasm. *Neurosurgery* 22:492–500, 1988.

33. Ljunggren B, Brandt L, Saveland H, et al: Outcome in 60 consecutive patients treated with early aneurysm operation and intravenous nimodipine. *J Neurosurg* 58:864–873, 1984.

34. Luessenhop AJ: Hypertensive intracerebral hemorrhage in the United States: Update on surgical treatment. In Mizukami M, Kogure K, Kanaya H, et al (eds): *Hypertensive Intracerebral Hemorrhage*. New York, Raven Press, 1983, pp 123–132.

35. Martin WRW, Baker RP, Grubb RL, et al: Cerebral blood volume, blood flow, and oxygen metabolism in cerebral ischemia and subarachnoid hemorrhage: An in vivo study using positron emission tomography. *Acta Neurochir (Wien)* 70:3–9, 1984.

36. Mayberg MR, Hauser OW, Sundt TM Jr: Ultrastructural changes in feline arterial endothelium following subarachnoid hemorrhage. *J Neurosurg* 48:49–57, 1978.

37. Mayberg MR, Okada T, Bark D: Cerebral arteriopathy and contractile changes after SAH are related to erythrocyte component of whole blood (abstract). *Stroke* 19:130, 1988.

38. Mee E, Dorrance D, Lowe D, et al: Controlled study of nimodipine in aneurysm patients treated early after subarachnoid hemorrhage. *Neurosurgery* 22:484–491, 1988.

39. Mizukami M, Tawaza T: Theoretical background for surgical treatments in hypertensive intracerebral hemorrhage. In Mizukami M, Kogure K, Kanaya H, et al (eds): *Hypertensive Intracerebral Hemorrhage*. New York, Raven Press, 1983, pp 239–248.

40. Nakagomi T, Kassell NF, Sasaki T, et al: Impairment of endothelium-dependent vasodilation induced by acetylcholine and adenosine triphosphate following experimental subarachnoid hemorrhage. *Stroke* 18:482–489, 1987.

41. Nakagomi T, Kassell NF, Sasaki T, et al: Effect of hypoxia on the contractile response to KCl, prostaglandin $F_{2\alpha}$, and hemoglobin. *J Neurosurg* 67:565–572, 1987.

42. Nath FP, Kelly PT, Jenkins A, et al: Effects of experimental intracerebral hemorrhage on blood flow, capillary permeability, and histochemistry. *J Neurosurg* 66:555–562, 1987.

43. Niizuma H, Suzuki J: Stereotactic aspiration of putamenal hemorrhage using a double-track aspiration technique. *Neurosurgery* 22:432–436, 1988.

44. Nosko M, Weir B, Krueger C, et al: Nimodipine and chronic vasospasm in monkeys. Part 1: Clinical and radiological findings. *Neurosurgery* 16:129–136, 1985.

45. Nosko M, Weir BK, Lunt A, et al: Effect of clot removal at 24 hours on chronic vasospasm after SAH in the primate model. *J Neurosurg* 66:416–422, 1987.

46. Ohman J, Heiskanen O: Effect of nimodipine on outcome of patients after aneurysmal subarachnoid hemorrhage and surgery. *J Neurosurg* 69:683–686, 1988.

47. Ohta T, Kajikawa H, Yoshikawa Y, et al: Cerebral vasospasm and hemoglobins: Clinical and experimental studies. In Wilkins RH (ed): *Cerebral Arterial Spasm*. Baltimore, Williams & Wilkins, 1980, pp 166–172.

48. Ojemann RG, Heros RC: Spontaneous brain hemorrhage. *Stroke* 14:468–475, 1983.

49. Petruk KC, West M, Mohr G, et al: Nimodipine treatment in poor-grade aneurysm patients. Results of a multicenter double-blind placebo-controlled trial. *J Neurosurg* 68:505–517, 1988.

50. Philippon J, Grob R, Dagreou F, et al: Prevention of vasospasm in subarachnoid hemorrhage. A controlled study with nimodipine. *Acta Neurochir (Wien)* 82:110–114, 1986.

51. Pickard JD, Murray GD, Illingworth R, et al: Effect of oral nimodipine on cerebral infarction and outcome after subarachnoid haemorrhage: British aneurysm nimodipine trial. *Br Med J* 298:636–642, 1989.

52. Poungvarin N, Bhoopat W, Viriyavejakul A, et al: Effects of dexamethasone in primary supratentorial intracerebral hemorrhage. *N Engl J Med* 16:1229–1233, 1987.

53. Sasaki T, Asano T, Takakura K, et al: Nature of the vasoactive substance in CSF from patients with subarachnoid hemorrhage. *J Neurosurg* 60:1186–1191, 1984.

54. Seiler RW, Grolimund P, Aaslid R, et al: Cerebral

vasospasm evaluated by transcranial ultrasound correlated with clinical grade and CT-visualized subarachnoid hemorrhage. *J Neurosurg* 64:594–600, 1986.

55. Seiler RW, Grolimund P, Zurbruegg HR, et al: Evaluation of the calcium-antagonist nimodipine for the prevention of vasospasm after aneurysmal subarachnoid hemorrhage. *Acta Neurochir (Wien)* 85:7–16, 1987.

56. Sinar EJ, Mendelow AD, Graham DI, et al: Experimental intracerebral hemorrhage: Effects of a temporary mass lesion. *J Neurosurg* 66:568–576, 1987.

57. Steinke DE, Weir BKA, Findlay JM, et al: A trial of the 21-aminosteroid U74006F in a primate model of chronic cerebral vasospasm. *Neurosurgery* 24:179–186, 1989.

58. Takayasu M, Bassett JE, Dacey RG: Effects of calcium antagonists on intracerebral penetrating arterioles in rats. *J Neurosurg* 69:104–109, 1988.

59. Tanabe Y, Sakata K, Yamada H, et al: Cerebral vasospasm and ultrastructural changes in cerebral arterial wall. *J Neurosurg* 49:229–238, 1978.

60. Taneda M: Effect of early operation for ruptured aneurysms on prevention of delayed ischemic symptoms. *J Neurosurg* 57:622–628, 1982.

61. Toffol GJ, Biller J, Adams HP Jr: Nontraumatic intracerebral hemorrhage in young adults. *Arch Neurol* 44:483–485, 1987.

62. Vinall PE, Simeone FA: Effects of oxygen and glucose deprivation on vasoactivity in isolated bovine middle cerebral arteries. *Stroke* 17:970–975, 1986.

63. Volpin L, Cerevellini P, Colombo F, et al: Spontaneous intracerebral hematomas: A new proposal about the usefulness and limits of surgical treatment. *Neurosurgery* 15:663–666, 1984.

64. Weir B: *Aneurysms Affecting the Nervous System.* Baltimore, Williams & Wilkins, 1987, pp 246–250.

65. Weir B: Antifibrinolytics in subarachnoid hemorrhage. Do they have a role? No. *Arch Neurol* 44:116–118, 1987.

66. Wilkins RH: Attempted prevention or treatment of intracranial arterial spasm: A survey. *Neurosurgery* 6:198–210, 1986.

67. Wilkins RH: Attempted prevention or treatment of intracranial arterial spasm: An update. *Neurosurgery* 18:808–825, 1986.

68. Yamakami I, Isobe K, Yamaura A, et al: Vasospasm and regional cerebral blood flow (rCBF) in patients with ruptured intracranial aneurysms: Serial rCBF studies with the xenon-133 inhalation method. *Neurosurgery* 13:394–401, 1983.

69. Yonas H, Wolfson SK Jr, Gur D, et al: Clinical experience with the use of xenon-enhanced CT blood flow mapping in cerebrovascular disease. *Stroke* 15:443–450, 1984.

70. Zervas NT, Liszczak TM, Mayberg MR, et al: Cerebrospinal fluid may nourish cerebral vessels through pathways in the adventitia that may be analogous to systemic vasa vasorum. *J Neurosurg* 56:476–481, 1982.

71. Zuccarello M, Marsch JT, Schmitt G, et al: Effect of the 21-aminosteroid U-74006F on cerebral vasospasm following subarachnoid hemorrhage. *J Neurosurg* 71:98–104, 1989.

CHAPTER EIGHTEEN

Hemodynamic Manipulation in the Treatment of Brain Ischemia

John R. Little, M.D.
Jeffrey V. Rosenfeld, M.D., F.R.A.C.S., F.R.C.S. Ed.
Gene H. Barnett, M.D.

Brain ischemia is a common pathophysiologic entity. In some circumstances, its role in producing a neurologic deficit is unequivocal, as in embolization from an ulcerated carotid atheroma to an intracranial artery or severe systemic hypotension from cardiac asystole. However, its impact spreads far beyond such obvious clinical disorders. Unrecognized brain ischemia probably contributes to the development of neurologic deficits in many other settings, such as an expanding intracerebral hematoma or other mass lesion and severely elevated intracranial pressure (ICP).

The treatment of acute brain ischemia continues to receive considerable attention from clinical and laboratory investigators. Although a comprehensive regimen for preventing brain infarction has not been defined, much has been learned that can improve the clinical outcome. The primary objectives of treatment are to improve blood flow to the ischemic area and to increase the resistance of brain tissue to metabolic injury. Improving circulation reduces the size of the ischemic area and enhances the delivery of agents intended to increase metabolic resistance to ischemia.

This chapter focuses on methods for increasing blood flow to ischemic areas. The primary emphasis is on the treatment of incomplete focal ischemia, the kind most often encountered clinically by neurologists and neurosurgeons.

BASIC PRINCIPLES OF BLOOD FLOW

Poiseuille's law states that volume flow rate is directly proportional to the product of the pressure differential between the ends of the tube and the fourth power of the radius of the tube, and is inversely proportional to the product of the length of the tube and the viscosity of the fluid. In simpler terms, this means that the volume flow rate can be altered by changing the driving pressure, the radius or length of the tube, or the viscosity of the fluid. Although Poiseuille's law generally applies to blood flow, it must be remembered that blood is a non-Newtonian fluid and that perfusion is normally pulsatile. Thus, blood viscosity varies with the velocity of flow (29). Furthermore, brain blood flow increases with conversion from nonpulsatile to pulsatile perfusion in the presence of a constant range of perfusion pressures (48).

Circulation of blood appears to be more complex in the microvasculature than in larger vessels. Fahraeus and Lindquist (12) found that Poiseuille's law did not accurately predict the flow of blood through tubes of progressively smaller diameter: As vessel diameter decreased to the 40 μm range (that of arterioles), blood viscosity decreased. They ascribed this phenomenon to a reduction in hematocrit. Dintenfass (11) subsequently found that when the radius of the tube was 5 to 7 μm (approximately that of capillaries), blood viscosity stopped decreasing; with further reductions, viscosity increased markedly.

Our understanding of the mechanisms that regulate intracranial circulation is incomplete. Under normal circumstances, the brain regulates blood flow in accordance with its metabolic needs (38). Regional blood flow is regulated by constriction or dilatation of precapillary arterioles; it increases or decreases in response to neuronal metabolic activity. These regional fluctuations are thought to be partly the result of changes in local pH, carbon dioxide tension, and tissue metabolite levels. Brain blood flow is also greatly influenced by changes in systemic arterial CO_2 (i.e. CO_2 reactivity). Under normal circumstances, brain blood flow remains within a constant range throughout the physiologic range of systemic arterial blood pressure. During severe ischemia, the mechanisms controlling blood flow break down as the arterial system reaches a state of maximal dilatation. As blood flow decreases, CO_2 reactivity and autoregulation are progressively impaired and cease when the ischemic threshold is crossed (2, 18). Impairment of CO_2 reactivity and autoregulation may persist in varying degrees for months or years after the ischemic event whether or not maximum vasodilatation persists (33, 44).

Methods of enhancing blood flow to ischemic areas are based on our knowledge of the principles of tubular flow and hemorrheology. It is currently possible to increase perfusion pressure, dilate conducting arteries, and alter blood viscosity. The results of some experimental studies support the validity of these approaches in the treatment of brain ischemia, but many questions remain regarding their effectiveness in reducing infarct size and their application in specific clinical settings.

HYPERTENSIVE THERAPY

Increasing systemic arterial blood pressure to raise cerebral perfusion pressure would appear to be a logical component of the treatment of brain ischemia. Arteries in an area of focal ischemia due to proximal vascular occlusion are connected, through collateral channels that vary greatly in size and number, to arteries in the nonischemic area. Despite the presence of these interconnecting vessels, perfusion pressure is lower in the ischemic area than in the nonischemic area (45). An increase in systemic arterial blood pressure would be expected to increase pressure in the collateral arterial conducting system proximal to the occluded artery and in surrounding areas, thereby increasing the pressure differential and augmenting flow into the ischemic area. Whether or not this phenomenon reduces the extent of ischemic tissue damage depends on the adequacy of the collateral circulation and the severity of the ischemia.

The effects of changes in systemic arterial blood pressure on the brain circulation in experimental ischemia have been investigated extensively, but the treatment of ischemia with hypertension has received surprisingly little attention. Waltz (49) studied the effects of varying systemic arterial blood pressure on cortical blood flow in cats undergoing acute middle cerebral artery (MCA) occlusion. In nonischemic cortex, blood flow remained relatively constant despite changes in systemic arterial blood pressure. In ischemic cortex, blood flow paralleled blood pressure at normotensive and hypotensive levels; at hypertensive levels (mean arterial blood pressure to 120 mm Hg), it increased but never reached the baseline levels of nonischemic cortex. With further increases in systemic arterial pressure, cortical blood flow decreased.

Symon et al (43) evaluated the effects of pharmacologically induced hypertension on cerebral blood flow (CBF) in baboons undergoing acute MCA occlusion. These studies clearly showed a link between the degree of ischemia and the extent of autoregulatory impairment. Autoregulation was partially preserved in ischemic areas with greater than 40% of basal flow (collateral zones) and was absent in areas with less than 20% of basal flow (core area of ischemia). Hypotension induced by exsanguination further reduced CBF in the ischemic zone, whereas pharmacologically induced hypertension increased flow. Like Waltz (49), Symon et al (43) found a limit to the favorable effects of hypertension on CBF. When the mean arterial blood pressure rose 50 mm Hg or more above normal preexisting pressure, CBF in the ischemic zone decreased.

Symon et al (43) made additional important observations during reperfusion. CBF was impaired during reperfusion after severe ischemia. CBF was also measured after restoration of normal systemic arterial blood pressure in baboons subjected to MCA occlusion followed by 2 hours of hypotension. CBF levels after restoration of blood pressure did not recover to levels observed immediately after MCA occlusion and before induction of hypotension; but CBF levels after restoration of blood pressure correlated with the severity of ischemia observed during the hypotensive period. Clearly, hypotension had an additive deleterious effect on blood flow during reperfusion. These findings confirmed the observations of others (1) that changes in the microcirculation in areas of severe ischemia may prevent adequate reperfusion. This secondary impairment in blood flow has been called the "no-reflow phenomenon" (43).

Hope et al (16) measured somatosensory evoked potentials and local CBF in baboons subjected to MCA occlusion. Increasing the mean systemic arterial blood pressure pharmacologically by an average of 40 mm Hg significantly improved the evoked potentials and local CBF. Hypertensive therapy elicited a similar response in a small group of patients with ischemic neurologic deficits after aneurysm surgery.

Denny-Brown (10) was probably the first to report that hypertensive therapy improved the neurologic function of patients with acute brain ischemia. Others have described similar observations, but most of the studies were uncontrolled, and the reports anecdotal. The effect of hypertensive therapy on acute focal brain ischemia has not yet been systematically evaluated in a clinical setting.

During the past few years, pharmacologically induced hypertension has become a major component in the treatment of ischemic neurologic deficit after subarachnoid hemorrhage (SAH) (*see* Chapter 17, this volume). The current tendency to operate on a ruptured intracranial aneurysm within hours or days of SAH has largely eliminated the potential risk of rebleeding due to hypertensive therapy. The results of studies in which hypertension has been used to treat this condition have been encouraging (4, 30, 34). In most of these reports, hypertension was combined with hypervolemia. Beneficial effects were not achieved in some patients until very high blood pressure levels (e.g. 240 mm Hg systolic blood pressure) were reached.

Careful monitoring and manipulation of systemic arterial blood pressure are essential in patients with acute brain ischemia. Allowing systemic arterial blood pressure to decrease below initially observed levels further reduces blood flow in ischemic areas and must be avoided. Although the role of hypertensive therapy is less well defined than in patients with SAH, the weight of the evidence strongly favors its application for patients with SAH. The guidelines for its use in patients with brain ischemia due to vascular occlusion have yet to be defined.

Hypertensive therapy is not without risk. For example, pharmacologically induced hypertension may not be tolerated in patients with heart disease and could precipitate rebleeding from an untreated intracranial aneurysm. Hypertensive therapy initiated after prolonged delay could worsen brain edema or produce hemorrhage, particularly if infarction has already occurred or if reperfusion is induced in a previously severely ischemic area, such as after dissolution of an embolism.

HYPERVOLEMIA

Total body blood volume varies with many factors including age, sex, body weight, fat content, activity, position, medications, and disease. Blood volume may be reduced in many persons already at risk for stroke. In patients with SAH, both red blood cell mass and total blood volume are often substantially reduced (27). These changes are thought to be partly the result of bed rest, supine diuresis, negative nitrogen balance, decreased erythropoiesis, and iatrogenic blood loss. Systemic secretion of vasoconstricting catecholamines that accompanies SAH is also considered an important factor in reducing intravascular volume. Most patients with acute ischemic stroke are hypovolemic at admission (13).

Maintaining intravascular volume appears to be an important factor in improving the outcome of patients with acute ischemia after a recent SAH. Hypovolemia increases the likelihood of relative or absolute systemic hypotension, which could further reduce blood flow in the ischemic area. However, the role of hypervolemia in treating brain ischemia has not yet been established. On the basis of Poiseuille's law, it is difficult to explain how hypervolemia per se would improve brain blood flow without a concomitant increase in perfusion pressure, dilatation of conducting arteries, or reduction of blood viscosity.

Some experimental studies (20) have related improved brain blood flow and outcome in ischemia to an increase in cardiac output induced by hypervolemia. In this setting, pulse pressure is augmented by the increased cardiac stroke volume. Raising pulse pressure might have favorable effects on blood flow in ischemic brain (48). However, another series of experimental studies showed that expanding intravascular volume without hemodilution did not improve cortical blood flow in areas of focal cerebral ischemia despite a significant rise in the cardiac output (51).

Decreased blood volume after SAH appears to increase the risk of symptomatic vasospasm. Solomon et al (37) found subnormal blood volume in 86% of patients with symptomatic vasospasm but in only 13% of patients with asymptomatic angiographic vasospasm. A number of clinical reports, although largely anecdotal, appear to show a considerable reduction of morbidity from vasospasm when aggressive steps are taken to increase intravascular volume (4, 30, 37). But there is no compelling evidence that hypervolemia is better than normovolemia in treating ischemic symptoms after SAH.

Systemic hypervolemia is unlikely to have any direct effect on blood volume in the ischemic area. Expansion of blood volume in the brain microcirculation is an early and consistent response to ischemia. When perfusion pressure and blood flow drop below the normal range, the brain arterial system dilates, spontaneously producing a state of reactive hypervolemia in the ischemic area. As blood flow approaches the ischemic threshold, vasodilatation and volume expansion of the microcirculation are already maximal and autoregulation and CO_2 reactivity are lost. Consequently, it is unclear what benefit systemic volume expansion would have on the microcirculation in and around an ischemic area of brain, except indirectly by its effect on blood pressure.

VASODILATATION

Cerebral arteries and arterioles in an ischemic area lose their autoregulatory capacity and CO_2 reactivity and become maximally dilated (38, 43). Conducting arteries in surrounding areas retain their reactivity either fully or partially depending on their proximity to the ischemic focus. These observations gave rise to the hypothesis that blood flow in the ischemic area could be enhanced by dilating the conducting collateral channels. The findings of subsequent studies, however, have not supported this hypothesis.

The early studies focused on the effects of CO_2 on the brain circulation in experimental and clinical ischemia. In 1968, Lassen and Palvolgyi (22) reported a further decrease in blood flow "in some brain regions in patients with acute cerebral vascular diseases." They attributed this response to a reduction in perfusion pressure in collateral vessels produced by arterial dilatation in nonischemic brain. This response was called the "intracerebral steal syndrome." They also observed an inverse response, the "Robin Hood" or "inverse steal" syndrome, where hypocapnia provoked an increase in blood flow shunted to poor ischemic areas in association with vasoconstriction and decrease in flow in rich nonischemic areas. Most subsequent reports have confirmed these observations.

Symon (41, 42) and Brawley and his associates (7, 8), measured the luminal pressure in arteries beyond the point of experimental occlusion of a major brain artery. During inhalation of CO_2, arterial pressure decreased. Using a thermocouple technique, Brawley et al (7, 8) also showed a concomitant further reduction of cortical blood flow in the ischemic area.

A few studies have shown improved blood flow in ischemic areas during CO_2 inhalation. For example, Yamamoto et al (52) performed fluorescein angiography and measured microregional CBF in dogs undergoing occlusion of a cortical artery. When the dogs breathed 5% CO_2 and 95% oxygen, collateral flow improved and the ischemic area was consistently reduced in size. Hyperventilation that lowered arterial CO_2 made the ischemic area larger by reducing collateral flow. Using autoradiography to study rats subjected to MCA occlusion, Jones* found a significant increase in cortical blood flow in the territory of the occluded vessel with high arterial CO_2 levels (i.e. 60 torr). The results of such studies indicate that the effects of elevated arterial CO_2 levels on the brain circulation in ischemia are variable and may be unpredictable. Clinical studies have never demonstrated significant benefit from induced hypercarbia.

Interest in the use of vasodilating agents to improve blood flow in ischemic brain was rekindled with the introduction of prostacyclin, a prostaglandin derivative, and the dihydropyridine group of calcium-entry blocking agents. Prostacyclin is a very potent vascular smooth muscle relaxant that is produced primarily in endothelial cells; it also reduces platelet adhesiveness. Intravenous injection or topical application to normal cortex causes intense arterial dilatation and a marked increase in blood flow. Unfortunately, prostacyclin has not consistently improved blood flow in experimental studies of brain ischemia (5), nor has it reduced the neurologic morbidity of ischemia in controlled clinical trials (17, 23, 28).

Nimodipine and nicardipine are dihydropyridine derivatives that have been extensively evaluated in experimental studies of ischemia. Both agents selectively dilate brain arteries and increase brain blood flow under normal circumstances. Their effects on blood flow during ischemia, however,

have varied; the most consistent benefit is seen during recirculation after temporary focal ischemia (6, 15). In studies of ischemia after SAH from aneurysm rupture (3, 26), nimodipine improved the clinical outcome despite the lack of any angiographic evidence of reduction in the severity of vasospasm. Nimodipine, it has been suggested, may exert a beneficial effect in brain ischemia by preventing toxic calcium accumulation in the cytoplasm of ischemic neurons and glia. The relative lack of binding affinity of dihydropyridine derivatives to neuronal and glial plasma membranes, however, reduces the likelihood of that possibility (36).

HEMODILUTION

Viscosity is a physical property of fluids that determines the internal resistance to shear forces. Blood viscosity is not constant (29). Blood is a non-Newtonian fluid: Its viscosity varies with the rate of flow. Slow-moving blood has a higher viscosity than the same blood moving rapidly. Hematocrit, erythrocyte rigidity, and plasma fibrinogen concentration also affect blood viscosity. Blood viscosity increases logarithmically with increasing hematocrit. Hematocrit, and consequently viscosity of blood, in the cerebral microcirculation is normally 70% to 80% of that in the large vessels (21).

Brain blood flow decreases with hematocrit levels above 50% and increases with hematocrit levels below 30% (14, 46). This compensatory increase allows adequate oxygen delivery in normal subjects even when hematocrit is as low as 20%. In a patient with an occluded brain artery and limited collateral circulation, a similar compensatory increase would not be possible; more severe impairment of oxygen delivery and greater tissue damage could result.

The relationship of blood viscosity to the pathogenesis and treatment of brain ischemia is of considerable interest. Studies have shown that a hematocrit level greater than 50% increases the risk of stroke (19, 47). Other clinical and experimental stud-

---

*SC Jones, personal communication, 1989.

ies have suggested that optimizing blood viscosity can limit tissue damage during an ischemic event (13, 50, 51). Hematocrit might also be a factor in the impairment of reperfusion after ischemia. Yield stress— the minimal force required to start blood flowing once it has been stationary—increases in relation to the third power of the hematocrit (29). Consequently, an elevation of hematocrit might prevent the restoration of blood flow after transient ischemia.

The optimal hematocrit for patients with brain ischemia has not been determined. Recent studies suggest that it is probably about 35% (13, 14, 29, 46, 50, 51). To achieve this level, hematocrit can be quickly reduced by the intravenous administration of low-molecular-weight dextran, albumin, or saline. Blood can be removed concomitantly by venesection if normovolemic hemodilution is desired. Transfusions of packed erythrocytes can be given to raise the hematocrit when it is below 35%.

Experimental studies have consistently demonstrated improved blood flow and reduced infarct size after treatment with low-molecular-weight dextran (50). These beneficial effects have been attributed to the lowering of blood viscosity through hemodilution and to the reduction of platelet adhesiveness. The clinical use of low-molecular-weight dextran in acute brain ischemia has many advocates, but most of the reports have been anecdotal.

The Scandinavian Stroke Study Group conducted a stratified randomized multicenter trial in 15 hospitals (35). Patients who had an acute ischemic stroke within 48 hours of admission and a hematocrit of 38% to 50% were randomized to hemodilution and control groups. The results showed no benefit from normovolemic hemodilution (mean hematocrit reduction, 6.9%) maintained by venesection and infusion of low-molecular-weight dextran. The failure to improve neurologic outcome does not mean that this form of therapy is without potential benefit in other situations. Undoubtedly, many of the patients treated in the Scandinavian study already had irreversible brain injury when treatment was initiated. Further studies are needed to evaluate this therapeutic approach in a more acute setting and to define potentially responsive subgroups of patients.

HYPEROSMOLARITY

Mannitol is the hyperosmolar agent used most frequently in the treatment of acute brain ischemia. Experimentally, this agent has been shown to have a beneficial effect on the microcirculation and infarct size when it is given early in the course of the ischemic event (24, 25). These favorable effects are not seen when mannitol is given after ischemic breakdown of the blood–brain barrier or irreversible brain injury has occurred.

Several mechanisms have been proposed to explain the action of mannitol. It increases blood osmolality, which appears to retard early brain swelling and maintain flow through the microcirculation (24, 25). Mannitol reduces erythrocyte rigidity and thereby enhances erythrocyte transit through the capillary bed (9). The rapid administration of mannitol transiently reduces blood viscosity by lowering the hematocrit. Lower viscosity would also improve flow in ischemic areas. Muizelaar and associates (31, 32) suggested that mannitol decreases blood viscosity and increases blood flow in nonischemic brain and that the arteries in nonischemic areas undergo secondary constriction to keep blood flow constant. They postulated that arterial constriction in nonischemic areas, rather than water conduction driven by an osmotic gradient, is primarily responsible for the reduction of ICP after mannitol infusion. These changes could also act to improve blood flow in ischemic areas by decreasing ICP and thereby increasing perfusion pressure and by producing an inverse steal syndrome.

Reports of the clinical efficacy of mannitol in brain ischemia are preliminary and anecdotal. It is unlikely, based on experimental evidence, that the delayed administration of mannitol would have a protective effect. The clinical applications for treatment of acute stroke therefore appear to be limited. Mannitol has frequently been given to patients by neurosurgeons when temporary artery occlusion is needed for clipping of an intracranial aneurysm. Suzuki et al (39, 40) have used mannitol extensively in combination with dexamethasone and vitamin E (the "Sendai cocktail") with good results in both experimental and uncontrolled surgical studies.

PERSPECTIVE

Brain ischemia is a frequently encountered problem. In the past, patients with impending or evolving infarction were generally believed to be beyond help and were managed supportively. Although it is difficult to prove a beneficial effect in any given patient, the findings of experimental and clinical studies suggest that the morbidity and mortality from acute ischemia might be reduced by optimizing systemic circulatory factors. Brain ischemia must be treated early if tissue necrosis is to be prevented or limited. In the usual clinical setting, treatment is often started too late to be effective. In patients undergoing cerebral vascular surgery with a potential risk of ischemia, the circulatory and hemodynamic state of the patient can be optimized in anticipation of the ischemic challenge.

References

1. Ames A, Wright RL, Kowada MD, et al: Cerebral ischemia. II. The no-reflow phenomenon. *Am J Pathol* 52:437–453, 1968.
2. Astrup J, Siesjö BK, Symon L: Thresholds in cerebral ischemia—the ischemic penumbra. *Stroke* 12:723–725, 1981.
3. Auer LM: Acute operation and preventative nimodipine improve outcome in patients with ruptured cerebral aneurysms. *Neurosurgery* 15:57–66, 1985.
4. Awad IA, Carter P, Spetzler RF, et al: Clinical vasospasm after subarachnoid hemorrhage: Response to hypervolemic hemodilution and arterial hypertension. *Stroke* 18:365–372, 1987.
5. Awad IA, Little JR, Lucas F, et al: Modification of focal cerebral ischemia by prostacyclin and indomethacin. *J Neurosurg* 58:714–719, 1980.
6. Barnett GH, Bose B, Little JR, et al: Effects of nimodipine on acute focal cerebral ischemia. *Stroke* 17:884–890, 1986.
7. Brawley BW: The pathophysiology in intracerebral steal following carbon dioxide inhalation (abstract). *Scand J Clin Lab Invest* 22 (Suppl 102):13B, 1968.
8. Brawley BW, Strandness DE, Kelly WA: The

physiologic response to therapy in experimental cerebral ischemia. *Arch Neurol* 17:180–187, 1967.
9. Burke AM, Quest DO, Chien S, et al: The effects of mannitol on blood viscosity. *J Neurosurg* 55:550–553, 1981.
10. Denny-Brown D: The treatment of recurrent cerebrovascular symptoms and the question of "vasospasm." *Med Clin North Am* 35:1457–1474, 1951.
11. Dintenfass L: Inversion of the Fahraeus-Lindquist phenomenon in blood flow through capillaries of diminishing radius. *Nature* 215:1099–1100, 1967.
12. Fahraeus R, Lindquist T: The viscosity of blood in narrow capillary tubes. *Am J Physiol* 96:562–568, 1931.
13. Grotta JC, Pettigrew LC, Allen S, et al: Baseline hemodynamic state and response to hemodilution in patients with acute cerebral ischemia. *Stroke* 16:790–795, 1985.
14. Haggendal E, Nilsson JN, Norback B: Effect of blood corpuscle concentration on cerebral blood flow. *Acta Chir Scand* Suppl 364:3–12, 1966.
15. Harris RJ, Branston NM, Symon L, et al: The effect of the calcium antagonist, nimodipine, upon physiological responses of the cerebral vasculature and its possible influence upon focal cerebral ischemia. *Stroke* 13:759–766, 1982.
16. Hope DT, Branston NM, Symon L: Restoration of neurological function with induced hypertension in acute experimental cerebral ischaemia. *Acta Neurol Scand* 56 (Suppl 64):506–507, 1977.
17. Huczynski J, Kostka-Trabka E, Sotowska W, et al: Double-blind controlled trial of the therapeutic effects of prostacyclin in patients with completed ischemic stroke. *Stroke* 16:810–814, 1985.
18. Jones TH, Morawetz RB, Crowell RM, et al: Thresholds of focal ischemia in awake monkeys. *J Neurosurg* 54:773–782, 1981.
19. Kannel WB, Gordon T, Wolf PA, et al: Hemoglobin and the risk of cerebral infarction: The Framingham Study. *Stroke* 3:409–420, 1972.
20. Keller TS, McGillicuddy JE, LaBond VA, et al: Modification of focal cerebral ischemia by cardiac output augmentation. *J Surg Res* 39:420–432, 1985.
21. Lammertsma AA, Brooks DJ, Beaney RP, et al: In vivo measurement of regional cerebral hematocrit using positron emission tomography. *J Cereb Blood Flow Metab* 4:317–322, 1984.
22. Lassen NA, Palvolgyi R: Cerebral steal during hypercapnia and the inverse reaction during hypocapnia observed by the xenon-133 technique in man. *Scand J Lab Clin Invest* Suppl 102:13D, 1968.
23. Linet O, Hsu CY, Faught RF, et al: Epoprostenol in acute stroke (abstract). *Stroke* 16:149, 1985.
24. Little JR: Modification of acute focal ischemia by treatment with mannitol and high-dose dexamethasone. *J Neurosurg* 49:517–524, 1978.
25. Little JR: Morphological changes in acute focal ischemia. Response to osmotherapy. *Adv Neurol* 28:443–457, 1980.
26. Ljungren B, Brandt L: Timing of aneurysm surgery. *Clin Neurosurg* 33:159–175, 1986.
27. Maroon JC, Nelson PB: Hypovolemia in patients with subarachnoid hemorrhage: Therapeutic implications. *Neurosurgery* 4:223–226, 1979.

28. Martin JF, Hamdy N, Nichole J, et al: Double-blind controlled trial of prostacyclin in cerebral infarction. *Stroke* 16:386–390, 1985.

29. Merrill EW: Rheology of blood. *Physiol Rev* 49:863–888, 1969.

30. Muizelaar JP, Becker DP: Induced hypertension for the treatment of cerebral ischemia after subarachnoid hemorrhage. *Surg Neurol* 25:317–325, 1986.

31. Muizelaar JP, Lutz HA, Becker DP: Effect of mannitol on ICP and CBF and correlation with pressure autoregulation in severely head-injured patients. *J Neurosurg* 61:700–706, 1984.

32. Muizelaar JP, Wei EP, Kontos HA, et al: Mannitol causes compensatory cerebral vasoconstriction and vasodilatation in response to blood viscosity changes. *J Neurosurg* 59:822–828, 1983.

33. Paulson OB: Regional cerebral blood flow in apoplexy due to occlusion of the middle cerebral artery. *Neurology* 20:63–77, 1970.

34. Ritchie WL, Weir B, Overton TR: Experimental subarachnoid hemorrhage in the cynomolgus monkey: Evaluation of treatment with hypertension, volume expansion and ventilation. *Neurosurgery* 6:57–62, 1980.

35. Scandanavian Stroke Study Group: Multicenter trial of hemodilution in acute ischemic stroke. I. Results in the total patient population. *Stroke* 18:691–699, 1987.

36. Snyder SH, Reynolds IJ: Calcium-antagonist drugs: Receptor interactions that clarify therapeutic effects. *N Engl J Med* 313:995–1002, 1985.

37. Solomon RA, Post KD, McMurtry JG: Depression of circulating blood volume in patients after subarachnoid hemorrhage: Implications for the management of symptomatic vasospasm. *Neurosurgery* 15:354–361, 1987.

38. Strandgaard S, Paulson OB: Cerebral autoregulation. *Stroke* 15:413–416, 1984.

39. Suzuki J, Fujimoto S, Mozoi K, et al: The protective effect of combined administration of antioxidants and perfluorocarbons on cerebral ischemia. *Stroke* 15:672–679, 1984.

40. Suzuki J, Yoshimoto T, Kayama T: Surgical treatment of middle cerebral artery aneurysms. *J Neurosurg* 61:17–23, 1984.

41. Symon L: Observations on the leptomeningeal collateral circulation in dogs. *J Physiol* 154:1–14, 1960.

42. Symon L: Experimental evidence for "intracerebral steal" following CO_2 inhalation (abstract). *Scand J Clin Lab Invest* 22 (Suppl 102):13A, 1968.

43. Symon L, Branston NM, Strong AJ: Autoregulation in acute focal ischemia. *Stroke* 7:547–554, 1976.

44. Symon L, Crockard HA, Dorsch NWC, et al: Local cerebral blood flow and vascular reactivity in a chronic stable stroke in baboons. *Stroke* 6:482–492, 1975.

45. Symon L, Ishikawa S, Meyer JS: Cerebral arterial pressure changes and development of leptomeningeal collateral circulation. *Neurology* 13:237–250, 1963.

46. Thomas DJ: Whole blood viscosity and cerebral blood flow. *Stroke* 12:285–287, 1982.

47. Tohgi H, Yamanouchi H, Murakami M, et al: Importance of the hematocrit as a risk factor in cerebral infarction. *Stroke* 9:369–374, 1978.

48. Tramner FI, Gross CE, Kindt GW, et al: Pulsatile versus nonpulsatile blood flow in the treatment of acute cerebral ischemia. *Neurosurgery* 19:724–731, 1986.

49. Waltz AG: Effect of blood pressure on blood flow in ischemic and non-ischemic cerebral cortex. *Neurology* 18:613–621, 1968.

50. Wood JH, Simeone FA, Fink EA, et al: Hypervolemic hemodilution in experimental focal cerebral ischemia. Elevations of cardiac output, regional cortical blood flow and ICP after intravascular volume expansion with low-molecular-weight dextran. *J Neurosurg* 59:500–509, 1983.

51. Wood JH, Snyder LL, Simeone FA: Failure of intravascular volume expansion without hemodilution to elevate cortical blood flow in regions of experimental focal ischemia. *J Neurosurg* 56:80–91, 1982.

52. Yamamoto YL, Phillips KM, Hodge P, et al: Microregional blood flow changes in experimental cerebral ischemia: Effects of arterial carbon dioxide studied by fluorescein angiography and xenon clearance. *J Neurosurg* 35:155–166, 1971.

CHAPTER NINETEEN

Protection from Cerebral Ischemia by Hyperoxygenation

Brian T. Andrews, M.D.
Philip R. Weinstein, M.D.

Hyperoxygenation of plasma during incomplete regional ischemia offers the theoretical advantage of maintaining adequate tissue levels of oxygen despite reduced cerebral blood flow (CBF). The potential use of hyperbaric oxygenation (HBO) to prevent cerebral injury caused by hypoxia and ischemia has been investigated since clinical application of the technique became possible in the 1940s (4, 17, 30). Experimental and clinical studies have shown that HBO can reverse neurologic deficits caused by acute ischemia and limit the extent and severity of cerebral infarction. HBO may also allow the viability of ischemic brain to be determined in potential candidates for cerebral revascularization. The early difficulties of monitoring patients during therapy have largely been overcome (32) and techniques for avoiding toxic side effects have been developed (1, 6, 32).

Intravenous administration of fluorocarbon emulsions, such as Fluosol-DA™ (FDA; Alpha Therapeutics, Los Angeles, CA), during inspiration of 100% oxygen also increases oxygen delivery to ischemic tissue (28, 34). The small size of FDA particles (average diameter, 0.1 micron) facilitates microcirculatory flow and decreases blood viscosity at low shear rates (25). With FDA, the total surface area accessible to gas exchange is 100 to 170 times that of blood. Oxygen is two times and carbon dioxide three times more soluble in FDA than in blood, and the oxygen content of FDA increases linearly with the partial pressure of oxygen (PO_2).

PHYSIOLOGIC EFFECTS OF HYPERBARIC OXYGENATION

Exposure to 100% oxygen at increased pressure increases the PO_2 of blood, cerebral spinal fluid (CSF), brain, and spinal tissue. In humans, arterial PO_2 rises from 73.5 torr in room air to 673 torr at 1.5 atmospheres (ATA) and to 902 torr at 2.0 ATA (13), perhaps in part because of the augmented oxygen content in plasma (36). The jugular venous PO_2 increases from 36 torr in room air to 47 torr at 1.5 ATA and to 55 torr at 2.0 ATA (13). The PO_2 of cisternal CSF rises from 66 torr in room air to 203 torr at 2.0 ATA (16). In cats, PO_2 of brain is 25 torr in room air and 250 torr in 100% oxygen at 6.5 ATA (5); in anesthetized rats, PO_2 in the spinal cord gray matter is 16 torr in room air and 608 torr at 5 ATA (27). After HBO is discontinued, PO_2 returns rapidly to normal (4, 5, 13, 16). The administration of 100% oxygen under normal pressure results in much smaller increases in arterial, venous, CSF, and tissue PO_2 (5, 13, 16).

In patients with ischemic or traumatic brain injury, Holbach et al (13) found that 1.5 ATA HBO for 35 to 40 minutes inhibited cerebral glycolysis, which decreased lactate production. HBO at 2.0 ATA for as little as 10 minutes, however, reduced cerebral glucose uptake and increased lactate production, possibly by inhibiting oxidative phosphorylation.

When autoregulation is intact, the increase in the PO_2 of brain tissue during

HBO results in moderate cerebral vasoconstriction through the direct effect of oxygen on arteriolar smooth muscle (4, 32, 33). This constriction can be reversed by an increase in arterial PCO_2 (4). Because HBO-induced vasoconstriction occurs selectively in normal brain, blood flow is diverted to vessels in the ischemic area, which remain persistently dilated (13, 35). Improved blood flow and increased oxygen availability are thought to prevent functional deterioration of the ischemic microcirculation (5, 35), including the "no-reflow" phenomenon (1, 2).

TOXIC EFFECTS OF HYPERBARIC OXYGENATION

At increased pressure, oxygen can interfere with mitochondrial enzyme systems. The toxic effects of HBO have been observed most often in the lung, eye, and central nervous system (2). Pulmonary toxicity similar to that caused by prolonged exposure to 100% oxygen at ambient pressure has been demonstrated both experimentally (6, 7, 20) and clinically (2, 7). High-pressure or prolonged HBO therapy may result in atelectasis, intraalveolar edema and hemorrhage, capillary thrombosis, and hyaline membrane formation and eventually leads to capillary proliferation and interstitial fibrosis (2). A direct proliferative effect of oxgen on the alveolar capillary wall is thought to be the primary mechanism of injury (2, 7). The clinical manifestations of pulmonary oxygen toxicity are progressive dyspnea and frothy pulmonary edema which may lead to death (2, 6, 10).

The ocular toxicities of HBO include retrolental fibroplasia, retinal necrosis, and segmental ganglion-cell degeneration (2, 24, 26). Retinal vasoconstriction induced by HBO may alter visual fields temporarily, but permanent retinal damage related to HBO therapy in adult patients has not been reported (2).

HBO may also cause seizures, selective necrosis of brain stem nuclei, and necrosis of the spinal cord (1–3, 24, 27). These side effects are probably caused by excessive tissue oxygenation and impaired enzymatic function (1). In rats, HBO at 2.5 to 3.0 ATA for as little as 15 minutes can cause seizures; longer exposure may lead to fatal status epilepticus (2). Patients treated with high-pressure or prolonged HBO therapy have suffered grand mal seizures, deafness, hyperactivity, and hallucinations (1). Jaundice and anemia due to hemolysis have also been reported (12).

The toxic side effects of HBO can be avoided by limiting the pressure to 1.5 ATA and the duration of therapy to 1 hour (2, 6). In gerbils, Burt et al (6) found that oxygen toxicity could be prevented by allowing the animals to breathe room air at normal pressure for 5 minutes every hour during up to 18 hours of 1.5 ATA HBO. The antioxidant alpha-tocopherol has been reported to retard oxygen toxicity during repeated HBO applications in rats (11) and has been used clinically as well, although without conclusive results (32). HBO therapy at lower pressure has not caused adverse effects in patients with cerebral ischemia (14, 16, 19, 21).

RESULTS OF HYPEROXYGENATION IN EXPERIMENTAL CEREBRAL ISCHEMIA

Early studies of the therapeutic efficacy of HBO therapy for acute cerebral ischemia yielded mixed results. Studies of cardiac arrest and global ischemia or anoxia suggested that HBO had favorable effects on neurologic function (17, 31) and on recovery of the electroencephalogram (EEG) (30) and helped to prevent cerebral infarction (18). In the only early study of regional cerebral ischemia, however, Jacobsen and Lawson (20) found that after permanent occlusion of the middle cerebral artery (MCA), dogs treated with HBO at 2.0 ATA had larger infarcts and more severe neurologic deficits than the untreated controls. CBF decreased during the treatment, and it was proposed that HBO induced vasoconstriction that lowered tissue PO_2.

Recent studies have shown a beneficial

effect of HBO therapy after the onset of global ischemia. Cats treated with 1.5 ATA HBO for $2\frac{1}{2}$ hours after 5 minutes of circulatory arrest had quicker recovery of the EEG and lower CSF lactate levels than controls treated with 100% oxygen at normal pressure (22).

HBO has also shown a beneficial effect in studies of regional ischemia. In gerbils subjected to permanent unilateral ligation of the common carotid artery, 2.0 ATA HBO for 1 hour preserved blood volume in the ischemic region and reduced the incidence of delayed ischemic neurologic deficit as compared with HBO at lower pressures or for shorter durations (8). Burt et al (6) used the same model to evaluate the effect of varying the duration of HBO therapy at 1.5 ATA. The rate of infarction was lowest when the gerbils breathed room air at normal pressure for 5 minutes every hour for 18 hours after the onset of ischemia. Despite breathing room air for an additional 18 hours after HBO, only 11% of the gerbils had histologically confirmed infarctions, as compared with 72% of the control group. These investigators proposed that HBO reduced the incidence of cerebral infarction by allowing time for collateral circulation to develop (6). Weinstein et al (36) have shown that HBO at 1.5 ATA during the first 15 minutes of temporary 20-minute bilateral ligation of the common carotid arteries in gerbils reduced the mortality rate from 100% to 16% and limited the extent of histologic ischemic damage.

Weinstein et al (35) also reported that 1.5 ATA HBO therapy for 40 minutes during the first or third hour of a 6-hour temporary occlusion of the MCA in unanesthetized cats improved neurologic function immediately. This effect persisted; at sacrifice 10 days later, the neurologic deficit was 94% less and the infarct size 58% less than in control animals. Treatment during the fourth hour of occlusion lessened the neurologic deficit but did not reduce the infarct size. In cats subjected to a 24-hour MCA occlusion, HBO during the fourth hour resulted in a persistent 74% decrease in neurologic deficit and a 41% reduction in infarct size compared with untreated controls. HBO therapy initiated after 6-hour or 24-hour MCA occlusion was of no benefit. These results demonstrate that HBO administered soon after the onset of temporary regional ischemia provided a significant protective effect.

The use of fluorocarbons to protect against cerebral ischemia has also been studied experimentally. In some studies, FDA increased oxygen availability and CBF in ischemic brain after permanent occlusion of the MCA in cats (28, 34). In another study, oxygen availability was increased by administration of FDA and oxygen before MCA occlusion and during reperfusion but not during ischemia (23). In cats given FDA before and during a 6-hour MCA occlusion followed by reperfusion for 7 days, however, Pereira et al (29) found a trend toward improvement in neurologic outcome only when mannitol was added to the treatment regimen. The infarct areas on coronal sections were 2.4 times larger in FDA-treated cats than in controls or in cats treated with FDA and mannitol. These results indicate that administration of FDA and 100% oxygen after the onset of ischemia aggravated the effects of reperfusion in cats after 6 hours of temporary MCA occlusion. The addition of mannitol and treatment before the onset of ischemia counteracted this effect but did not improve on the outcome observed in the control group.

CLINICAL APPLICATIONS OF HYPERBARIC OXYGENATION

Acute Ischemia

In 1965, Ingvar and Lassen (19) treated two patients with acute strokes using 2.0 to 2.5 ATA HBO for up to $2\frac{1}{2}$ hours. The EEG and clinical status improved immediately in both patients. In one, the recovery did not persist after therapy was discontinued; the late outcome for the other was not reported.

Heyman et al (12) treated 15 patients with HBO at 2.0 ATA to 3.0 ATA within

1 to 7 hours after the onset of major acute ischemic neurologic deficits. The exposure time was less than 1 hour at 3.0 ATA or up to 5 hours at 2.0 ATA. Four patients had complete or almost complete reversal of their deficits beginning during the first 10 minutes of therapy. In two patients, the beneficial effect persisted after treatment; in the other two, the deficits recurred after each of two HBO exposures. Six patients had favorable temporary responses to HBO. HBO had no significant effect in five patients.

A potentially valuable use of HBO is to assess the viability of marginally oxygenated neural tissue in patients with acute cerebral ischemia. If HBO can improve neural function temporarily, surgical revascularization may provide a permanent increase in oxygen supply. HBO therapy might also maintain the viability of ischemic tissue during diagnostic studies and while preparations are made for surgery, effectively lengthening the period during which revascularization may be beneficial (9, 33).

Another use for HBO is to supplement surgical revascularization (21). In one patient, exposure to 1.5 ATA for 2 hours rapidly reversed an acute hemiplegia caused by embolic occlusion of the MCA. An embolectomy was performed immediately. Afterward, there was mild weakness on the involved side, but normal strength returned over the next 2 weeks. The second patient became hemiplegic after clipping of an internal carotid artery aneurysm. The clip was repositioned immediately, but the carotid artery remained occluded. An extracranial-intracranial (EC–IC) arterial bypass was performed. Postoperatively, the patient was hemiplegic and received HBO at 1.5 ATA twice daily for 5 days. Progressive neurologic recovery was observed. Subsequently, angiography showed that the superficial temporal artery had enlarged and was supplying the entire middle cerebral complex. Although the patient might have recovered spontaneously, it is also possible that HBO protected the viable but ischemic brain while the bypass enlarged to provide adequate collateral perfusion.

Chronic Ischemia

Several prospective studies have evaluated the ability of HBO therapy to reverse neurologic and electrophysiologic deficits weeks or months after stroke. In 1976, Holbach et al (14) treated 40 such patients with 1.5 ATA HBO for 40 minutes daily for 10 to 15 days. Twenty patients were treated within 4 weeks and 20 patients more than 4 weeks after the onset of neurologic deficits. Angiography demonstrated an occlusion of either the MCA or the internal carotid artery in each patient. After HBO, 27% of the patients had marked improvement and 53% had moderate improvement in the ipsilateral EEG; only 20% of patients had no change in EEG abnormalities. These findings correlated well with the neurologic changes, but no details of neurologic improvement were given. HBO had a favorable effect on both subacute and chronic deficits.

The ability of HBO to reverse neurologic deficits after chronic stroke caused by occlusion of the internal carotid artery has also been studied. Fifteen of 35 patients reported by Holbach et al (15) had a major lessening of their neurologic deficits during HBO therapy and underwent EC–IC bypass surgery. In each case, the neurologic deficits continued to resolve after revascularization. Five patients in whom HBO had no apparent effect also underwent EC–IC bypass surgery. No improvement was observed. Fifteen patients with little or no change after HBO therapy who did not undergo bypass surgery had little spontaneous neurologic improvement 12 months later. These results suggest that HBO can be used to assess the reversibility of ischemic deficits in order to select patients who are likely to benefit from revascularization.

We have used HBO to treat 10 patients with cerebral ischemia. In three patients with acute major strokes and in five with mild or moderate fixed deficits, HBO had no effect on the EEG or on the results of neurologic examination. In two patients with normal CT scans and subacute fluctuating deficits, functional improvement persisted for 1 to 2 hours after HBO treatment and was maintained after superficial temporal artery–MCA bypass surgery.

PERSPECTIVE

HBO may have a role in assessing, limiting, or temporarily reversing the effects of cerebral ischemia. Application of HBO is currently hindered by logistics and the limited availability of treatment chambers. The potential toxic side effects of HBO are dose dependent and may be avoided by limiting the pressure and duration of therapy. Recent experimental data and preliminary clinical reports suggest that HBO may be useful for treating acute regional cerebral ischemia and identifying patients with viable yet nonfunctional ischemic brain who might benefit from cerebral revascularization.

References

1. Ames A III, Wright RL, Kowada MD, et al: Cerebral ischemia II: The no-reflow phenomenon. *Am J Pathol* 52:437–453, 1968.
2. Ballantine JD: Pathologic effects of exposure to high oxygen tensions. *N Engl J Med* 275:1038–1040, 1966.
3. Balentine JD, Gutsche BB: Central nervous system lesions in rats exposed to oxygen at high pressure. *Am J Pathol* 48:107–127, 1966.
4. Bean JW: Cerebral O_2 in exposures to O_2 at atmospheric and higher pressure, and influence of CO_2. *Am J Physiol* 201:1192–1198, 1961.
5. Bicher HI, Bruley DF, Reneau DD, et al: Autoregulation of oxygen supply to microareas of brain tissue under hypoxic and hyperbaric conditions. *Bibl Anat* 11:526–531, 1973.
6. Burt JT, Kapp JP, Smith RR: Hyperbaric oxygen and cerebral infarction in the gerbil. *Surg Neurol* 28:265–268, 1987.
7. Cedergren B, Gyllensten L, Wersall J: Pulmonary injury caused by oxygen poisoning: Electron microscopic study in mice. *Acta Paediatr Scand* 48:477–494, 1959.
8. Corkill G, Van Housen K, Hein L, et al: Video-densitometric estimation of the protective effect of hyperbaric oxygen in the ischemic gerbil brain. *Surg Neurol* 24:206–210, 1985.
9. Crowell RM, Olsson Y: Effect of extracranial–intracranial vascular bypass graft on experimental acute stroke in dogs. *J Neurosurg* 38:26–31, 1973.
10. Fuson RL: Clinical hyperbaric oxygen with severe oxygen toxicity: Report of a case. *N Engl J Med* 273:415–417, 1965.
11. Hart GB, Lee WS, Rasmussen BD, et al: Compli-

cations of repetitive hyperbaric therapy. In Trapp WG, Banister EW, Davidson AJ, et al (eds): *O_2: Fifth International Hyperbaric Congress Proceedings, 1973.* Burnaby, British Columbia, Simon Fraser University, 1974, pp 867–873.
12. Heyman A, Saltzman HA, Whalen RE: The use of hyperbaric oxygenation in the treatment of cerebral ischemia. *Circulation* (Suppl 2) 33:20–27, 1966.
13. Holbach KH, Caroli A, Wassmann H: Cerebral energy metabolism in patients with brain lesions at normo- and hyperbaric oxygen pressures. *J Neurol* 217:17–30, 1977.
14. Holbach KH, Wassmann H, Hoheluchter KL: Reversibility of the chronic post-stroke state. *Stroke* 7:296–300, 1976.
15. Holbach KH, Wassmann H, Hoheluchter KL, et al: Differentiation between reversible and irreversible post-stroke changes in brain tissue: Its relevance for cerebrovascular surgery. *Surg Neurol* 7:325–331, 1977.
16. Hollin SA, Espinosa OE, Sukoff MH, et al: The effect of hyperbaric oxygenation on cerebrospinal fluid oxygen. *J Neurosurg* 29:229–235, 1968.
17. Illingworth C: Treatment of arterial occlusion under oxygen at two-atmospheres pressure. *Br J Med* 2:1271–1275, 1962.
18. Illingworth CFW, Smith G, Lawson DD, et al: Surgical and physiological observations in an experimental pressure chamber. *Br J Surg* 49:222–227, 1961.
19. Ingvar DH, Lassen NA: Treatment of focal cerebral ischemia with hyperbaric oxygenation: Report of 4 cases. *Acta Neurol Scand* 41:92–95, 1965.
20. Jacobsen I, Lawson DD: The effect of hyperbaric oxygen on experimental cerebral infarction in the dog. *J Neurosurg* 20:849–859, 1963.
21. Kapp JP: Hyperbaric oxygen as an adjunct to acute revascularization of the brain. *Surg Neurol* 12:457–461, 1979.
22. Kapp JP, Phillips M, Markov A, et al: Hyperbaric oxygenation after circulatory arrest: Modification of postischemic encephalopathy. *Neurosurgery* 11:496–499, 1982.
23. Kolluri S, Heros RC, Hedley-White ET, et al: Effect of fluosol on oxygen availability, regional cerebral blood flow, and infarct size in a model of temporary focal cerebral ischemia. *Stroke* 17:976–980, 1986.
24. Margolis G, Brown IW Jr: Hyperbaric oxygenation: The eye as a limiting factor. *Science* 151:466–468, 1966.
25. Naito R, Kokoyama K: Physical and chemical properties of Fluosol-DA after mixing with Annex solution. In Naito F, Yokoyama K (eds): *Perfluorochemical Blood Substitutes.* Osaka, Japan, Green Cross Corp, 1978, pp 73–79.
26. Noell WK: Effect of high and low oxygen tension on the nervous system. In Shaefer KE (ed): *First International Symposium on Submarine and Undersea Medicine.* New York, Macmillan, 1958, pp 3–18.
27. Ogilvie RW, Balentine JD: Oxygen tension in spinal cord gray matter during exposure to hyperbaric oxygen. *J Neurosurg* 43:156–161, 1975.
28. Peerless SJ, Ishikawa R, Hunter G, et al: Protec-

tive effect of Fluosol-DA in acute cerebral ischemia. *Stroke* 12:558–563, 1981.

29. Pereira BM, Weinstein PR, Rodriguez y Baena R: Effect of treatment with fluosol and mannitol during temporary middle cerebral artery occlusion in cats. *Neurosurgery* 23:139–142, 1988.

30. Smith G, Lawson DD, Renfrew S, et al: Preservation of cerebral cortical activity by breathing oxygen at two atmospheres of pressure during cerebral ischemia. *Surg Gynecol Obstet* 113:13–16, 1961.

31. Smith G, Ledingham IM, Sharp GR, et al: The treatment of coal-gas poisoning with oxygen at 2 atmospheres pressure. *Lancet* 1:816–819, 1962.

32. Sukoff MH, Ragatz RE: Hyperbaric oxygenation for the treatment of acute cerebral edema. *Neurosurgery* 10:29–38, 1982.

33. Sundt TM, Grant WC, Garcia JH: Restoration of middle cerebral artery flow in experimental infarction. *J Neurosurg* 31:311–322, 1969.

34. Sutherland GR, Farrar JK: Changes in oxygen availability induced by Fluosol-DA. *J Cereb Blood Flow Metab* (Suppl 1) 3:S662–S663, 1983.

35. Weinstein PR, Anderson G, Telles DA: Results of hyperbaric oxygen therapy during temporary middle cerebral artery occlusion in unanesthetized cats. *Neurosurgery* 20:518–524, 1987.

36. Weinstein PR, Hameroff SR, Johnson PC, et al: Effect of hyperbaric oxygen therapy or dimethyl sulfoxide on cerebral ischemia in unanesthetized gerbils. *Neurosurgery* 18:528–532, 1986.

CHAPTER TWENTY

Pharmacologic Attenuation of Cellular Excitation

Roger P. Simon, M.D.

Neuronal damage found after anoxia–ischemia is characterized by injury to certain "selectively vulnerable" cell groups: the Purkinje and basket cells of the cerebellum, small pyramidal neurons in lamina III of the cerebral cortex, and the pyramidal neurons in CA1 and CA3–4 regions of the hippocampus. Although exceptions exist (1), the similar distribution of injury of these cell groups and their similar morphologic appearance following ischemic injury, status epilepticus, and hypoglycemia have led to the suggestion that a common pathophysiologic process produces cell death in these conditions (4).

THE CONCEPT OF SELECTIVE VULNERABILITY

The concept that neurons with specific metabolic characteristics might be selectively vulnerable to ischemia and anoxic injury was introduced over 60 years ago (37). One shared characteristic of these cells is a tendency to excitation-induced burst firing, probably because of a high density of excitatory (glutamate-containing or aspartate-containing) synapses on dendritic trees. The selectively vulnerable CA3 pyramidal neurons of hippocampus also display the paroxysmal depolarization shift, a membrane characteristic which predisposes the cells to calcium (Ca^{2+}) accumulation via voltage-dependent channels during the depolarizing phase of the paroxysmal depolarization shift and during burst firing. It has been proposed that in ischemia followed by reperfusion, the enhanced neuronal firing rate (34) and the restoration of extracellular Ca^{2+} concentrations from plasma permit excessive Ca^{2+} influx through voltage-dependent channels. These observations have thus suggested that neuronal calcium toxicity resulting, at least in part, from excessive excitation is a potential explanation for the mechanism of ischemic injury in selectively vulnerable cells (8, 21, 22, 29).

INTRACELLULAR CALCIUM TOXICITY

Farber (11) has attributed the coagulation necrosis that occurs in a similar manner in many tissues following various forms of cellular injury to a failure of intracellular CA^{2+} homeostasis. We have recently developed evidence to support a role for CA^{2+} toxicity in cell death and in the phenomenon of selective vulnerability, using the calcium pyroantimonate method for localization of intracellular Ca^{2+} accumulation. In models of ischemia (31) and status epilepticus (16, 17), we have demonstrated massive Ca^{2+} accumulation in distended mitochondria of selectively vulnerable neurons (Fig. 20.1) and have also shown that this process is partially reversible in cells that survive the insult. Deshpande et al (9) have shown that elevations in the regional brain Ca^{2+} concentration precede neuronal damage in selectively vulnerable hippocampal neurons, and Chen et al (6) have correlated postischemic cortical accumulation of Ca^{2+} with infarct volume in a model of focal ischemia. Uematsu et al (36) have recently correlated electroencephalographic recovery following global ischemia with an attenuation in the ischemia-induced increase in intracellular Ca^{2+}

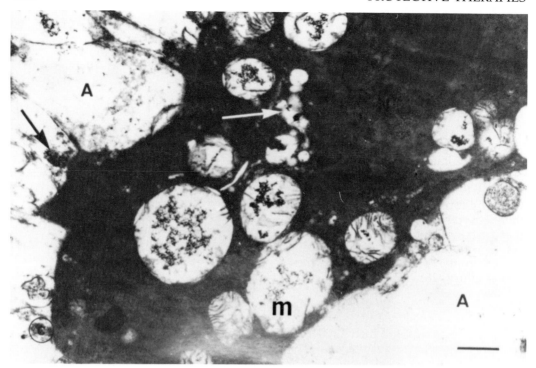

Figure 20.1. Electron micrograph shows a portion of an ischemic dentate granule cell from an adult rat following 30 minutes of ischemia and 30 minutes of reperfusion using the calcium (CA^{2+}) pyroantimonate technique for intracellular Ca^{2+} localization. The cell is extremely electron dense with a barely distinguishable nucleus. Vacuoles are identified as swollen mitochondria (m) and Golgi apparatus *(white arrow)* and contain CA^{2+} pyroantimonate deposits. The cell is surrounded by swollen astrocytic processes (A). An axosomatic nerve terminal is indicated on the left *(black arrow)*. Bar indicates 1 μm. (From Simon RP, Griffiths T, Evans MC, et al: Calcium overload in selectively vulnerable neurons of the hippocampus during and after ischemia: An electron microscopy study in the rat. *J Cereb Blood Flow Metab* 4:350–361, 1984.)

The role of Ca^{2+} toxicity in excitatory amino-acid-induced neuronal injury has been questioned on the basis of recent in vitro studies indicating that passive chloride (Cl^-) flux might explain acute neuronal injury (27). Choi (7, 8) has clarified these issues by demonstrating that both Cl^- and Ca^{2+} are operative in "excitotoxicity," but that the effect of each ion predominates at a different stage of cell injury. Cl^- flux is responsible for acute swelling and Ca^{2+} for late cell death. Further evidence of a link between excitatory neurotransmission and neuronal death is the observation that removal of extracellular Ca^{2+} markedly reduces neuronal loss in tissue cultures exposed to the putative excitatory neurotransmitter glutamate (7).

EXCITATORY AMINO ACIDS IN NEURONAL INJURY

Excitatory (glutaminergic) postsynaptic receptors have been categorized pharmacologically according to their preferential agonists: N-methyl-D-aspartate (NMDA), quisqualate, and kainate. Burst firing can be experimentally induced in selectively vulnerable cells by the iontophoresis of agonist compounds acting at the NMDA-preferring receptor (10); excitatory amino acids acting on the quisqualate- or kainate-preferring receptor do not produce a comparable pattern of burst firing (18). This difference supports a central role for the NMDA receptor in neuronal death from an acute injury state such as ischemia. The ultrastructural cytopathology found after such excitotoxic lesions is similar to that seen in cerebral ischemia followed by reperfusion, in that postsynaptic dendritic and somatic structures are affected (31). Moreover, extracellular fluid concentrations of glutamate and aspartate rise rapidly following ischemia (2), and lesioning intrinsic excitatory pathways to the hippocampus protects selectively vulnerable neurons there against injury following transient forebrain ischemia (19). All of these observations support the hypothesis that excitatory amino acids, probably those acting at the NMDA receptor, are central factors in the pathogenesis of ischemic neural injury (28).

ATTENUATION OF NEURONAL INJURY BY ANTAGONISTS OF EXCITATORY AMINO ACIDS

A logical extension of the theory of excitatory amino acid involvement in ischemic injury is that at least some of the harmful effects of ischemic injury to neurons might be prevented by blocking the action of excitatory amino acids at the NMDA receptor site. Antagonists of excitation at the NMDA receptor are available and include compounds that are both highly potent and highly selective for that receptor (38). Our initial studies in a rat model of global ischemia followed by reperfusion demonstrated a marked protective effect for 2-amino-7-phosphonoheptanoic acid (AP-7), a potent and specific NMDA receptor blocking agent (32). In these experiments, AP-7 was directly administered into the region of the selectively vulnerable cells of the hippocampus prior to the induction of global ischemia; the contralateral region injected with the diluent served as a control (Fig. 20.2).

These initial studies have been confirmed and extended by others. Boast et al (3) used systemic AP-7 in the gerbil bilateral carotid occlusion model; ischemic hippocampal damage was reduced and motor performance improved at 4 days following

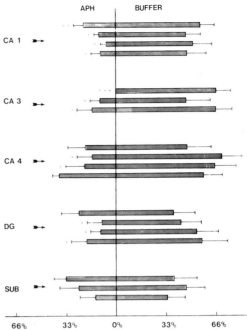

Figure 20.2. Protection by 2-amino-7-phosphonoheptanoic acid (AP-7) against ischemic cell change in rats ($n = 7$). The bars represent mean percentages ($\pm$ standard error of the mean) of neurons showing ischemic damage (scored on a 3-point percentage scale for each: 0 = normal; 1 = one-third or less neurons affected; 2 = two-thirds or less; 3 = all neurons affected) for the indicated type of cell. *Arrows* indicate the injection site (4.5 mm anterior to the intraaural line, 2.0 mm lateral to the midline, and 3.5 mm below the cortical surface). Bars above arrows refer sequentially to histologic sections 4.7 and 5.7 mm anterior, and bars below arrows to sections 3.7 and 2.7 mm anterior. Statistically significant differences between AP-7 and buffer-infused hippocampi are indicated by asterisks: * = $p<0.05$, ** = $p<0.01$, and *** = $p<0.001$ (paired two-tailed t test). DG = dentate granule cells; SUB = pyramidal neurons of subiculum. (From Simon RP, Swan JH, Griffiths T, et al: Blockade of N-methyl-D-aspartate receptors may protect against ischemic damage in the brain. *Science* 226:850–852, 1984.)

global ischemia. Gill et al (14), using the NMDA antagonist MK-801, presented similar data in the gerbil model and Gerhardt et al (12) reported similar results in the gerbil with systemic administration of the NMDA antagonist 3-3(2-carboxypiperazine-4-yl)propyl-1-phosphonic acid. Swan et al (35) have shown that the protective effect of acute AP-7 administration is sustained; a significant protection is seen at 7 days following global ischemia and reperfusion.

Because the NMDA receptor is coupled to a receptor-gated calcium channel (20), one likely mechanism for the reduction of ischemic neuronal injury by NMDA antagonists is by the inhibition of calcium flux through NMDA-gated channels. Some NMDA antagonists, such as dextrorphan, inhibit voltage-dependent calcium flux in neuronal preparations (5). In addition, NMDA antagonists interact with second messenger systems coupled to intracellular Ca^{2+} mobilization (33). However, th.. is not the only possible explanation for the protective effect of NMDA antagonists because there are a family of voltage-dependent calcium channels which are physiologically distinct from the NMDA-gated channel and also mediate the influx of extracellular Ca^{2+} into neurons (15).

Thus, a growing body of evidence supports the theory of excitation-induced neuronal injury and the usefulness of excitatory amino acid antagonists in the attenuation of such injury. A number of questions are as yet incompletely answered, however. Are NMDA antagonists the only effective agents? Can these drugs be administered after the ischemic insult, and, if so, what is the time window of their effectiveness? And perhaps most important, can these studies in models of global ischemia and reperfusion be extended to models of permanent focal ischemia, and thus bring hope for the development of effective pharmacologic therapies for stroke in humans?

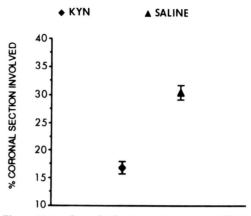

Figure 20.3. Size of infarction in kynurenate (KYN)-pretreated animals and controls (saline). Data are expressed as mean ± standard error of the mean and represent the percentage of coronal section infarcted ($p<0.001$). (From Germano IM, Pitts LH, Meldrum BS, et al: Kynurenate inhibition of cell excitation decreases stroke size and deficits. *Ann Neurol* 22:730–734, 1987.)

EXCITATORY AMINO ACID ANTAGONISTS IN FOCAL ISCHEMIA

There are as yet only a few studies in the use of excitatory amino acid antagonists in the setting of permanent focal ischemia, but the results so far are promising. Our initial studies in this area used kynurenic acid—an inhibitor of excitatory amino acid neurotransmission that is nonspecific as to receptor type—in a model of permanent middle cerebral artery (MCA) occlusion in the rat. We showed a significant

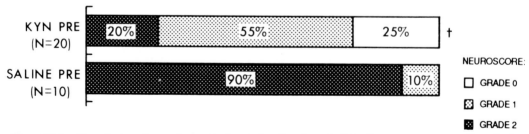

Figure 20.4. Neurologic outcome (percent of each functional grade 0 to 2) versus treatment. Neurologic score assessed at 24 hours following ischemia: 0 = no deficit; 1 = reflex forelimb flexion; 2 = reflex forelimb flexion and decreased resistance to lateral push. KYN PRE = kynurenate pretreatment; SALINE PRE = controls. (From Germano IM, Pitts LH, Meldrum BS, et al: Kynurenate inhibition of cell excitation decreases stroke size and deficits. *Ann Neurol* 22:730–734, 1987.)

reduction in both infarct size and motor deficit when the drug was administered systemically in three doses at 0, 4, and 10 hours following ischemia (13) (Figs. 20.3 and 20.4). More recently, we have performed similar experiments using both AP-7 and kynurenate, withholding the first administration of the drug until 15 minutes after occlusion (30). A significant attenuation of infarct size and motor deficit was shown with AP-7, but not with kynurenate. Ozyurt et al (24) have also reported a reduction of focal ischemic brain damage using pretreatment with the NMDA blocker MK-801 in a cat model of MCA occlusion. The cats, which were killed at 6 hours, showed a significantly reduced area of ischemic damage. Park et al (25) administered MK-801 30 minutes following permanent MCA occlusion in rats. The rats, studied 3 hours following MCA occlusion, showed attenuation of ischemic cell changes in cortex, but not caudate–putamen.

These studies empirically suggest that the excitotoxic hypothesis of ischemic injury is operative in situations of permanent focal ischemia as well as in conditions of global ischemia and reperfusion and, further, that at least some delay in the administration of a drug following the ischemic insult can be tolerated without losing the pharmacologic effect. As in the case of the global ischemia and reperfusion experiments, many questions still remain about the types of effective drugs and the dosing schedules needed to achieve optimal neuroprotection.

CELL EXCITATION IN THE ISCHEMIC PENUMBRA

Because global ischemia and reperfusion and permanent focal ischemia represent different physiologic situations, the question of the underlying pathophysiologic events and the mechanism of action of the pharmacologic antagonists in the model of focal ischemia becomes even more pertinent. Some recent data suggest an increased metabolism in the "penumbra" surrounding an area of focal ischemia.

Nedergaard and Astrup (23) and Peek et al (26), using the 2-deoxyglucose (2-DG) technique in the rat MCA occlusion model, have shown a rim of increased metabolism encompassing nearly 50% of the eventual volume of the infarct. This is similar to the degree of attenuation of infarct volume that our laboratory and that of Ozyurt et al (24) have demonstrated using pharmacologic inhibition of excitatory amino acids. Although the increase of 2-DG metabolism may be a result of events other than cell excitation, excitation within the penumbra and its inhibition by excitatory amino acid antagonists would explain the effects of infarct attenuation which have been demonstrated (13, 24).

References

1. Auer RN, Siesjö BK: Biological differences between ischemia, hypoglycemia and epilepsy. *Ann Neurol* 24:699–707, 1988.
2. Beneveniste H, Drejer J, Schousboe A, et al: Elevation of the extracellular concentrations of glutamate and aspartate in rat hippocampus during transient cerebral ischemia monitored by intracerebral microdialysis. *J Neurochem* 43:1369–1374, 1984.
3. Boast CA, Gerhardt SC, Janak P: Systemic AP7 reduces ischemic brain damage in gerbils. In Hicks TP, Lodge D, McLennan H (eds): *Excitatory Amino Acid Transmission*. New York, Alan R. Liss, 1987, pp 249–252.
4. Brierley JB, Graham D: Hypoxia and vascular disorders of the central nervous system. In Adams JH, Corsellis JAN, Duchen LW (eds): *Greenfield's Neuropathology*, ed. 4. New York, John Wiley & Sons, 1984, pp 125–207.
5. Carpenter CL, Marks SS, Watson DL, et al: Dextromethorphan and dextrorphan as calcium channel antagonists. *Brain Res* 439:372–375, 1988.
6. Chen ST, Hsu CY, Hogan EL, et al: Brain calcium content in ischemic infarction. *Neurology* 37:1227–1229, 1987.
7. Choi DW: Ionic dependence of glutamate neurotoxicity. *J Neurosci* 7:369–379, 1987.
8. Choi DW: Glutamate neurotoxicity and diseases of the nervous system. *Neuron* 1:623–634, 1988.
9. Deshpande JK, Siesjö BK, Wieloch T: Calcium accumulation and neuronal damage in the rat hippocampus following cerebral ischemia. *J Cereb Blood Flow Metab* 7:89–95, 1987.
10. Dingledine R: N-methyl aspartate activates voltage-dependent calcium conductance in rat hippocampal pyramidal cells. *J Physiol* 343:385–405, 1983.
11. Farber JL: The role of calcium in cell death. *Life Sci* 29:1289–1295, 1981.
12. Gerhardt SC, Bernard P, Pastor G, et al: Effects of systemic administration of the NMDA antag-

onist, CPP, on ischemic brain damage in gerbils. *Neurosci Abs* 12:59, 1986.

13. Germano IM, Pitts LH, Meldrum BS, et al: Kynurenate inhibition of cell excitation decreases stroke size and deficits. *Ann Neurol* 22:730–734, 1987.

14. Gill R, Foster AC, Woodruff GN: MK-801 is neuroprotective in gerbils when administered during the post-ischaemic period. *Neuroscience* 25:847–855, 1988.

15. Greenberg DA: Calcium channels and calcium channel antagonists. *Ann Neurol* 21:317–330, 1987.

16. Griffiths T, Evans MC, Meldrum BS: Intracellular calcium accumulation in rat hippocampus during seizures induced by bicuculline or L-allylglycine. *Neuroscience* 10:385–395, 1983.

17. Griffiths T, Evans MC, Meldrum BS: Status epilepticus: The reversibility of calcium loading and acute neuronal pathological changes in the rat hippocampus. *Neuroscience* 12:557–567, 1984.

18. Herrling PL, Morris R, Salt TE: Effects of excitatory amino acids and their antagonists on membrane and action potentials of cat caudate neurones. *J Physiol* 339:207–222, 1983.

19. Jorgensen MB, Johansen FF, Diemer NH: Removal of the entorhinal cortex protects hippocampal CA-1 neurons from ischemic damage. *Acta Neuropathol* 73:189–194, 1987.

20. MacDermott AB, Mayer ML, Westbrook GL, et al: NMDA-receptor activation increases cytoplasmic calcium concentration in cultured spinal cord neurones. *Nature* 321:519–522, 1986.

21. Meldrum BS: Metabolic effects of prolonged epileptic seizures and the causation of epileptic brain damage. In Rose FC (ed): *Metabolic Disorders of the Nervous System*, London, Pitman, 1981, pp 175–187.

22. Meldrum BS: Metabolic factors during prolonged seizures and their relation to nerve cell death. *Adv Neurol* 34:261–275, 1983.

23. Nedergaard M, Astrup J: Infarct rim: Effect of hyperglycemia on direct current potential and [^{14}C]2-deoxyglucose phorphorylation. *J Cereb Blood Flow Metab* 6:607–615, 1986.

24. Ozyurt E, Graham DI, Woodruff GN, et al: Protective effect of the glutamate antagonist MK-801 in focal cerebral ischemia in the cat. *J Cereb Blood Flow Metab* 8:138–143, 1988.

25. Park CK, Nehls DG, Graham DI, et al: The glutamate antagonist MK-801 reduces focal ischemic brain damage in the rat. *Ann Neurol* 24:543–551, 1988.

26. Peek KE, Izumiyama M, Lockwood AH, et al:

27. Rothman SM: The neurotoxicity of excitatory amino acids is produced by passive chloride influx. *J Neuorsci* 5:1483–1489, 1985.

28. Rothman SM, Olney JW: Glutamate and the pathophysiology of hypoxic–ischemic brain damage. *Ann Neurol* 19:105–111, 1986.

29. Siesjö BK: Cell damage in the brain: A speculative synthesis. *J Cereb Blood Flow Metab* 1:155–185, 1981.

30. Simon RP, Bartkowski H, Roman R: Attenuation of infarct size by pharmacologic inhibition of excitatory amino acid neurotransmission by specific NMDA antagonist administered 15 minutes after stroke (abstract). *Neurology* 38(Suppl 1):146, 1988.

31. Simon RP, Griffiths T, Evans MC, et al: Calcium overload in selectively vulnerable neurons of the hippocampus during and after ischemia: An electron microscopy study in the rat. *J Cereb Blood Flow Metab* 4:350–361, 1984.

32. Simon RP, Swan JH, Griffiths T, et al: Blockade of N-methyl-D-aspartate receptors may protect against ischemic damage in the brain. *Science* 226:850–852, 1984.

33. Sladeczek F, Pin J-P, Recasens M, et al: Glutamate stimulates inositol phosphate formation in striatal neurones. *Nature* 318:717–719, 1985.

34. Suzuki R, Yamaguchi T, Choh-Luh L, et al: The effects of 5-minute ischemia in mongolian gerbils: II. Changes of spontaneous neuronal activity in cerebral cortex and CA$_1$ sector of hippocampus. *Acta Neuropathol* 60:217–222, 1983.

35. Swan JH, Evans MC, Meldrum BS: Long-term development of selective neuronal loss and the mechanism of protection by 2-amino-7-phosphonoheptanoate in a rat model of incomplete forebrain ischaemia. *J Cereb Blood Flow Metab* 8:64–78, 1988.

36. Uematsu D, Greenberg JH, Reivich M, et al: In vivo measurement of cytosolic free calcium during cerebral ischemia and reperfusion. *Ann Neurol* 24:420–428, 1988.

37. Vogt C, Vogt O: Erkrankungen der groszhirnrinde im lichte der topistik, pathoklise und pathoarchitektonik. *J Psychol Neurol* 28:1–171, 1922.

38. Watkins JC, Evans RH: Excitatory amino acid transmitters. *Ann Rev Pharmacol Toxicol* 21:165–204, 1981.

Acidosis corresponds with excess glucose utilization in ischemic penumbra (abstract). *Ann Neurol* 22:160, 1987.

CHAPTER TWENTY-ONE

Anticoagulants and Antiplatelet Aggregation Agents

Carmela M. Picone, M.D.
Daniel M. Rosenbaum, M.D.
L. Creed Pettigrew, M.D.
Frank M. Yatsu, M.D.

ANTICOAGULANTS

Anticoagulation has been available clinically since 1937 (45, 49), but the indications for its use and its efficacy in treating ischemic cerebral vascular disease remain controversial despite numerous clinical trials. Most of the studies were performed in the 1960s, before computerized tomography (CT) became available, and were not conducted in randomized, double-blind fashion. Thus, their results and interpretation may be subject to criticism. Nonetheless, anticoagulation is a widely used, well-accepted treatment for certain types of cerebral vascular ischemia. This chapter begins by reviewing the mechanism of action of heparin and warfarin and presenting the rationale and recommendations for their use in various stroke syndromes.

Heparin has three major mechanisms of action on the coagulation cascade. First, the activated coagulation factors IXa, Xa, XIa, and XIIa have serine residues that cause esterification of the arginyl residue on antithrombin III, which inhibits the coagulation factors (20, 36, 37). Heparin reversibly binds to an epsilon–aminolysyl residue on antithrombin III, causing a conformational change in antithrombin III's molecular structure. This process exposes the arginine residue and enhances antithrombin III's ability to inhibit the coagulation factors IX, X, XI, and XII. Second, at higher concentrations, heparin inhibits thrombin by heparin cofactor II. Thrombin is the only protease known to be inhibited by heparin cofactor II (36, 37). The third mechanism is a recent discovery that has

been found only in vitro. In the absence of antithrombin III in vitro, heparin can inhibit the activation of prothrombin by factor Xa. This mechanism was described by Walker and Esman (68) and confirmed by Hirsch and colleagues, but its clinical relevance at this time is not known (36, 37).

Heparin also affects platelets, by both inhibiting and enhancing their aggregation. Inhibition of platelet function has been suggested as one of the mechanisms by which heparin suppresses coagulation. This is supported by the finding that bleeding times increase in normal subjects given heparin (36). Paradoxically, heparin can also cause thrombocytopenia and thromboembolism. Heparin-associated thrombocytopenia and thrombosis is an uncommon but well-defined entity with a rate of occurrence of 3% to 30%; in a pooled analysis of 1,500 patients, the incidence was 6% (40). Although thrombocytopenia and thrombosis can occur with both porcine and bovine heparin preparations (49), among four prospective studies two have shown a significant increase in heparin-associated thrombocytopenia and thrombosis with bovine heparin, and two have shown a trend toward an increased occurrence (3, 43). Heparin-induced thrombocytopenia and thrombosis is attributed to immunologic factors. Heparin-dependent antibody, an immunoglobulin G antibody, has been isolated in the plasma of patients with heparin-induced thrombocytopenia (2, 37, 40, 49). Cines and Tannenbaum (16) showed that this antibody cross-reacts with endothelial cells, which suggests that injury to a vessel may be an initiating factor for thrombosis.

Low-molecular-weight heparin and synthetic heparinoids are new agents currently being investigated. Their mechanism of action is mediated by heparin cofactor II, which inhibits thrombin (36, 37). Low-molecular-weight heparin has been reported to have less platelet aggregation activity than heparin; however, Kelton and Levine (40) demonstrated no difference in platelet aggregation between low-molecular-weight heparin and bovine or porcine preparations of heparin. The heparinoid ORG 10172 was shown to not induce platelet aggregation in another study (49). In five patients who suffered intracerebral hemorrhage and who later developed systemic thromboses, Ten Cate et al (65) found that ORG 10172 prevented propagation of the clot without hemorrhagic complications or a decrease in platelet concentration or function.

The most commonly used oral anticoagulant is warfarin, a vitamin K antagonist. Warfarin competitively inhibits the effects of vitamin K on the postribosomal step of hepatic synthesis of factors II, VII, IX, and X. It is almost completely absorbed in the gastrointestinal tract and is 99% protein bound. The 1% free fraction of warfarin in plasma is the active component. Because warfarin can be easily displaced from protein, caution should be used when prescribing other protein-bound agents (Table 21.1). Also, a diet high in vitamin K can override the effects of warfarin and decrease prothrombin time. Warfarin crosses the placenta and is excreted in milk; therefore, it should not be prescribed for pregnant women or nursing mothers (36, 45).

Anticoagulants are contraindicated in patients with hemorrhage at any site of the body, thrombocytopenia, coagulopathy, or hypersensitivity to the anticoagulant. Relative contraindications should also be excluded. These include pregnancy (for warfarin), impending surgery, inability to obtain adequate coagulation studies, patient compliance, and the patient's general physical condition (alcohol abuse, ataxia, etc.) (45).

It is recommended that heparin be ad-

Table 21.1. Drugs That Increase Warfarin's Action on Prothrombin Time

alcohol[a]	indomethacin
allopurinol	influenza vaccine
amiodarone	methyldopa
antibiotics	metronidazole
aspirin	miconazole
Bactrim[b]	monoamine oxidase
Bromelains	inhibitor
chloral hydrate[a]	nalidixic acid
chlorpropamide	naproxen
chymotrypsin	oxyphenbutazone
cimetadine	pentoxifylline
cinchophen	phenylbutazone
clofibrate	phenytoin
dextran	quinidine
dextrothyroxine	quinine
diazoxide	ranitidine[a]
disulfiram	steroids
diuretics[a]	sulfinpyrazone
ethacrynic acid	sulfonamides
fenoprofen	sulindac
glucagon	thyroid supplements
ibuprofen	tolbutamide

[a]Has been reported to both increase and decrease prothrombin time in patients taking warfarin.
[b]Trimethoprim and sulfamethoxazole.

ministered as a continuous intravenous infusion. Heparin therapy is monitored indirectly, by the partial thromboplastin time (PTT). The PTT should be measured daily and kept at a level of 1.5 to 2 times control. Platelets should also be monitored closely to avoid heparin-induced thrombocytopenia. Warfarin is given orally; therapy is guided by the prothrombin time and should be evaluated frequently during the first few months and at least every 6 months during long-term therapy (44).

Transient Ischemic Attacks

Transient ischemic attacks (TIAs) are defined as the acute onset of a focal neurologic deficit that is completey resolved within 24 hours. Most last less than 1 hour, and many less than 15 minutes (10, 51). TIAs are found in the carotid, vertebral, or retinal artery distributions. These attacks are attributed to microemboli from atherosclerotic plaques in major extracranial vessels (i.e. cervical carotid or vertebral arteries) or, less frequently, to a decrease in cardiac output causing a reduction in perfusion distal to a stenotic lesion (11). Epidemiologic studies have demonstrated that a patient with TIAs has a 5% to 6% per year risk of stroke, with a 1% per month incidence in the first 6 months, and an equal risk of cardiac disease resulting in death (55).

Whether heparin is beneficial in the acute therapy of TIAs has not been definitively answered by the studies that have been performed to date. Most clinical trials have examined long-term rather than acute therapy. Recently, an open trial was reported by Putman and Adams (58) in which 74 patients who presented with TIAs were treated with intravenous heparin within 72 hours; the PTT was maintained at 1.5 to 2.5 times control. Analysis of the outcome according to the onset, crescendo characteristics, and anatomic distribution of the TIAs showed no evidence that heparin therapy was beneficial to these subgroups. A 15% cerebral infarction rate occurred in the crescendo TIA group; the

overall rate for cerebral infarction was 6.8% and for recurrent TIAs was 16.2%. The authors of this study suggested that the frequency of cerebral infarction and TIAs might have been higher if heparin had not been used (58). However, the reverse argument may be made that a control group or a group treated with antiplatelet agents would have done as well as or better than patients who received heparin.

Other studies of anticoagulation for patients with TIAs were designed to evaluate long-term therapy. Most of them were conducted before CT was available and did not require arteriography to exclude other potential etiologies for TIA-like events. Some were prospective studies, and others were retrospective, with and without controls. None of the studies were randomized, double-blind, controlled trials. Table 21.2 lists some of the aspects of the major studies conducted in the 1960s and 1970s (4, 5, 47, 56, 72). Weksler and Lewin (70) reviewed 969 patients who were reported in the literature and followed over 14

Table 21.2. Results of Anticoagulation in Patients with Transient Ischemic Attacks

Study	Number of patients	Number of controls	Number of angiographies	Results
Baker et al[a] (prospective)	30	30	10	Nonsignificant decrease in TIAs and cerebral infarcts. Increase in mortality in treated group.
Link et al[b]	31	0	31	0% TIA and 0% cerebral infarct while on therapeutic anticoagulants. Four of 31 had complications related to anticoagulant.
Olsson et al[c] (prospective)	112 TIA 66 TIA-IR	0 0	70% of TIA 82% of TIA-IR	21% repeat TIAs; 5% repeat TIAs-IR; 0% cerebral infarction; 17.4% complications.
Whisnant et al[d]	130	69	?	No significant difference in overall treatment group. Vertebral basilar significantly better than controls. Complications treated three times as intracranial hemorrhages. Ages 55–74 in treated group had eight times as many intracranial hemorrhages.

TIA = transient ischemic attack; IR = incomplete recovery.
[a]Data from Baker RN, Broward JA, Fang HC, et al: Anticoagulant therapy in cerebral infarction. *Neurology* 12:823–835, 1962; Baker RN, Schwartz WS, Rose AS: Transient ischemic strokes: A report of a study of anticoagulant therapy. *Neurology* 16:841–847, 1966.
[b]Data from Link H, Lebram G, Johansson I, et al: Prognosis in patients with infarction and TIA in carotid territory during and after anticoagulant therapy. *Stroke* 10:529–532, 1979.
[c]Data from Olsson JE, Müller R, Berneli S: Long-term anticoagulant therapy for TIAs and minor strokes with minimum residuum. *Stroke* 7:444–451, 1976.
[d]Data from Whisnant JP, Niall EF, Cartlidge MB, et al: Carotid and vertebral basilar transient ischemic attacks: Effect of anticoagulants, hypertension and cardiac disorders on survival and stroke occurrence–a population study. *Ann Neurol* 3:107–115, 1978.

months. No differences were found in the rates of recurrent TIAs and cerebral infarction in patients treated with anticoagulants, antiplatelet agents, or surgery. The highest mortality rate was among patients who received anticoagulants.

Although anticoagulation therapy has never been shown unequivocally to be of benefit for TIAs, it is recommended for patients with TIAs who do not respond to antiplatelet therapy and those in whom a cardiac etiology is present or suspected. Anticoagulation is also recommended for vertebral basilar TIAs to prevent catastrophic basilar artery thrombosis. It is not recommended that anticoagulation be used in every case of crescendo TIAs or every first-time TIA. Randomized, double-blind, placebo-controlled studies are needed to determine if anticoagulation is an effective treatment for patients with TIAs.

Stroke-in-Evolution

Progressive cerebral infarction, or stroke-in-evolution, is defined as a focal neurologic deficit that develops in a stepwise fashion as a result of an enlarging intraarterial thrombus. The rationale for anticoagulation in this setting is to stop propagation of the thrombus and thereby prevent occlusion and halt neurologic deteriora-

tion. The studies evaluating heparin therapy for stroke-in-evolution are open to the same criticisms as those evaluating anticoagulation for TIAs. They were conducted in the 1960s and 1970s, before CT was available, and were not prospective, randomized, double-blind trials. Nevertheless, the earlier studies show a trend toward a decrease in the progression of cerebral infarction but not in the mortality rate among patients who received anticoagulants. Table 21.3 summarizes the findings of older prospective studies (4, 5, 13, 25, 52).

Recently, a randomized, double-blind, placebo-controlled study of the effects of intravenous heparin in preventing cerebral infarction in 225 patients with minor, stable neurologic deficits was reported (17). The patients in the heparin and control groups were matched for age, sex, hypertension, diabetes, smoking, carotid bruits, and arrhythmias. The heparin-treated group had a 26.6% improvement rate, and the placebo group had a 24.3% improvement rate. Nineteen (17%) of 112 patients treated with heparin progressed, compared with 22 (19.5%) of 113 patients in the control group. The differences between groups were not statistically significant.

Thus, the data acquired to date show that heparin does not have a statistically significant beneficial effect for strokes in

Table 21.3. Results of Anticoagulation in Patients with Stroke-in-Evolution

Study	Number of patients	Number of infarcts	Hemorrhagic complications	Deaths
Baker et al[a]	61 treated	8	22 (2 severe)	13 (2 from hemorrhage)
(prospective, randomized)	67 controls	21	2	17
Carter[b]	38	9	?	3
(prospective, randomized)	38	12	?	7
Fisher[c]	49 treated	7	20 (2 fatal, 1 severe)	10
(prospective, randomized)	51 controls	14	? (8 in total study of 184)	9 (2 from hemorrhage)
Millikan & McDowell[d]	181	37	?	?
	60	32	?	?

[a]Data from Baker RN, Broward JA, Fang HC, et al: Anticoagulant therapy in cerebral infarction. *Neurology* 12:823–835, 1962; Baker RN, Schwartz WS, Rose AS: Transient ischemic strokes: A report of a study of anticoagulant therapy. *Neurology* 16:841–847, 1966.
[b]Data from Carter AB: Anticoagulant treatment in progressing stroke. *Br Med J* 2:70–73, 1961.
[c]Data from Fisher CM, Miller MD: Anticoagulant therapy in cerebral thrombosis and cerebral embolism: A National Cooperative Study, Interim Report. *Neurology* 11:119–131, 1961.
[d]Data from Millikan CH, McDowell FH: Treatment of transient ischemic attacks. *Stroke* 9:299–300, 1978.

progress. In most studies, however, heparin appeared to prevent the progression of fluctuating neurologic deficits. No studies comparing heparin, antiplatelet drugs, and placebo have been conducted in patients with stroke-in-evolution. Until more definitive data are available, heparin is recommended for stroke-in-evolution in the absence of absolute and relative contraindications.

Completed Thrombotic Stroke

A completed stroke is defined as an acute focal neurologic deficit that is static; that is, without evidence of progression or improvement. Older studies of completed thrombotic stroke have shown that anticoagulation is not beneficial (Table 21.4) (4, 5, 25, 67). It neither prevents further infarction nor reduces the mortality rate and is therefore not recommended.

Embolic Strokes of Cardiac Origin

Cardiogenic emboli can cause cerebral infarction. The most common etiology of cardiac emboli is atrial fibrillation; other etiologies include atrial myxoma, myocardial infarction (MI), and mitral valve prolapse (MVP) (28). Determining the cause of infarction in a patient with a potential cardiac source of emboli may be difficult because these patients often have atherosclerotic cerebral vascular disease as well. The sudden occurrence of a neurologic deficit that is maximal at or near its onset suggests stroke from cardiogenic embolus; however, 20% of patients with embolic strokes of cardiac origin have stepwise or progressive deficits (26). Cardiac emboli can also cause TIAs (28) or lacunar infarcts (61). The patient's age is a further clue, because younger patients have less atherosclerotic disease. Cardiogenic emboli are the cause of stroke in one-third to one-half of patients younger than 45 years (28). Evidence of systemic emboli also suggests a cardiac cause of stroke. This etiology is uncommon, occurring in about 3% of patients (53). A hemorrhagic infarct demonstrated by CT suggests a cardiac source but is not pathognomonic (14).

Cardiac arrhythmias predispose to the formation of cardiac thrombus, which can result in embolization to the brain. Atrial fibrillation was the etiology of cerebral infarction in 27% of patients in the Michael Reese Stroke Registry (12) and 31% of patients in the Harvard Cooperative Stroke Registry (53). The Framingham Study showed that with the onset of atrial fibrillation there is a clustering of central ischemic events and that as the duration of atrial fibrillation increases, so does the likelihood of stroke (75). Recurrent stroke within 6 months is twice as common in patients with atrial fibrillation as in those without atrial fibrillation. Retrospective studies have shown that 10% to 20% of patients have a recurrent brain embolism

Table 21.4. Results of Anticoagulation in Patients with Completed Strokes

Study	Number of patients	New stroke progression	Hemorrhages	Deaths
Baker et al[a]	72 treated	12	31	18
	60 control	5	2	15
Fisher[b]	112 treated	12 (1 hemorrhage)	52 (6 fatal, 7 severe)	19
	113 control	9	?	18
VA Cooperative	56 treated	3	?	12
Study[c]	62 control	4	?	7

[a]Data from Baker RN, Broward JA, Fang HC, et al: Anticoagulant therapy in cerebral infarction. *Neurology* 12:823–835, 1962; Baker RN, Schwartz WS, Rose AS: Transient ischemic strokes: A report of a study of anticoagulant therapy. *Neurology* 16:841–847, 1966.
[b]Data from Fisher CM, Miller MD: Anticoagulant therapy in cerebral thrombosis and cerebral embolism: A National Cooperative Study, Interim Report. *Neurology* 11:119–131, 1961.
[c]Veterans Administration Cooperative Study of Atherosclerosis, Neurology Section: An evaluation of anticoagulant therapy in the treatment of cerebrovascular disease. *Neurology* 11:132–144, 1961.

within 2 weeks (28, 48); the long-term risk is 5% per year (28).

In a study by the Cerebral Embolism Study Group (14), 24 eligible randomized treated patients were compared with 21 eligible randomized controls. The numbers in each group were too small to reach statistical significance, but a definite trend favoring anticoagulation therapy was observed. A similar trend was demonstrated in a retrospective study of recurrent embolism in patients with nonvalvular atrial fibrillation by Hart et al (Table 21.5) (33). Several other studies support the use of anticoagulation therapy for patients with cardiac emboli who have no signs of hemorrhage (19, 34, 48).

The issue of when to administer anticoagulants, either acutely or subacutely, is controversial. Koller studied 44 patients who had atrial fibrillation and their first cerebral infarct (42). Only 15 of the 44 patients received anticoagulants within the first 48 hours. Eleven of the 44 patients suffered recurrent emboli, four within the first 2 weeks. Ten of the 11 patients were not receiving anticoagulants; the remaining patient was taking warfarin but not a therapeutic dose (42). Other studies have also shown that anticoagulants reduce recurrent emboli (Table 21.4) (4, 5, 25, 67).

Lodder and van der Lugt (48) reported 21 patients with cardiogenic embolic stroke who began receiving therapeutic doses of anticoagulants within 21 hours after the initial event. Only one patient had an intracranial hemorrhage; the patient had required ventilatory support and died of pulmonary embolism. The authors concluded that early anticoagulation in patients without impaired consciousness or mass effect was safe.

It is recommended that anticoagulation therapy be instituted as early as possible for embolic strokes of cardiac origin from atrial fibrillation as long as the patient has mild to moderate neurologic deficit, no mass effect or hemorrhage on CT, and no absolute contraindications to the treatment. In patients with large infarctions, CT scanning should be repeated in 3 to 5 days to rule out hemorrhagic transformation of the infarct. If the infarct remains bland, anticoagulation therapy may be instituted; if not, anticoagulation should be postponed for approximately 6 weeks (76).

Another cause of cardiogenic embolic stroke is ischemic MI that results in mural thrombi. Autopsy studies of patients with MIs have shown that systemic infarcts due to cardiac embolization occur in 45% to 60% of the cases; in half of them, the infarct is cerebral. Survivors of MI have a 3% to 5% risk of cerebral infarction; the majority of infarcts occur within the first 3 weeks. Patients with anterior or anteroseptal MI are at the greatest risk for developing mural thrombi and therefore embolic strokes (34). One study has shown a beneficial effect of anticoagulants in patients with transmural MI (69). Forty-three patients with mural thrombi were followed for 15 months: 25 patients received anticoagulants, and 18 did not. No embolic phenomenon occurred in the treated group, but seven embolic events occurred in the controls, all within 4 months after MI.

MVP, another cause of embolic stroke

Table 21.5. Results of Early Anticoagulation in Patients with Atrial Fibrillation

Study	Number of patients	Follow-up (days)	Percent recurrence
Cerebral Embolism Study Group[a]	25 randomized to anticoagulation within 32 h	14	0
	20 no anticoagulation for first 14 days	14	10
Hart et al[b]	12 immediate <48 h	14	0
	23 no treatment with anticoagulation	14	13

[a]Data from Cerebral Embolism Study Group: Immediate anticoagulation of embolic stroke: A randomized trial. *Stroke* 14:668–676, 1983.
[b]Data from Hart RG, Coull BM, Hart D: Early recurrent embolism associated with nonvalvular atrial fibrillation: A retrospective study. *Stroke* 14:688–693, 1983.

(6, 7), results from redundant mitral leaflet tissue. MVP can be associated with Marfan's syndrome, Ehlers-Danlos syndrome, and pseudoxanthoma elasticum (9). In a study comparing 60 patients younger than 45 years of age who had cerebral infarction with 60 age-matched controls, 40% of the patients, but only 6.8% of the controls, had MVP. The treatment of emboli from MVP is uncertain because the pathophysiology is poorly understood. These emboli may arise from platelet aggregation or thrombus formation. The treatment of choice for platelet aggregation would be antiplatelet therapy, whereas anticoagulants would be used for thrombus formation (28). Anticoagulation should be used only if the patient has recurrent episodes of emboli while receiving antiplatelet therapy.

THROMBOLYTIC AGENTS

The use of thrombolytic agents, such as streptokinase, urokinase, and, more recently, tissue-type plasminogen activator, t-PA, is still controversial and experimental. This form of therapy is reviewed in detail by Zivin (see Chapter 22, this volume).

ANTIPLATELET AGGREGATION AGENTS

Acute Therapy

Clinical trials of eicosanoids for treating acute ischemic cerebral infarction have focused primarily on prostacyclin (PGI$_2$). The biochemistry and mechanism of action of PGI$_2$ have been described previously. Because it has both antiplatelet and vasodilator properties, PGI$_2$ has been used in ischemic vascular disorders, including peripheral arterial disease, angina pectoris, Raynaud's phenomenon, and central retinal vein thrombosis (54). Three open-label trials of PGI$_2$ have shown beneficial effects in patients with acute strokes (30, 31, 50). Three double-blind, placebo-controlled studies (32, 35, 38), however, demon-

strated that PGI$_2$ is no more effective than placebo in the treatment of acute ischemic strokes. The negative results may stem from a type II error, nonoptimal doses of PGI$_2$, delay in initiating therapy, or hypoperfusion of the infarct area as a result of systemic hypotension (15). Possibly, earlier treatment with synthetic analogues of PGI$_2$ that are less hypotensive may prove more effective. This issue is reviewed in detail in the chapter by Black and Hoff (see Chapter 27, this volume).

Secondary Prevention

The term *secondary prevention* refers to therapeutic measures undertaken to prevent recurrent episodes of cerebral ischemia. Since the observation by Fisher (23) of platelet-fibrin emboli in retinal arteries during transient monocular blindness, the use of antiplatelet aggregating agents to treat TIAs and stroke has become more widespread. This section focuses primarily on clinical trials of aspirin in patients with cerebral ischemia.

Transient Ischemic Attacks

Five prospective randomized trials have evaluated the use of aspirin to treat TIAs. Each study had flaws in design or patient numbers. The first of these investigations, the United States trial (21, 22), compared aspirin (1,300 mg/day) with placebo in patients with TIAs in the carotid distribution. This study was conducted in two stages: (a) medical stage, in which aspirin was compared with placebo in patients who did not undergo surgery; and (b) surgical stage, in which patients who had undergone endarterectomy were randomized to aspirin or placebo arms of the study. In the medical stage of the trial, 88 patients were randomized to the treatment arm and 90 were randomized to the placebo arm. Each group was similar with respect to risk factors, and the compliance rate, determined by urine salicylate concentrations and platelet function studies, was high. The end points of the study were: absolute (i.e. mortality, stroke) and construct for unfavorable events (i.e. TIA, stroke, and death). Life-table analysis of the endpoints mortality, cerebral ischemia and infarction, and retinal infarction showed no statistically significant difference between groups. However, there was a statistically significant difference between subgroups for infarction and death among patients with multiple TIAs, especially those who had appropriate carotid lesions on angiography. Construct analysis showed a statistically significant decrease in unfavorable events in the treatment group.

The next study to assess this problem was the Canadian Cooperative Study (11) of 585 patients with TIAs in the carotid or vertebral basilar artery territory. The patients were randomized to four treatment groups: aspirin (1,300 mg/day, four times a day), sulfinpyrazone (800 mg/day), aspirin plus sulfinpyrazone (1,300 mg and 800 mg/day, respectively), and placebo. At the conclusion of the trial, TIA, stroke, and death were reduced by 19%, and stroke and death by 31%, in the two groups that received aspirin compared with the two that did not. These differences were statistically significant but were limited to males: Separate analysis showed a 48% decrease in stroke and death among men who received aspirin.

The Heidelberg study (60) consisted of 58 patients who had TIAs in both carotid and vertebral basilar territories but whose angiograms were normal or showed a nonsurgical lesion. Half of the patients received aspirin (1,500 mg/day), and half received placebo. The end point was a cerebral ischemic episode. At the conclusion of the trial, the aspirin group had fewer cerebral ischemic episodes, but the difference was not statistically significant. A statistical difference was seen when only patients with TIAs in the carotid territory were considered.

The Danish study (62) enrolled 203 patients who had transient deficits lasting less than 72 hours in the carotid or vertebral basilar territory. One hundred one patients received aspirin (1,000 mg/day); 102 received placebo. Only 75% of patients completed the study, and no statistical difference in ischemic events was observed.

The largest study evaluating the use of aspirin in cerebral vascular disease is the United Kingdom TIA trial (66). This study was made up of 35 study centers and included patients with TIA or reversible ischemic neurologic deficits. Patients were randomized to three groups: aspirin (1,200 mg/day), aspirin (300 mg/day), and placebo. Risk factors were equally distributed among the groups. Compliance was measured by random testing of urine samples for aspirin (ferric chloride test). These patients were followed for a period of about 5 years. At the start of the trial, major stroke, MI, and death were selected as the end points; about 2 years into the trial, disabling stroke and vascular death were added. No difference was seen between high- and low-dose aspirin groups. Benefit was seen when both aspirin groups were compared with the placebo group; nonvascular deaths decreased about 40% in the aspirin-treated group, but only in males (Table 21.6) (8, 11, 21, 22, 29).

Completed Stroke

Two studies have addressed the issue of antiplatelet agents (aspirin) in preventing recurrent strokes in patients with completed strokes. The French study (8) was a prospective, double-blind, 3-year trial of 604 patients with ischemic stroke (84%) and TIAs (16%) in both the carotid and vertebral basilar territories. One hundred ninety-eight patients were randomized to aspirin (1,000 mg/day), 202 to aspirin (1,000 mg/day) and dipyridamole (225 mg/day), and 204 to placebo. No statistically significant difference was seen between the aspirin group and the aspirin/dipyridamole group. The aspirin-treated groups had a statistically significant reduction of recurrent cerebral infarctions compared with the placebo group. When reductions of death and stroke were taken together, no statistical difference was found between groups.

The second study on the effect of aspirin on completed stroke was the Swedish study (64). The study was a multicenter, double-blind, randomized, 2-year trial of 505 patients with completed cerebral infarction; 253 received aspirin (1,500 mg/day), and 252 received placebo. Randomization was

Table 21.6. Effect of Aspirin on the Incidence of Stroke in Three Studies[a]

	Number of subjects		Number of infarctions or deaths			
			Aspirin group		Placebo group	
Study	Aspirin group	Placebo group	n	Percent	n	Percent
Accidents Ischemiques Cérébraux Leis à l'Atherosclérose[b]	400	204	53	13	38	19
Canadian Cooperative Study Group[c]	290	295	46	16	68	23
Aspirin in Transient Ischemic Attacks[d]						
Medical	88	90	13	15	19	21
Surgical	65	60	8	12	8	13
Total (mean %)	843	649	120	14	133	20

[a] Adapted by permission from Grotta JC: Current medical and surgical therapy for cerebrovascular disease. *N Engl J Med* 317:1505–1516, 1987.
[b] Data from Bousser MG, Eschwege, E, Haguenau M, et al: AICLA: Controlled trial of aspirin and dipyridamole in the secondary prevention of athero-thrombotic cerebral ischemia. *Stroke* 14:5–14, 1983.
[c] Data from Canadian Cooperative Study Group: A randomized trial of aspirin and sulfinpyrazone in threatened stroke. *N Engl J Med* 299:53–59, 1978.
[d] Data from Fields WS, Lemak NA, Frankowski CF, et al: Controlled trial of aspirin in cerebral ischemia. *Stroke* 8:301–314, 1977; Fields WS, Lemak NA, Frankowski CF, et al: Controlled trial of aspirin in cerebral ischemia. Part II: Surgical group. *Stroke* 9:309–319, 1977.

fairly even except that there were more men in the aspirin group (67%) than in the placebo group (58%). The primary end points were recurrent cerebral infarction or death. The dropout rate was about 30% in both groups. No difference was seen in the rate of stroke or death between the two groups. Similar conclusions were reached for the secondary end points (i.e. TIA and MI), and subgroup analysis showed no difference by age or sex.

Aspirin

When the data from all the above studies are taken together the following conclusions can be drawn:

Dose

Theoretically, the aspirin doses used in most of the trials were too high (at least 1 g per day). Aspirin blocks the production of thromboxane A_2 in platelets (a beneficial effect) as well as PGI_2 in the vessel (a negative effect). The platelet system appears to be more sensitive (in vitro) to this aspirin effect and doses as low as 75 mg/day (71) would probably be enough, whereas the vessel wall system is less sensitive and probably requires higher doses to inhibit PGI_2 synthesis. The United Kingdom TIA trial showed convincingly that there is no difference between high- and low-dose aspirin therapy; the low dose was 300 mg/day (66). Therefore, for stroke prophylaxis, one can recommend aspirin at a dose of 300 mg/day, which is better tolerated and has fewer adverse side effects.

Sex

Clinical and laboratory evidence suggests that aspirin's beneficial effects may be limited to males. The Canadian study (11) showed no statistical difference between women who received aspirin and those who did not despite the major decrease in stroke and death in men who received aspirin. Using iodine-125-labeled fibrin to quantitate injury-induced jugular vein thrombosis in rabbits, Kelton et al (39) found that aspirin reduced the size of thrombi only in male rabbits. A possible explanation for these sex differences may be the small number of events and the benign nature of the disease (18). Studies of a larger group of women followed for a longer period of time would be necessary to show a statistically significant difference. The conclusion that can be reached from clinical studies, however, is that aspirin has not been shown to be effective in women, but it has not been shown to be ineffective either (i.e. statistical type II error).

Transient Ischemic Attack Versus Stroke

The results of clinical trials suggest that aspirin is effective in the secondary prevention of TIAs in men. Aspirin has not been shown to be beneficial in patients with completed stroke, nor has it been shown to be ineffective (type II error).

Other Antiplatelet Agents

Sulfinpyrazone or dipyridamole does not offer any advantage over aspirin alone or in combination (1, 46). Ticlopidine is a promising agent that prevents platelet aggregation through a direct effect on the platelet membrane. It does not seem to affect arachidonate metabolism and, in particular, does not inhibit the production of prostacyclin (56). Large randomized trials of ticlopidine in patients with TIAs and completed stroke are currently in progress (57). Specific inhibitors of thromboxane A_2 synthase, such as imidazole, are in the initial stage of development (27, 57).

Subarachnoid Hemorrhage

After aneurysmal subarachnoid hemorrhage (SAH), narrowing of the major cerebral arteries at the base of the brain can lead to cerebral ischemia and infarction (24). This narrowing, commonly referred to as vasospasm, remains one of the most devastating complications of SAH, occurring in about 30% of patients (73). The narrowing is caused by a spasmogenic substance released by blood in the cerebral spinal fluid; the exact pathologic mechanisms are unknown. However, among the agents that have been implicated in the pathogenesis of vasospasm (73), the eicosanoids appear to be important (41). In several animal studies, manipulation of prostaglandin metabolites has influenced vasospasm. PGI_2 was effective in decreasing vasospasm (59) in cats with oxyhemoglobin-induced vasospasm (59). In another study involving dogs pretreated with nonsteroidal antiinflammatory drugs, a reduction in experimental vasospasm as well as associated behavioral changes were noted (74). A recent clinical study (63) showed improved outcome in patients treated with trapidil (a platelet antagonist and selective inhibitor of thromboxane A_2 synthesis). Despite this, the pathophysiology of vasospasm remains unknown, and the role of eicosanoids is therefore unknown.

Acknowledgments—A portion of this work was funded by the Clayton Foundation of Research.

References

1. American-Canadian Co-Operative Study Group: Persantine aspirin trial in cerebral ischemia. Part II: Endpoint results. *Stroke* 16:406–415, 1985.
2. Ansell J, Deykin D: Heparin-induced thrombocytopenia and recurrent thromboembolism. *Am J Hematol* 8:325–332, 1980.
3. Ansell J, Slepchuk N Jr, Jumar R, et al: Heparin induced thrombocytopenia: A prospective study. *Thromb Haemost* 43:61–65, 1980.
4. Baker RN, Broward JA, Fang HC, et al: Anticoagulant therapy in cerebral infarction. *Neurology* 12:823–835, 1962.
5. Baker RN, Schwartz WS, Rose AS: Transient ischemic strokes: A report of a study of anticoagulant therapy. *Neurology* 16:841–847, 1966.
6. Barnett HJ, Boughner DR, Taylor DW, et al: Further evidence relating mitral-valve prolapse to cerebral ischemic events. *N Engl J Med* 302:139–144, 1980.
7. Barnett HJM: Embolism in mitral valve prolapse. *Ann Rev Med* 33:489–507, 1982.
8. Bousser MG, Eschwege E, Haguenau M, et al: AICLA: Controlled trial of aspirin and dipyramole in the secondary prevention of atherothrombotic brain infarction. *Stroke* 14:5–14, 1983.
9. Braunwald E: Valvular heart disease. In Adams RD, Braunwald E, Petersdorf R, et al (eds): *Harrison's Principles of Internal Medicine,* ed. 9. New York, McGraw-Hill, 1980, p 1103.
10. Brust JCM: Transient ischemic attacks: Natural history and anticoagulation. *Neurology* 27:701–707, 1977.
11. Canadian Cooperative Study Group: A randomized trial of aspirin and sulfinpyrazone in threatened stroke. *N Engl J Med* 299:53–59, 1978.
12. Caplan LR, Hier DB, D'Cruz I: Cerebral embolism in the Michael Reese Stroke Registry. *Stroke* 14:530–536, 1983.
13. Carter AB: Anticoagulant treatment in progressing stroke. *Br Med J* 2:70–73, 1961.
14. Cerebral Embolism Study Group: Immediate anticoagulation of embolic stroke: A randomized trial. *Stroke* 14:668–676, 1983.
15. Chen ST, Hsu CY, Hogan EL, et al: Thromboxane, prostacyclin and leukotrienes in cerebral ischemia. *Neurology* 36:466–470, 1986.

16. Cines D, Tannebaum S: Immune endothelial cell injury in heparin associated thrombocytopenia. Clin Res 336A, 1985.

17. Duke RJ, Bloch RF, Turpie AGG, et al: Intravenous heparin for the prevention of stroke progression in acute partial stable stroke. Ann Intern Med 105:825–828, 1986.

18. Dyken ML: Anticoagulant and platelet-antiaggregating therapy in stroke and threatened stroke. Neurol Clin 1:223–242, 1983.

19. Easton JD, Sherman DG: Management of cerebral embolism of cardiac origin. Stroke 11:433–442, 1980.

20. Fareed J, Walenga JM, Williamson K, et al: Studies on the antithrombotic effects and pharmacokinetics of heparin fractions and fragments. Semin Thromb Hemost 11:56–74, 1985.

21. Fields WS, Lemak NA, Frankowski CF, et al: Controlled trial of aspirin in cerebral ischemia. Stroke 8:301–314. 1977.

22. Fields WS, Lemak NA, Frankowski CF, et al: Controlled trial of aspirin in cerebral ischemia. Part II: Surgical group. Stroke 9:309–319, 1977.

23. Fisher CM: Observations of the fundus oculi in transient monocular blindness. Neurology 9:333–347, 1959.

24. Fisher CM, Kistler JP, Davis JM: Relation of cerebral vasospasm to SAH visualized by CT scanning. Neurosurgery 6:1–9, 1980.

25. Fisher CM, Miller MD: Anticoagulant therapy in cerebral thrombosis and cerebral embolism: A National Cooperative Study, Interim Report. Neurology 11:119–131, 1961.

26. Fisher CM, Pearlman A: The nonsudden onset of cerebral embolism. Neurology 17:1025–1032, 1967.

27. Fisher M. Weiner B, Ockene IS, et al: Selective thromboxane inhibition: A new approach to antiplatelet therapy. Stroke 15:813–816, 1984.

28. Gates PC, Barnett HJM, Silver MD: Cardiogenic stroke. In Barnett HJM, Mohr JP, Stein BM, et al (eds): Stroke: Pathophysiology, Diagnosis and Management. New York, Churchill Livingstone, 1986, p 1085.

29. Grotta JC: Current medical and surgical therapy for cerebrovascular disease. N Engl J Med 317:1505–1516, 1987.

30. Gryglewski RJ, Nowak S, Kostka-Trabka E, et al: Treatment of ischemic stroke with prostacyclin. Stroke 14:197–202, 1983.

31. Hakim A, Pokrupa RP, Wolfe LS: Preliminary report on the effectiveness of prostacyclin in stroke. Can J Neurol Sci 11:409, 1984.

32. Handy NAT, Martin JF, Nicholl J, et al: Controlled trial of prostacyclin in acute cerebral infarction (abstract). Clin Sci 66:48, 1984.

33. Hart RG, Coull BM, Hart D: Early recurrent embolism associated with nonvalvular atrial fibrillation: A retrospective study. Stroke 14:688–693, 1983.

34. Hart RG, Sherman DG, Miller VT, et al: Diagnosis and management of ischemic stroke. Part II: Selected controversies. Curr Prob Cardiol 8(7):1–77, 1983.

35. Hass WK, Kamm B: The North American ticlopidine aspirin stroke study: Structure, stratifica-

36. Hirsch J: Mechanism of action and monitoring of anticoagulants. Semin Thromb Hemost 12:1–9, 1986.

37. Hirsch J, Ofosu F, Buchanan M: Rationale behind the development of low-molecular-weight heparin derivatives. Semin Thromb Hemost 11:13–16, 1985.

38. Huczynski J, Kostka-Trabka E, Sotowska W, et al: Double-blind controlled trial of the therapeutic effects of prostacyclin in patients with completed ischaemic stroke. Stroke 16:810–814, 1985.

39. Kelton JG, Hirsch J, Carter CJ, et al: Sex differences in the antithrombotic effects of aspirin. Blood 52:1073–1076, 1978.

40. Kelton J, Levine M: Heparin-induced thrombocytopenia. Semin Thromb Hemost 12:59–62, 1986.

41. Kiwak KJ, Coughlin SR, Moskowitz MA: Arachidonic acid metabolism in brain blood vessels. Implications for the pathogenesis and treatment of cerebrovascular disease. In Barnett HJM, Mohr JP, Stein BM, et al (eds): Stroke: Pathophysiology, Diagnosis and Management. New York, Churchill Livingstone, 1986, pp 141–164.

42. Koller RL: Recurrent embolic cerebral infarction and anticoagulation. Neurology 32:283–285, 1982.

43. Kwaan HC, Kampmier PA, Gomez HJ: Incidence of thrombocytopenia during therapy with bovine lung and porcine mucosal heparin preparation (abstract). Thromb Haemost 46:680A, 1981.

44. Levine M, Hirsch J: Hemorrhagic complications of long-term anticoagulant therapy for ischemic cerebral vascular disease. Stroke 17:111–116, 1986.

45. Levine W: Anticoagulant, antithrombotic and thrombolytic drugs. In Goodman LS, Gilman A, Koelle GB (eds): The Pharmacological Basis of Therapeutics. New York, MacMillan, 1975, pp 1350–1368.

46. Linet O, Hsu CY, Faught RE, et al: Epo-prostenol in acute stroke. Stroke 16:149, 1985.

47. Link H, Lebram G, Johansson I, et al: Prognosis in patients with infarction and TIA in carotid territory during and after anticoagulant therapy. Stroke 10:529–532, 1979.

48. Lodder J, van der Lugt PJM: Evaluation of the risk of immediate anticoagulant treatment in patients with embolic stroke of cardiac origin. Stroke 14:42–46, 1983.

49. Makhoul R, Greenberg CS, McCann RL: Heparin-associated thrombocytopenia and thrombosis: A serious clinical problem and potential solution. J Vasc Surg 4:522–528, 1986.

50. Miller VT, Coull BM, Yatsu FM, et al: Prostacyclin infusion in acute cerebral infarction. Neurology 34:1431–1445, 1984.

51. Millikan CH, McDowell FH: Treatment of transient ischemic attacks. Stroke 9:299–300, 1978.

52. Millikan CH, McDowell FH: Treatment of progressing stroke. Stroke 12:397–409, 1981.

53. Mohr JP, Caplan LR, Melski JW, et al: The Harvard Cooperative Stroke Registry: A prospective registry. Neurology 28:754–762, 1978.

54. Moufaruj NA, Little JR, Skrinska V, et al: Thromboxane synthetase inhibition in acute focal cere-

bral ischemia in cats. *J Neurosurg* 61:1107–1112, 1984.

55. Olsson JE, Muller R, Berneli S: Long-term anti-coagulant therapy for TIAs and minor strokes with minimum residum. *Stroke* 7:444–451, 1976.

56. Panak E, Maffrand JP, Picard-Fraire C, et al: Ticlopidine: A promise for the treatment of thrombosis and its complications. *Haemostasis* 13 (Suppl 1):1–54, 1983.

57. Pettigrew LC, Grotta JC, Hall ER, et al: 1-Ben-zylimidazole inhibits thromboxane synthesis in experimental ischemia (abstract). *Ann Neurol* 18:125. 1985.

58. Putman SF, Adams HP Jr: Usefulness of heparin in initial management of patients with recent transient ischemic attacks: *Arch Neurol* 42:960–962, 1985.

59. Quintana L, Konda R, Ishibashi Y, et al: The effect of prostacyclin on cerebral vasospasm. *Acta Neurochir (Wien)* 62:187–193, 1982.

60. Ruether R, Dorndorf W: Aspirin in patients with cerebral ischemia and normal angiograms of non-surgical lesions. The results of a double-blind trial. In Breddin K, Dorndorf W, Loew D, et al (eds): *Acetylsalicylate Acid in Cerebral Ischemia and Coronary Heart Disease*. Stuttgart, Schuttauer, 1978, p 97.

61. Santamaria J, Graus F, Rubio F, et al: Cerebral infarction of the basal ganglia due to embolism from the heart. *Stroke* 14:911–914, 1983.

62. Sorenson PS, Pederson H, Marquardsen J, et al: Acetylsalicylic acid in the prevention of stroke in patients with reversible cerebral ischemic attacks. A Danish Cooperative Study. *Stroke* 13:15–22, 1983.

63. Suzuki S, Sobata E, Iwabuchi T: Prevention of cerebral ischemic symptoms in cerebral vaso-spasm with trapidil, an antagonist and selective synthesis inhibitor of thromboxane A2. *Neurosurgery* 9:679–685, 1981.

64. Swedish Cooperative Study: High dose acetyl-salicylic acid after cerebral infarction. *Stroke* 18:325–334, 1986.

65. Ten Cate H, Henny CP, Buller HR, et al: Use of a heparinoid in patients with hemorrhagic stroke and thrombolic disease. *Ann Neurol* 15:268–270, 1984.

66. UK-TIA Study Group: United Kingdom Transient Ischemic Attack (UK-TIA) Aspirin Trial: Interim results. *Br Med J* 296:316–320, 1988.

67. Veterans Administration Cooperative Study of Atherosclerosis, Neurology Section: An evalua-tion of anticoagulant therapy in the treatment of cerebrovascular disease. *Neurology* 11:132–144, 1961.

68. Walker FJ, Esman CT: Interaction between hep-arin and Factor Xa inhibition of prothrombin activation. *Biochem Biophys Acta* 585:504–515, 1979.

69. Weinreich DJ, Burke JF, Pauletto FJ: Left ventric-ular mural thrombi complicating acute myocar-dial infarction. Long-term follow-up with serial echocardiography. *Ann Intern Med* 100:789–794, 1984.

70. Weksler BB, Lewin M: Anticoagulation in cere-bral ischemia. *Stroke* 14:658–663, 1983.

71. Weksler BB, Pett BB, Alonso D, et al: Differential inhibition by aspirin of vascular and platelet prostaglandin synthesis in atherosclerotic pa-tients. *N Engl J Med* 308:800–805, 1983.

72. Whisnant JP, Cartlidge MB, Elveback LR: Carotid and vertebral basilar transient ischemic attacks: Effect of anticoagulants, hypertension and car-diac disorders on survival and stroke occur-rence—a population study. *Ann Neurol* 3:107–115, 1978.

73. White RP, Hagen AA, Morgan H, et al: Experi-mental study on the genesis of cerebral vaso-spasm. *Stroke* 6:52–57, 1975.

74. White RP, Hagen AA, Robertson JT: Effect of nonsteroidal anti-inflammatory drugs on SAH in dogs. *J Neurosurg* 51:164–171, 1979.

75. Wolf PA, Dawber TR, Thomas HE Jr, et al: Epi-demiologic assessment of chronic atrial fibrilla-tion and risk of stroke: The Framingham Study. *Neurology* 28:973–977, 1978.

76. Yatsu FM, Hart RG, Mohr JP, et al: Anticoagu-lation of embolic strokes of cardiac origin: An update. *Neurology* 38:314–316, 1988.

CHAPTER TWENTY-TWO

Thrombolytic Therapy for Stroke

Justin A. Zivin, M.D., Ph.D.

Thrombosis and embolism are responsible for approximately 80% of strokes in the United States (14), and in cases of stroke caused by thrombosis or embolism, thrombolysis would appear to be a useful form of therapy. Several years ago, the exogenous thrombolytic agents streptokinase and urokinase were used in clinical trials of stroke therapy. The results were generally disappointing because of hemorrhagic side effects and a lack of unequivocal proof of therapeutic efficacy. Although those investigations were only preliminary studies, the difficulties that were encountered discouraged further work, and a consensus developed that the thrombolytic agents available at that time should not be used in stroke patients (18).

Recently tissue-type plasminogen activator (t-PA), the normal endogenous initiator of thrombolysis, has been produced through molecular biology technology and it is now available in quantities that permit pharmacologic investigation. It is effective in the treatment of coronary artery thrombosis, and successful results with an agent that may produce fewer side effects than streptokinase or urokinase suggest that the value of thrombolytic therapy for stroke should be reconsidered.

THROMBOLYSIS

Our current knowledge about fibrinolysis has been well reviewed (3, 15) and needs only be summarized here. During clot formation, circulating plasminogen binds to fibrin and to platelets throughout the thrombus. Thus, the clot contains the seeds of its own destruction. Subsequently, when dissolution of thrombus begins, circulating plasminogen activators (either t-PA or exogenous activators such as streptokinase or urokinase) catalyze plasmin formation from the bound plasminogen. Plasmin release causes fibrin degradation, producing fibrin fragments ("split products") and removal of the clot. Under normal circumstances, fibrinolytic activity is initiated by the release of plasminogen activator from vascular endothelium. The plasminogen activator can contact only the plasminogen on the surface of the thrombus. The plasminogen sequestered within the clot is activated as the clot dissolves and the outer layers are removed. Therefore, the rate of clot dissolution is related to the concentration of circulating plasminogen activator and the surface area of the clot (4).

The main complication of the use of thrombolytic agents is hemorrhage. Excessive levels of the drug may deplete circulating fibrinogen and coagulation factors V and VIII (1, 16). These losses prevent formation of thrombus at the sites of new injuries. All existing clots are subject to thrombolytic actions of the agent which may cause bleeding to resume at sites of old damage. Also, downstream from a thromboembolic occlusion the vessel wall may have become devitalized. When the thrombus or embolus is dissolved, blood under arterial pressure reenters the damaged vessel and may cause the wall to rupture, causing hemorrhage into the tissue surrounding the damaged vessel. Hemorrhagic destruction then may extend beyond the initially infarcted zone (6). Streptokinase and urokinase are thought to be particularly likely to produce hemorrhage because, as compared with t-PA, these exogenous agents cause prolonged depletion of clotting factors (21).

HISTORY OF EXOGENOUS THROMBOLYTIC THERAPY FOR STROKE

During the past 30 years, several evaluations of streptokinase and urokinase for stroke therapy have been conducted (5, 17). Of the clinical trials, two are more frequently cited than the others. Meyer and his associates (12, 13) described the effects of streptokinase administered intravenously to patients within 72 hours after the onset of neurologic symptoms of stroke. These patients were simultaneously treated with heparin and coumarin. Four of 36 control subjects died, whereas 13 of 37 treated patients died, a statistically significant worsening of outcome with treatment. Most of the deaths in the treated group were attributable to intracerebral hemorrhages. There was no evidence of clinical improvement in the treated group relative to the untreated control group, although the observers rating improvement were not blinded to the therapy each patient received. Thus, streptokinase therapy apparently afforded no therapeutic benefit and placed treated patients at an increased risk of fatal cerebral hemorrhage.

Urokinase proved to be somewhat less toxic than streptokinase for the treatment of some thrombotic problems in noncerebral vascular systems. Fletcher et al (7) used intravenous urokinase, administered for 10 to 12 hours, in the treatment of 31 patients who had moderate to severe strokes 8 to 31 hours after the onset of their symptoms. They detected no instance of improvement in neurologic function. Intracerebral hemorrhages were observed in all four of their patients who underwent autopsy (8); however, of those patients, it is possible that at least one showed signs consistent with the onset of hemorrhage before the initiation of therapy. Because the frequency of intracerebral hemorrhage in patients with stroke is estimated to be approximately 18% (14), about five of the 31 patients could be expected to have intracerebral hemorrhages. The total of four hemorrhages does not differ significantly from the expected total, although it is not known how many in the series had clinically undetectable hemorrhages. Considering the small sample of patients studied, one could reliably assume that hemorrhages were significantly increased by treatment only if more than 14 of the 31 patients had developed hemorrhages.

A variety of factors complicated the interpretation of the results of these earlier studies. Most of the patients were not treated until several days after the onset of ischemia and few, if any, were treated within the first 8 hours. Because irreversible damage to ischemic brain tissue begins within 1 hour after the stroke (9), it is unlikely that any substantial functional recovery could be expected when treatment did not begin until much later. Because strokes are so variable in their presentation, and because relatively small numbers of patients were tested in the earlier series, it is not surprising that functional improvements were not apparent. Also, most of the patients showed severe injury from the stroke. Even if there were substantial preservation of cerebral tissue, the improvements might not have been detectable clinically. Because the investigations were conducted without the benefit of computerized tomography (CT) scans, it is not known how many of the patients selected for thrombolytic therapy had existing intraparenchymal hemorrhages before initiation of drug therapy. Because the patients did not have repeated arteriography immediately after treatment, it is not certain how many vessels were reopened (5). Thus, it is not known whether the patients were given sufficient doses of thrombolytic agents or whether excessive doses were administered. Many of the patients were simultaneously treated with anticoagulants, which may have caused interactions with the thrombolytic agents. Thus, the risk of hemorrhage as a complication may have been substantially overestimated. There was no appropriately blinded assessment of the clinical efficacy of therapy and there was no attempt to select patients who might have been most able to benefit from therapy—

those with mild to moderate deficits. Therefore, it is not possible to arrive at any definite conclusions about the efficacy of streptokinase or urokinase therapy from these reports.

STUDIES WITH TISSUE PLASMINOGEN ACTIVATOR

Experimental Investigations

In the past few years, two major cooperative studies of the effects of streptokinase and t-PA in the treatment of acute coronary thrombosis have been conducted. The thrombolysis in myocardial infarction (TIMI) trial in the United States was initially designed to compare the effects of streptokinase and t-PA (19). In phase I, the unequivocal superiority of t-PA resulted in an early termination of the streptokinase trial and the selection of t-PA alone for further investigation. In the TIMI study, heparin was administered to prevent the clots from reforming at sites of damage in the arterial system until the injury was repaired (19). The European Cooperative Study Group for Recombinant Tissue-Type Plasminogen Activator (21) reported that intravenous t-PA was superior to streptokinase in reopening occluded coronary arteries and produced fewer bleeding episodes. Subsequent studies have further confirmed the value of t-PA therapy for a variety of thromboembolic disorders (10).

Several groups have initiated investigations of the effects of t-PA in experimental stroke models and have published some preliminary results (17, 22). So far, our group at the University of California, San Diego has conducted the most extensive studies in animals, using two types of embolic stroke models to examine the effects of t-PA in rabbits. In our preliminary experiments, we used a multiple cerebral embolism model (24). Blood from a donor rabbit was allowed to clot, then was fragmented into small pieces and filtered through screens so that the clot particles ranged between 100 and 250 μm in diameter. We anesthetized each recipient rabbit, surgically exposed and ligated one external carotid artery, and cannulated the common carotid artery. Each rabbit was allowed to recover from anesthesia, after which a quantity of the small clots was injected into the carotid system. The small clots dispersed throughout the cerebral circulation, producing small embolic occlusions at various locations throughout the brain. When only a small number of clots had been injected into the rabbit, no behavioral alterations were observed. When large numbers of clots had been injected, the rabbit developed severe encephalopathy or died. Observers who graded the rabbits were blinded to the quantity of clots and the treatment that each animal received. Using a quantal dose–response data analysis technique (23, 24), we were able to determine the amount of clots that produced irreversible neurologic damage in 50% of a group of rabbits. Treatments that produced neurologic improvement shifted the dose–response curve to the right of the control curve. The neurologic grading system was highly simplified for each rabbit and consequently there was almost no intraobserver variability. Despite its simplicity, the test was sensitive for determining therapeutic efficacy.

Our second technique involved a large clot model. Rabbits were cannulated in essentially the same fashion as in the small clot model. Each rabbit was injected with only one relatively large clot (4 to 5 mg), which usually produced one large infarction in the distribution of the middle cerebral artery. In the untreated control group, approximately 20% of the rabbits developed hemorrhages within the infarction. The advantages of this model as compared with the small clot model are that it simulates a more common neurologic problem and allows us to evaluate hemorrhage rates, the principal side effect of concern. The large clot model also has disadvantages. As is true of all such embolic infarction models, it is impossible to predict the extent or precise location of the damage that will occur. Also, because there is poor correlation between the extent of loss of neurologic function and the size of the infarction, the large clot model is insensitive, as compared with the small clot model, for assessing an agent's therapeutic efficacy in improving neurologic function.

In the small clot model, we found that intravenous administration of t-PA within 2 minutes after the onset of ischemia significantly reduced the injury response and no drug-induced hemorrhages were found (24). In subsequent experiments using the small clot model, we found improved neurologic function when treatment was delayed for as long as 45 minutes after clot administration (25). However, by 60 minutes after embolization, even a high dose of t-PA (2 mg/kg) did not produce neurologic improvement. Using the large clot model, we found no increase in the frequency of hemorrhages when t-PA was administered at doses as high as 5 mg/kg up to 8 hours after the onset of embolization, regardless of whether or not the clot dissolved (11). These results suggest that t-PA has the potential to produce neurologic improvement if it is administered rapidly after the onset of embolic stroke, and it appears to be safe to administer the drug in reasonably high doses for several hours.

Several questions remain unanswered. We do not know whether larger doses of t-PA can dissolve very large clots rapidly enough to produce significant neurologic improvement without danger of inducing hemorrhages. At low doses, t-PA is comparatively clot specific and at high doses it can deplete circulating clotting factors (21); higher doses of t-PA will dissolve larger clots but there may be an increased risk of hemorrhage. Whether primary intracranial hemorrhage is a contraindication to t-PA therapy, as is presumed, has not been investigated. Moreover, the interactions between t-PA and other drugs such as heparin, coumarin, and other agents that might be used concomitantly have not been explored. Although the drug appears to be promising for use in previously healthy animals, it may act differently in patients with stroke, who frequently are elderly and hypertensive. Clinical efficacy studies are essential to resolve these questions.

Clinical Stroke Trials

Since spring of 1987, two clinical trials have been in progress to determine the safety and efficacy of t-PA in the treatment of patients with stroke. In the first of these, sponsored by the National Institutes of Health (Bethesda, MD), phase I is to determine the dose range within which t-PA is safe for therapeutic use in humans (2). Patients selected for study are treated with t-PA within 90 minutes after the onset of stroke symptoms; they are given no anticoagulants. Among patients who are not selected, the principal reason for rejection is the presence of hemorrhage observed on the CT scans of the head which are made before treatment is begun. Although the investigators recognize that some patients with transient ischemic attacks (TIAs) will be treated under this protocol, no hazard to their safety is anticipated as preliminary work indicates that t-PA should not be harmful to patients who have TIAs. From the results of these phase I trials, it should be possible to identify an appropriate t-PA dose for subsequent trials designed to establish potential efficacy of treatment.

The other clinical trial, sponsored by the Burroughs Wellcome Company (Research Triangle Park, NC), is also designed to be a two-phase study, the first phase of which is similarly to determine an effective and safe dose of t-PA (20). Patients who have the abrupt onset of focal neurologic deficits are examined and a CT scan is done to exclude from the trial patients who have intracranial hemorrhage. Then, cerebral angiography is performed to ascertain that patients selected for study show occlusion of a vessel in a location that is consistent with their neurologic signs. These evaluations must be completed within 8 hours of the onset of symptoms. The selected patients then receive t-PA. Immediately after t-PA treatment, arteriography is repeated to determine if the vascular occlusion has altered and then CT scans are done to assess whether there has been any intracerebral hemorrhage. Heparin is administered only during angiography in the minimal amounts required to ensure that the initial catheterization is safely accomplished. As the study proceeds, successive patients receive t-PA in progressively higher increments until a dose is found that is both safe and effective in opening thrombosed vessels. t-PA at that dose level will be used in phase II of the investigation, which is an efficacy study.

SPECULATION ABOUT FUTURE PROSPECTS

t-PA may prove to be of value in the treatment of some forms of thromboembolic strokes. Its potential utility will be determined by two factors that have not as yet been adequately evaluated: (a) how rapidly therapy can be initiated; and (b) the risk of side effects. So far, in tests of t-PA used to treat various disorders, such as myocardial infarction, pulmonary embolism, and deep venous thrombosis of the legs, no major side effects other than hemorrhage have been reported. When hemorrhage has occurred, it has not always been possible to decide whether its cause was t-PA therapy, itself, or concomitant anticoagulant therapy. Hemorrhage is a likely consequence if t-PA is administered for prolonged periods at excessively high doses or if therapy is delayed too long after the onset of ischemia, but it is not yet apparent whether hemorrhage occurs at the lower doses that produce clot dissolution.

Clinical availability of a thrombolytic agent such as t-PA may cause a marked change in the treatment of many stroke patients. Currently, we have no specific treatment for many common types of strokes—most therapeutic approaches are based on the prevention of secondary damage and future strokes. There is usually no reason to arrive at a definitive diagnosis of stroke with any urgency because, other than general support, little can be done. In contrast, if thrombolytic therapy is shown to be effective for a sizable fraction of patients, it will be essential to treat most strokes as acute medical emergencies. Even if a patient is not eligible for this form of treatment, the decision will have to be made quickly. Much as the general public has been made aware of the symptoms of myocardial infarction, people will require education about the importance of an abrupt onset of neurologic deficit and the urgent need to seek medical attention rapidly for the acute stroke victim. Physicians, in turn, will have to reorganize the emergency medical system so that timely decisions about the diagnosis and treatment of stroke can be made, as they are currently in cases of cardiac arrest.

Because the brain has a high metabolic rate and low energy stores, rapid initiation of therapy is essential. If methods can be designed to allow paramedics to administer the drug before the patient is brought to the hospital, the potential value of treatment may be substantially increased. It may be possible to design protocols for use in the field that will reasonably assure that patients with definite or suspected intracranial hemorrhages can be identified and excluded, assuming that studies show intracranial hemorrhage to be the contraindication to t-PA therapy it is presumed to be.

The biologic half-life of intravenously administered t-PA is approximately 3 minutes (4), making it a reasonably safe drug for acute administration because treatment can be terminated rapidly if problems develop. It is reasonable to assume that, after a clot initially is dissolved, reformation of the clot will have to be prevented, as the site of vascular damage will not heal immediately. Various alterations of the t-PA molecule allow it to act for longer periods, and the longer-acting forms of t-PA may be more effective than heparin or coumarin in preventing repeated vascular occlusions.

The rate of clot lysis depends on the concentration of t-PA that can be delivered to the site of the clot. Because the rate of blood flow is reduced in an occluded vessel, direct injection of t-PA into that vessel might improve thrombolysis. The ability to lyse small clots rapidly through intravenous t-PA administration is a major advantage, but after the initial intravenous therapy is administered it may be useful to selectively catheterize the obstructed vessel and administer the drug locally to treat larger clots.

A major focus of experimental stroke research in recent years has concerned the identification of methods for reducing neurologic damage after the onset of ischemia. Various classes of drugs have been explored and such agents as glutamate antagonists, opiate antagonists, serotonin antagonists, and calcium channel blockers have been shown, in various studies, to have some potential for reducing such damage. Because these drugs exert their actions by mechanisms unrelated to clot lysis, they may be useful adjuvants to t-PA therapy. In addition, early t-PA therapy may increase the possibility that some patients will benefit from subsequent surgical procedures.

References

1. Agnelli G, Buchannan MR, Fernandez F, et al: A comparison of the thrombotic and hemorrhagic effects of tissue-type plasminogen activator and streptokinase in rabbits. *Circulation* 72:178–182, 1985.
2. Brott T, Haley EC, Levy DE, et al: The investigational use of t-PA for stroke. *Ann Emerg Med* 17:1202–1205, 1988.
3. Collen D: On the regulation and control of fibrinolysis: Edward Kowalski Memorial Lecture. *Thromb Haemost* 67:77–89, 1980.
4. Collen D, Strassen JM, Marafino BJ, et al: Biological properties of human tissue-type plasminogen activator obtained by expression of recombinant DNA in mammalian cells. *J Pharmacol Exp Ther* 231:146–152, 1984.
5. Del Zoppo GJ, Zuemer H, Harker LA: Thrombolytic therapy in stroke: Possibilities and hazards. *Stroke* 17:595–607, 1986.
6. Fisher CM, Adams RD: Observations on brain embolism with special reference to the mechanism of hemorrhagic infarction. *J Neuropathol Exp Neurol* 10:92–93, 1951.
7. Fletcher AP, Alkjersig N, Lewis M, et al: A pilot study of urokinase therapy in cerebral infarction. *Stroke* 7:135–142, 1976.
8. Hanaway J, Torack R, Fletcher AP, et al: Intracranial bleeding associated with urokinase therapy for acute ischemic hemispheral stroke. *Stroke* 7:143–146, 1976.
9. Hossmann KA, Kleihues P: Reversibility of ischemic brain damage. *Arch Neurol* 29:375–382, 1973.
10. Loscalzo J, Braunwald E: Drug therapy: Tissue plasminogen activator. *N Engl J Med* 319:925–931, 1988.
11. Lyden PD, Zivin JA, Clark WA, et al: Tissue plasminogen activator mediated thrombolysis of cerebral emboli and its effect on hemorrhagic infarction in rabbits. *Neurology,* 39:703–708, 1989.
12. Meyer JS, Gilroy J, Barnhart MI, et al: Therapeutic thrombolysis in cerebral thromboembolism: Randomized evaluation of intravenous streptokinase. In Millikan CH, Siekert RG, Whisnant JP (eds): *Cerebrovascular Diseases (Fourth Princeton Conference).* New York, Grune & Stratton, 1965, pp 200–213.
13. Meyer JS, Herndon RM, Gotoh F, et al: Therapeutic thrombolysis. In Millikan CH, Siekert RG, Whisnant JP (eds): *Cerebrovascular Diseases (Third Princeton Conference).* New York, Grune & Stratton, 1961, pp 160–177.
14. Mohr JP, Caplan LR, Melski JW, et al: The Harvard Cooperative Stroke Registry: A prospective registry. *Neurology* 28:754–762, 1978.
15. Sharma GVRK, Cella G, Parisi AF, et al: Thrombolytic therapy. *N Engl J Med* 306:1268–1276, 1982.
16. Sherry S. Tissue plasminogen activator (t-PA): Will it fulfill its promise? *N Engl J Med* 313:1014–1017, 1985.
17. Sloan MA: Thrombolysis and stroke: Past and future. *Arch Neurol* 44:748–768, 1987.
18. Thrombolytic therapy in thrombosis: A National Institutes of Health consensus development conference. *Ann Intern Med* 93:141–144, 1980.
19. TIMI Study Group: Special Report: The thrombolysis in myocardial infarction (TIMI) trial: Phase I findings. *N Engl J Med* 312:932–936, 1985.
20. t-PA–Acute Stroke Study Group: An open multicenter study of the safety and efficacy of various doses of rt-PA in patients with acute stroke: Preliminary results (abstract). *Stroke* 19:134, 1988.
21. Verstraete M, Bernard R, Bory M, et al: Randomised trial of intravenous recombinant tissue-type plasminogen activator versus intravenous streptokinase in acute myocardial infarction. Report from the European Cooperative Study Group for Recombinant Tissue-Type Plasminogen Activator. *Lancet* 1:842–847, 1985.
22. Watson BD, Prado R, Dietrich WD, et al: Mitigation of evolving cortical infarction in rats by recombinant tissue plasminogen activator following photochemically induced thrombosis. In Powers WJ, Raichle ME (eds): *Cerebrovascular Diseases (Fifteenth Research [Princeton] Conference).* New York, Raven Press, 1987, pp 317–330.
23. Waud DR: On biological assays involving quantal responses. *J Pharmacol Exp Ther* 183:577–607, 1972.
24. Zivin JA, Fisher M, DeGirolami U, et al: Tissue plasminogen activator reduces neurological damage after cerebral embolism. *Science* 230:1289–1292, 1985.
25. Zivin JA, Lyden PD, DeGirolami U, et al: Tissue plasminogen activator: Reduction of neurologic damage after experimental embolic stroke. *Arch Neurol* 45:385–391, 1988.

CHAPTER TWENTY-THREE

Optimal Anesthetic Techniques for Patients at Risk of Cerebral Ischemia

Robert W. McPherson, M.D.
Jeffrey R. Kirsch, M.D.
Richard J. Traystman, Ph.D.

Ischemic cerebral injury is a complex phenomenon probably representing a combination of factors, such as the type of insult (global versus regional ischemia), duration of insult, and level of cerebral metabolic demand relative to the cerebral oxygen supply. Mechanisms of ischemic injury that have been suggested include energy failure, excessive lactic acid production, free fatty acid production (72), excitatory neurotoxin production, and the production of oxygen-derived free radicals (37, 119). As the exact pathophysiology of ischemic injury has not yet been exactly defined, it is difficult to determine a priori what the optimal anesthetic technique should be in operations on patients at risk of neurologic injury from ischemia. Differences in the severity of ischemic injury may relate to the anesthetic technique used (99), but in fact there are probably a series of acceptable anesthetic techniques depending on the patient's specific requirements. This chapter addresses direct brain effects of alterations of cerebral blood flow (CBF) and the cerebral metabolic rates of oxygen ($CMRO_2$) and glucose, direct hemodynamic effects, and the impact on other aspects of clinical management using anesthetic drugs that may alter neurologic outcome.

Perioperative cerebral infarction occurs in less than 1% of all surgical procedures, and cardiac emboli are the most frequent cause (33). In patients with predisposing factors such as atherosclerosis, 83% of perioperative strokes in a recent study occurred in the postoperative period, and the neurologic injury appeared to be unrelated to intraoperative events such as hypotension (38). Little information is available concerning the relationship of specific anesthetic drugs to neurologic outcome because the exact moment the neurologic injury occurs is usually unknown. Thus, beneficial or adverse effects of specific agents may be masked by the concomitant effects of other drugs or surgical maneuvers. Although some anesthetic drugs are protective in animal models of cerebral hypoxia or ischemia, specific drugs or specific drug doses may be inappropriate for clinical anesthesia; studies in animals frequently use supraanesthetic doses. The choice of anesthetic agents and anesthetic management may affect neurologic outcome by effects on CBF and cerebral metabolism and effects on the ability of neural tissue to withstand oxygen deprivation.

Attention must be given to drug doses, specifically doses that have been shown to be protective during cerebral ischemia in animal studies. Higher than anesthetic doses shown to have a protective effect in animals are not clinically useful because hemodynamic effects, such as hypotension, may limit beneficial cerebral effects and may even increase neurologic injury in humans. Thiopental (90 mg/kg), for example, has been shown to be protective in animals, but cardiopulmonary bypass is required to support the blood pressure (59). Lesser doses of thiopental, probably with lesser degrees of cerebral protection, are used in clinical anesthesia.

The divergence of results in animal experiments and subsequent clinical studies may be due to the cause and type of ischemic insult, for example, global versus focal or complete versus incomplete ischemia. We discuss the practice of anesthesia as it relates to cerebral ischemia on the basis of results of studies of both animals and humans.

OVERVIEW OF ANESTHETIC MANAGEMENT

Modern neuroanesthesia combines volatile anesthetic gases, intravenous agents, neuromuscular blocking agents, and vasoactive agents to maintain unconsciousness while maintaining cardiovascular stability in the patient. The anesthetic plan, devised before surgery, incorporates important aspects of the patient's medical history and specific surgical requirements. It is then modified during surgery depending on the patient's initial reactions to the anesthetic drugs. Anesthesia may influence ultimate neurologic outcome by depressing the level of consciousness after surgery, which makes neurologic examination difficult or impossible. At the end of the procedure, residual anesthesia effects may make the detection of potentially reversible injury difficult by masking changes in the neurologic examination; conversely, neurologic alterations observed may be mistakenly attributed to residual anesthesia. Anesthetic agents may transiently alter the neurologic examination, even in neurologically normal patients; transient hyperreflexia, Babinski reflex, and sustained clonus commonly occur during awakening from general anesthesia in patients with no central nervous system lesions (89). Such abnormalities occur while the patient is poorly responsive to verbal commands, but findings on the neurologic examination return to normal as the level of consciousness increases.

Airway management is extremely important in patients with neurologic deterioration or who are at immediate risk of cerebral ischemia. The airway may be secured by oral intubation under direct vision or by nasal intubation either without direct vision or using fiberoptic bronchoscopy. Each method may be used successfully in patients at risk of neurologic injury, but the technique should be individualized for each patient. By far the most important part of airway management is recognition and correction of airway obstruction. Neurologic injury not only may be increased by respiratory insufficiency, but it also predisposes the patient to respiratory insufficiency because of reduced respiratory drive and diminished upper airway reflexes. If rapid intubation is indicated, we recommend oral intubation as the technique of choice.

Endotracheal intubation usually causes arterial hypertension that may increase intracranial pressure (ICP) (9). Lidocaine (1.5 mg/kg intravenously) (9), vasoactive drugs (20, 52), repeated doses of thiopental (50% of induction dose) (110), intravenous fentanyl (15), esmolal (an ultrashort-acting β-blocker) (20), and labetatol (combined α- and β-adrenergic blocker) (84) have been used to blunt the hemodynamic and intracranial hypertensive response to intubation.

CIRCUMSTANCES OF INCREASED RISK OF CEREBRAL ISCHEMIA

Neurodiagnostic Procedure

Neurodiagnostic procedures, including cerebral angiography, computerized tomography (CT) scan, and magnetic resonance (MR) imaging, are frequently performed in patients at risk of cerebral ischemia. Immobilization during the procedure is required and optimal positioning may require head flexion, which increases the risk of upper airway obstruction. Airway obstruction is particularly important because the combination of hypoxia and hypercapnia is especially detrimental to the regulation of brain blood flow (55). Patients with a depressed level of consciousness frequently have a diminished ability to maintain an adequately patent upper airway, and thus may be placed at great risk of respiratory failure because of depressed respiratory reflexes and head flexion. Continuous monitoring of respiratory function should be undertaken with pulse oximetry and end-tidal carbon dioxide (CO_2) determinations.

Intravenous sedation may be used to facilitate cooperation of the patient during neurodiagnostic studies. Patients with a depressed level of consciousness may become agitated and respond violently to normal levels of stimulation such as catheter insertion for angiography. In such circumstances, increasing sedation does little to enhance cooperation and may lead to respiratory depression and airway obstruction. Undiagnosed hypoxia may increase agitation which then may be incorrectly treated with additional sedative drugs. In patients with depressed levels of consciousness, general anesthesia with endotracheal intubation may decrease the risk of cerebral injury by control of arterial oxygen tension (PaO_2) and carbon dioxide tension ($PaCO_2$) levels. Regardless of anesthetic technique used (sedation or general), appropriate hemodynamic and neurophysiologic monitoring must be employed so that decreased cerebral perfusion or early evidence of ischemia may be treated promptly. Anesthesia management during diagnostic procedures is clearly a circumstance in which improvement in neurologic outcome can be accomplished by appropriate anesthetic management.

Intracranial Hypertension

The goal of management in patients with intracranial hypertension is to induce anesthesia, control ventilation, and perform decompression surgery without decreasing cerebral perfusion pressure (CPP) or CBF. These aims may be accomplished with general anesthesia alone or by a technique which uses systematically administered vasoactive agents combined with basal anesthesia. In the latter technique, anesthesia is induced using small doses of anesthetics to avoid arterial hypotension and to blunt the hypertensive systemic and intracranial response to endotracheal intubation by blocking upper airway reflexes with local anesthesia, either by intravenous injection or injection near somatic nerves. Numerous other intravenous drugs have been given to attempt to blunt this response with only partial success compared to the results with the application of local anesthesia (9, 15, 20, 52, 84). In patients with intracranial hypertension, intravenous anesthetics that have minimal direct effects on ICP should be used to reduce the amount required of volatile anesthetic gases that increase ICP until the intracranial cavity is decompressed.

Cerebral Vascular Operations

During operations for intracranial aneurysm, arteriovenous malformation, and cartoid endarterectomy, focal cerebral ischemia by surgical reduction of regional CBF may be produced from vessel occlusion and tissue retraction, resulting in decreases in CPP due to hypoperfusion. The ability to determine the onset, duration, and circumstances of impairment of function is eliminated during anesthesia unless cerebral ischemia is detected by electroencephalogram (EEG) or somatosensory evoked potential monitoring. Because the onset and severity of ischemia may not be apparent, the entire anesthetic period should be managed in such a way as to minimize the risk of infarction.

There is little information concerning the effects of specific anesthetic agents on collateral blood flow in the brain. Blood flow to ischemic brain through brain collateral vessels may not be controlled by autoregulation and CPP should be maintained at normal levels by using vasoactive agents, if necessary. Several agents have been recommended on the basis of laboratory results for use in patients at risk for ischemic injury during neurovascular surgery including ketamine (1 to 2 mg/kg) to increase CBF and thiopental (4 to 6 mg/kg) administered immediately before temporary vessel occlusion to reduce cerebral metabolism. However, neither of these drugs has been shown to be protective when administered in these doses in controlled clinical studies.

Use of an anesthetic technique that permits prompt awakening after surgery is particularly important in patients undergoing neurovascular operations. Serial neurologic examination during the immediate postoperative period continues to be the most sensitive indicator of postoperative changes in neurologic function that might signify occurrence of a treatable complication. Prolonged unconsciousness following operation may lead to unnecessary diagnostic procedures or may mask neurologic changes such as those due to development of a hematoma or thrombosis of a vessel repair.

ANESTHESIA INDUCTION AGENTS

Barbiturates

Thiopental (4 mg/kg by intravenous bolus) rapidly induces anesthesia (within 30 to 45 seconds) and mean arterial blood pressure (MABP) is well maintained in normotensive, normovolemic patients (average decrease in MABP, 15 mm Hg) (19). However, a greater decrease in MABP may occur in hypertensive patients (80) or in patients who are hypovolemic. Hypovolemia is frequently unappreciated in neurologic patients treated with diuretics for control of elevated ICP and it may predispose those patients to a decrease in CPP following thiopental administration. In a study of focal ischemia in animals, barbiturates were shown to be more protective than halothane, which increased infarct size beyond that which occurred without anesthesia (99), or as compared to use of nitrous oxide with fentanyl or to isoflurane anesthesia (71). In that study, the extent of cerebral infarction observed in animals receiving nitrous oxide with fentanyl was double, and in those receiving isoflurane was triple, the extent observed in animals receiving thiopental. Even in very short episodes of ischemia, barbiturates limit the degree of neuronal damage observed (31). Many studies in animals show protective effects of barbiturates during cerebral oxygen deprivation (59, 61, 100), but information about humans at risk of neurologic injury is limited. In fact, only one clinical study, which involved cardiopulmonary bypass, shows neurologic protection by thiopental (74).

In patients sustaining global ischemia during cardiac arrest, thiopental does not appear to protect from ischemic injury (68). In 262 patients, treatment with high-dose thiopental (30 mg/kg) did not decrease the death rate, improve neurologic recovery, or increase the number of patients who survived, even with poor neurologic outcome (12). In an earlier study, 53 patients received thiopental and were compared to a historical group of similar size. The mortality rate was similar for the two groups and the mortality rate was higher in patients with ischemic heart disease who received thiopental (68).

The apparent protective effects of barbiturates have resulted in their use in high doses for anesthesia. Thiopental (75 mg/kg over 60 minutes) (108) and methohexital (24 mg/kg over 60 minutes) (107) produced an isoelectric EEG and a reduction of $CMRO_2$ by 50%, with reduction of MABP to 87% of control, increase in heart rate to 116% of control, and reduction of cardiac output to 87% of control. Deep barbiturate anesthesia for long operations (10 to 20 hours) prolongs awakening for 48 to 72 hours (108) and may cause seizures (107). There is little evidence that this type of anesthesia is advantageous in protecting the brain from ischemia, particularly considering its interference with hemodynamic stability and with assessment of electrophysiologic function intraoperatively and neurologic function postoperatively.

Although there is substantial evidence from experiments in animals that thiopental is protective under isolated, controlled circumstances, results in studies of humans do not support the use of barbiturates at doses that produce detrimental hypotension or dramatically prolong awakening following operation. Results with an alternative barbiturate anesthetic protocol have been described by Spetzler and colleagues (see Chapter 24, this volume).

Etomidate

Etomidate is a nonbarbiturate intravenous agent that maintains MABP during induction of anesthesia, even in elderly patients. Etomidate can be used to maintain anesthesia by continuous infusion or it can be used to induce anesthesia (bolus injection, 0.3 to 0.4 mg/kg). In dogs, etomidate reduces $CMRO_2$ to 48% of control at the level of isoelectric EEG (64). Etomidate, even when given as a single dose (0.35 mg/kg bolus intravenously) to induce anesthesia, blocks the adrenal stress response to surgery for several hours postoperatively (29). However, since most patients at risk of neurological injury receive exogenous steroids, this effect is of little consequence in determining the use of etomidate in patients at risk of ischemia. Thus, etomidate is an acceptable anesthesia induction agent in such patients.

Findings in studies with animals regarding neural protection with etomidate are ambiguous. Protection was shown during global ischemia (35, 118), but not during regional ischemia (111). Despite there having been only a few studies in animals, observation of cerebral metabolic depression and minimal cardiac toxicity with etomidate led to its clinical use during temporary vessel occlusion for clipping of giant intracranial aneurysms (8). In that study, etomidate was administered until burst suppression was shown on the EEG (0.4 to 0.5 mg/kg) in 14 anesthetized patients; 71% of those patients had a good neurologic outcome. The authors attributed the good results to protection of the brain by etomidate during vessel temporary occlusion. However, there was no control group in that study.

Ketamine

Ketamine (1 to 2 mg/kg bolus intravenously) is a dissociative anesthetic that is used infrequently because it causes hallucinations postoperatively. However, its anesthetic properties are of considerable theoretical interest. Ketamine maintains cardiovascular stability by release of endogenous catecholamines and supports spontaneous respiration but with increased $PaCO_2$ at surgical levels of anesthesia (101). However, upper airway reflexes may be reduced and hypoxia or hypercapnia may occur when airway con-

trol is lost. Ketamine does not alter CBF unless $PaCO_2$ is altered (95); however, ketamine administered intravenously usually causes increases in $PaCO_2$ and CBF.

Ketamine is functionally related to the N-methyl-D-aspartate (NMDA) receptor that is found in brain regions most susceptible to ischemia. It inhibits the action of the excitatory amino acids glutamate and aspartate; thus, theoretically it may protect the brain from injury during ischemia. Wieloch (119) presented evidence that areas of the brain selectively vulnerable to ischemic insult receive a dense excitatory aminoacidergic innervation. During global ischemia, excessive amounts of glutamate were released and transsection of glutamate-containing nerves reduced the amount of postischemic injury. Whereas other specific NMDA receptor inhibitors, such as MK-801, protect the brain from ischemia (76), ketamine does not. Moreover, ketamine appears to block the beneficial effects of the cyclooxygenase inhibitor indomethacin in the cat middle cerebral artery (MCA) occlusion model (21). Ketamine lacks the protective effect of depressing metabolic processes that is afforded by barbiturates during regional ischemia. Thus, ketamine at present is not recommended in patients at risk of neurologic injury. However, synthesis of related anesthetic drugs in the future may provide agents that block specific mechanisms of neural injury and provide anesthesia.

Neuromuscular Blocking Agents

Neuromuscular blocking agents facilitate endotracheal intubation and prevent nonpurposeful movement during light levels of anesthesia. In addition to effects on the myoneural junction, neuromuscular blocking drugs cause hemodynamic and other systemic effects that may be important in preventing neurologic injury.

Succinylcholine produces paralysis in 30 to 45 seconds and permits rapid control of the airway and rapid initiation of hyperventilation. Succinylcholine directly increases ICP (17, 50), probably by stimulation of afferent fibers in systemic muscle (50). Prior administration of a nondepolarizing drug, such as pancuronium, blocks the increase in ICP (66). The average increase in ICP in patients with brain tumors who receive succinylcholine is 5 mm Hg, but 50% of patients have an increase in ICP of more than 10 mm Hg (66). The increase in ICP caused by succinylcholine is greater in circumstances of intracranial hypertension (17). Succinylcholine increases CBF by 77% of control within 3 minutes without a change in $CMRO_2$ (50). An additional disadvantage of succinylcholine is occurrence of life-threatening hyperkalemia which can occur as early as 1 week after denervation injury of the musculature (43, 67).

Nondepolarizing neuromuscular blocking drugs such as pancuronium and vercuronium (Norcuron, Organon Pharmaceuticals, West Orange, NJ) appear to have no direct effect on the cerebral circulation. A potential disadvantage of these drugs as compared to succinylcholine is the greater time necessary for complete paralysis to develop in order to allow intubation or manual hyperventilation. In patients with intracranial pathology, CPP decreases less when pancuronium is used for neuromuscular blockade than when succinylcholine is used (54).

Atracurium (Tracrium, Burroughs-Wellcome, Research Triangle Park, NC) is a short-acting, nondepolarizing agent that does not increase ICP in patients with intracranial masses, even when given in doses sufficient to cause rapid paralysis (87). However, it has a metabolite—laudanosine—that may alter CBF and that, in high concentrations, may reverse general anesthesia (34).

Neuromuscular blockade is a universal component of intraoperative care in patients at risk of neurologic injury. Thus, the question is not whether to produce neuromuscular blockade, but which drug should be used. Complications are sufficiently high with succinylcholine to suggest that this drug has little use in patients at risk of neurologic injury. Although pancuronium has a relatively long duration of action (about 1 hour) and has a slow onset as compared to succinylcholine (2 to 3 minutes for complete muscle relaxation), it probably should be considered the neuromuscular blocking agent of choice for neurosurgical patients.

Narcotics

Narcotics are major components of general anesthesia, particularly in patients at risk of neurologic injury, because their hemodynamic and respiratory effects are easily reversed by a narcotic antagonist, naloxone. Because synthetic narcotics do not cause hemodynamic instability, they maintain CPP near normal. Doses of fentanyl of less than 50 μg/kg do not block the stress response to surgery (36). However, at higher doses (100 μg/kg), fentanyl blocks the increase in cortisol, epinephrine, and norepinephrine observed during surgery and thus prevents potentially damaging hyperglycemia (48). Morphine (2 mg/kg intravenously) produces clinical anesthesia and does not alter cerebral autoregulation (42); however, it may cause hypotension and increased ICP as a result of histamine release (3). Synthetic narcotics such as fentanyl and its analogues, alfentanil and sufentanil, do not cause histamine release and are preferable to morphine because they produce a lesser degree of hypotension. Both fentanyl and alfentanil preserve cerebral homeostatic mechanisms such as autoregulation responses to hypoxia and changes in $PaCO_2$ (56, 57). The direct effect of synthetic narcotics on CBF is uncertain, there being reports of lack of change in CBF (57) and decreases in CBF (by about 53%) and $CMRO_2$ (by about 40%) (14, 46) after their administration. These effects are probably a consequence of differences in the experimental models used. There is no evidence that synthetic narcotics increase CBF or ICP.

The efficacy of naloxone in humans with neurologic injury has not been established, although there are reports of at least transient improvement of neurologic function after naloxone administration (1, 10, 24). There is little evidence of permanent improvement in neurologic outcome. However, since studies in both animals and humans show that naloxone, a narcotic antagonist, decreases ischemic injury or improves neurologic function (32), the potential that narcotic administration may contribute to neurologic injury has been raised. However, hemodynamic stability during high-dose narcotic anesthesia (112) makes it a desirable anesthetic technique in patients who are hypovolemic from dehydration by mannitol. Moreover, it has been suggested that certain opiate agonists (e.g. U50,488H, a κ-opiate receptor agonist) may offer protection from cerebral ischemia (104).

The role of an opiate receptor mechanism as a mediator of ischemic brain injury has been suggested by Sandor et al (92), who found that cortical blood flow decreased in the ischemic hemisphere but not in the normal hemisphere following injection of the opiate agonist (D-Met 2, Pro 5)-enkephalinamide. In their cat model, naloxone (1 mg/kg intravenously) doubled CBF and increased cerebral blood volume (CBV) (92). In a recent review of naloxone in cerebral ischemia, however, the role of increased CBF in neurologic benefit was questioned (32) (*see also* Chapter 26, this volume).

Despite the results of these studies, we feel that there is no need to avoid narcotic anesthesia because the benefits of hemodynamic stability it affords probably outweigh any direct effects of the opiate receptor in aggravating neurologic injury. Furthermore, the ability to reverse narcotic anesthesia quickly makes it a desirable agent. Additional studies are required to resolve this issue.

A disadvantage of high-dose narcotic anesthesia is that the anesthesia level cannot be easily reversed without using a narcotic antagonist. Care must be taken in administering naloxone to postoperative patients who have received narcotic anesthesia because temporary reversal of neurologic deficit may occur simultaneously with reversal of the narcotic effect. Thus, presence of alteration in the level of consciousness or neurologic function may be incorrectly attributed to persistence of narcotic anesthesia, and presence of a treatable lesion may be masked. Finally, abrupt reversal of narcotic anesthesia may produce life-threatening hypertension and cardiac arrhythmias. Therefore, naloxone

should be given slowly in increments of 1.5 g/kg.

Anesthetic Gases

Nitrous Oxide

Nitrous oxide is frequently a primary component of general anesthesia. It is often compared with other agents experimentally rather than with a nonanesthetized control group, or it is combined with other anesthetic drugs so that the contribution of nitrous oxide to observed cerebral effects cannot be ascertained (105). Nitrous oxide is a nonvolatile agent that has direct cerebral effects and produces an increase in CBF by 32% when added to halothane anesthesia (91). In the awake goat model, Pelligrino et al (77) found that nitrous oxide increased CBF to a maximum of 165% of the control level after 15 minutes. Much of the CBF increase was confined to cerebral cortex (188% to 246% of control) and was associated with an increase of $CMRO_2$ to 170% of the control level. The effect on ICP was less clear. In patients with normal cerebral spinal fluid (CSF) pressure, nitrous oxide does not increase CSF pressure but in the presence of decreased intracranial compliance, nitrous oxide would be expected to increase ICP because of its effects on CBF.

The use of nitrous oxide decreases the concentration of volatile anesthetic gases (halothane, isoflurane) necessary to maintain adequate anesthesia. At present, it is unclear which anesthetic technique—a combination of nitrous oxide with volatile anesthetic gas in a relatively low dose, or volatile anesthetic gas alone in a higher dose—is more detrimental to the ischemic brain.

Volatile Anesthetics

The concentration of volatile anesthetics required to prevent hemodynamic changes following surgical stimulation is 50% greater than that necessary to prevent purposeful movement to stimulation (minimal alveolar concentration) (86). Thus, hypertension frequently occurs in response to surgical stimulation unless high inspired anesthetic concentrations are administered. Volatile anesthetic gases cause concentration-dependent increases in CBF and concentration-dependent decreases in the efficiency of autoregulation, so that the hypertensive response to stimulation may cause an increase in CBF and ICP.

Halothane

In the past few years, the use of halothane has declined because of the potential for hepatic toxicity associated with it. Halothane continues to be used in pediatric patients because it causes little or no airway irritation, and in adults with asthma to reduce or treat intraoperative bronchospasm. Induction of halothane anesthesia by mask is frequently used in children because of the difficulty of venous cannulation in the awake child, but this induction technique may increase ICP even in children who are not excited or have no airway obstruction (102). Therefore, if ICP is an important consideration, an alternative technique such as intravenous induction should be used, even in children.

Halothane produces more cerebral vasodilation than does either enflurane or isoflurane (106), as shown in a study in which halothane produced a greater increase in ICP and brain swelling in cats receiving equal anesthetic doses of the three drugs (22). Halothane increases CBF and decreases $CMRO_2$ by 50% (47), and causes a dose-dependent failure of autoregulation (65). Even in patients who are hyperventilated, ICP remains elevated for more than 5 minutes after the initiation of halothane or enflurane anesthesia (102).

The cerebral vascular response to volatile anesthetics appears to be time dependent. Albrecht et al (2) showed that although CBF increases with halothane to 210% of the control level, flow returns to control levels following 2.5 hours of anesthesia. Warner et al (113) found that CBF decreased during 7 hours of halothane anesthesia, with the flow at 7 hours being 47% of the value at 2 hours.

In a model of focal cerebral ischemia, greater neural injury occurred in the animals receiving halothane in a high concentration, with or without hypotension, than in those receiving light halothane anesthesia or those operated without general anesthesia (99). Hypotension caused by volatile anesthetic agents such as halothane has variable effects on CBF in patients with subarachnoid hemorrhage and at risk of vasospasm (78). Patients who experienced an increase in CBF with halothane had a good neurologic outcome, whereas those patients (25%) who had a decrease in CBF had a poor outcome.

Thus, we do not recommend halothane in neuroanesthesia. If it is used for anesthesia induction, other agents such as isoflurane should be substituted as soon as possible.

Enflurane and Isoflurane

Enflurane and isoflurane are isomers that have apparently dissimilar effects on the cerebral circulation despite their similar chemical composition.

In patients with normal preoperative EEGs who receive enflurane anesthesia, EEG slowly occurs postoperatively (13, 49), as manifested by a decrease in the alpha frequency for 2 to 6 days. In approximately 66% of patients, posterior delta activity persists for 6 to 30 days after exposure to enflurane. Seizures beginning 6 to 8 days following an apparently uneventful course of anesthesia with enflurane have been reported (75). The increased metabolic demand associated with seizures might be detrimental to a patient. The induction of abnormal EEG activity with enflurane anesthesia occurs at concentrations higher than those most often used clinically, but hyperventilation increases the risk of EEG abnormalities at clinical levels of the drug (88).

Patients receiving enflurane show less extensive cerebral vasodilation than those receiving halothane, and 2% enflurane does not increase ICP in patients with intracranial tumors (69). Unlike enflurane, isoflurane does not cause seizure activity (23) but it does significantly lower CPP.

In patients, 1% isoflurane does not increase ICP or change CBF but it does cause decreased CPP because of a decrease in MABP. However, 2% isoflurane causes a further reduction in CPP and increases ICP without a change in CBF (53). Isoflurane causes a dose-dependent effect on cerebral autoregulation: Autoregulation is preserved with 1.4% isoflurane but absent with 2.8% isoflurane (58). Michenfelder et al (60) found that, during clamping of the carotid artery, the critical CBF (i.e. flow that produces an ischemic EEG pattern) is less in patients receiving isoflurane (10 ml/ 100 g/minute) than in those given either halothane or enflurane anesthesia (25 ml/ 100 g/minute). These results are consistent with a cerebral metabolic depression caused by isoflurane and the authors have interpreted their data as being consistent with a protective role for isoflurane (73).

In a nonhuman primate model of regional ischemia, isoflurane did not reduce infarct size whereas thiopental was protective (71). With isoflurane, as with halothane anesthesia, CBF appears to decrease over time (11). Isoflurane does not prevent ischemic cell necrosis in a rat model of transient forebrain ischemia (115) and, in comparison with halothane, is not protective in preventing the edema that follows temporary brain ischemia (93). Scheller et al (93) found that unlike halothane, isoflurane does not prevent increases in ICP due to cerebral edema produced by brain injury induced with a cold probe.

Although the effect of volatile anesthetics on cerebral autoregulation has been emphasized as an important aspect of their use with enflurane and isoflurane, the emphasis properly should be placed on achieving and maintaining a stable level of CBF at a specific CPP. In Figure 23.1, the effects of increasing concentrations of isoflurane on autoregulation are shown as CPP is altered by hemorrhage or increased ICP. Whereas 2.8% isoflurane completely abolishes autoregulation, autoregulation is intact at 1.4%. At all levels of CPP below 90 mm Hg, oxygen delivery to the brain with 2.8% isoflurane is greater than or equal to that with 1.4% isoflurane.

VASOACTIVE AGENTS

Nitroprusside and Nitroglycerin

Vasoactive agents, both vasodilators and vasoconstrictors, are frequently used to regulate MABP during anesthesia to optimize CPP. Blood pressure control can be accomplished by increasing doses of anesthetic, as all anesthetics decrease blood pressure when given in sufficiently high doses, or by use of vasoactive agents. After a surgical level of anesthesia is achieved, increasing the additional anesthesia dose to control blood pressure may be undesir-

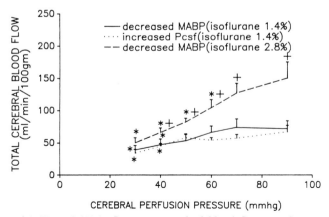

Figure 23.1. Effects of 1.4% or 2.8% isoflurane on cerebral blood flow are shown as cerebral perfusion pressure was decreased by hemorrhage ($n=6$), intracranial hypertension ($n=6$), or increased cerebral spinal fluid pressure (Pcsf; $n=6$). $^*=p<.05$ compared to flow at cerebral perfusion pressure of 90 mm Hg; $+=p<.05$ compared to 1.4% isoflurane; MABP = mean arterial blood pressure. (From McPherson RW, Traystman RJ: Effects of isoflurane on cerebral autoregulation in dogs. *Anesthesiology* 69:493–499, 1988.

able in neurosurgical patients because it may retard their awakening after surgery.

Nitroprusside causes an initial cerebral hyperemia as MABP is reduced from control values to about 65 mm Hg; at lower levels CBF decreases. In patients, this produces an initial increase in ICP with a small depression in MABP followed by a decrease in ICP (109). This hyperemia and an associated increase in CBV may increase the risk of brain herniation. During nitroprusside-induced hypotension, autoregulation is abolished (26, 41). When hypertension follows nitroprusside-induced hypotension, ICP is increased as a result of the residual direct vasodilatory effect of nitroprusside (103) (Fig 23.2). Simultaneous administration of nitroprusside and neosynephrine has been suggested for treating vasospasm, but this drug combination does not increase CBF in the presence of cerebral vasospasm (90).

Nitroglycerin is also used to produce intraoperative hypotension, particularly because the associated coronary vasodilation that occurs may prevent myocardial ischemia. Nitroglycerin is less effective than nitroprusside in producing hypotension (120) and produces significant increases in ICP (85), probably owing to increased CBV from venous dilatation. Thus, if a vasodilator must be used, nitroprusside is more desirable then nitroglycerin. However, in the spontaneous hypertensive rat, nitroprusside causes a decrease in CBF and

$CMRO_2$, with only moderate hypotension, whereas nitroglycerin decreases CBF slightly less and maintains $CMRO_2$ better (39, 40). This difference suggests that nitroprusside might be less desirable for use in the chronically hypertensive patient.

Longer-acting intravenous agents, such as trimethaphan and hydralazine, are alternative drugs to control CPP that do not allow precise minute-to-minute titration of MABP, but do allow a stable decrease in CPP for long periods of time. Michenfelder and Theye (62) found that trimethaphan decreases CBF more than nitroprusside does at a MABP of 50 mm Hg and results in cerebral metabolic alterations. Trimethaphan decreases CBF as MABP falls, although $CMRO_2$ is maintained, whereas nitroprusside does not decrease CBF at the same level of MABP (98). Metabolic derangement as a result of trimethaphan hypotension is partially blocked by the metabolic depression that results from administering high levels of anesthetic gases (47). In the rat, hydralazine maintains CBF as MABP is decreased from 138 mm Hg to 50 mm Hg (7). Hydralazine increases CBF by about 22% in normal humans without a change in MABP (94).

Exogenous vasopressors do not appear to alter CBF directly. However, this does not mean that vasopressor administration does not affect CBF and ICP. Subcutaneous local anesthesia blunts the hemodynamic response to scalp incision. Epi-

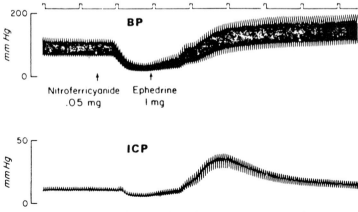

Figure 23.2. Effects of nitroferricyanide followed by ephedrine on intracranial pressure (ICP) and arterial blood pressure. Time = 1 tick/minute. BP = blood pressure. (From Stullken EH, Sokoll MD: Intracranial pressure during hypotension and subsequent vasopressor therapy in anesthetized cats. *Anesthesiology* 42:425–431, 1975.)

nephrine may be safely combined with local anesthesia to reduce scalp blood loss. Rapid absorption of epinephrine may unmask the β-adrenergic effects of epinephrine (hypotension, increased cardiac output, and increased $PaCO_2$) which may injure the brain by decreasing MABP at a time when ICP is increased by elevated $PaCO_2$. During halothane anesthesia in dogs, phenylephrine does not alter CBF (16).

Phenylephrine is useful in increasing MABP and increasing CBF in patients who have cerebral vasospasm following subarachnoid hemorrhage, possibly associated with regional impairment of autoregulation. In one study, phenylephrine increased CBF by about 50% and was associated with improvement of neurologic function (70). Hypertension therapy effectively treats cerebral vasospasm in approximately 70% of patients after subarachnoid hemorrhage (45). Vasoactive agents appear to produce major effects on CBF and metabolism by their hemodynamic effects rather than their direct cerebral effects.

Other Intravenous Drugs

Benzodiazepines

Diazepam has been used for its long-lasting effect in reducing anxiety and to produce perioperative amnesia. In the elderly, the sedative effect may be prolonged (44). Thus, diazepam is best avoided because of the possibility of prolonged postoperative somnolence or disorientation. Diazepam decreases $CMRO_2$ by 21% and CBF by 15%; this effect is reversed by a specific benzodiazepine antagonist, Ro15-1788 (Hoffman-LaRoche, Inc., Nutley, NJ) (82). Survival following cerebral ischemia in hyperglycemic rats is enhanced by either pentobarbital or diazepam (97). Midazolam (0.15 mg/kg bolus intravenously) decreases CBF by 35%. Midazolam is a much shorter-acting benzodiazepine and increases cerebral vascular resistance by 40%, with a slight decrease in MABP (28). The specific antagonist, Ro15-1788, reverses effects of midazolam on both CBF and $CMRO_2$ (27).

Lidocaine

Lidocaine (1.5 mg/kg bolus intravenously) has been used to treat intracranial hypertension in response to surgical stimulation. Bedford et al (9) found that this dose of lidocaine decreased ICP by 16 mm Hg without a decrease in MABP. In similar circumstances, thiopental (3 mg/kg bolus intravenously) decreased ICP to a similar degree, but decreased MABP by 26 mm Hg, thus producing a lower CPP

A specific cellular protective effect has been reported for lidocaine due to membrane stabilization in high doses (160 mg/kg; supraseizure dose) (5), which also induce cardiac arrest requiring cardiopulmonary bypass. This potentially protective effect is due to reduction of cellular energy metabolism normally required to support sodium–potassium pump activity that appears to occur in addition to the reduction of $CMRO_2$ associated with induction of severe hypothermia (4, 5). Recent animal studies suggest that lidocaine in doses that are tolerated without cardiac effects offers minimal cerebral protection. Warner et al (116) found that nontoxic doses of lidocaine have no effect on postischemic brain injury. Milde and Milde (63) found that lidocaine (15 mg/kg) had little effect on $CMRO_2$ or CBF when administered together with 3% isoflurane. Lidocaine in doses sufficient to produce an isoelectric EEG is not protective in focal ischemia, even when given before injury (96). However, Evans and Kobrine (25) found that lidocaine blunts the intracranial hypertension response to embolic injury and may be useful in reducing intracranial hypertension.

FLUID MANAGEMENT

Fluid management in patients at risk of neurologic injury is regulated to maintain hemodynamic stability while maintaining cerebral dehydration. Although Ringer's lactate solution with dextrose is the most commonly used intraoperative fluid, it is inappropriate for patients at risk of ischemic neurologic injury for several reasons.

First, use of diuretics (e.g. mannitol, furosemide) causes a loss of potassium ions that must be replaced. Second, administration of glucose aggravates the hyperglycemia produced by the normal stress response to surgery.

Systemic dehydration appears to be effective in producing brain dehydration, and diuresis is frequently used in patients at risk of cerebral ischemia from increased ICP. Both osmotic and loop diuretics may be used to dehydrate the brain. However, mannitol draws water into the vascular system and may lead to vascular overload, a paradoxical increase in ICP, and congestive heart failure if the rate of intravascular water entry is higher than the rate of renal water loss. Roberts et al (83) found that mannitol decreases ICP in a dose-dependent manner (83) but that it also may increase CBV by as much as 25%. Thus, ICP will decrease only after the dehydration effect has counteracted the increase in brain bulk caused by the initial increase in CBV (81). An intravenous infusion administered slowly over a period of 15 to 30 minutes will provide rapid onset of diuresis without causing an increase in ICP due to increased CBV which may be produced if the mannitol is given rapidly as a bolus. Intraoperatively, the mannitol infusion is begun with the surgical incision so that peak diuresis will have occurred by the time of dural incision (usually 45 minutes later). Furosemide can provide a reduction in ICP similar to that produced by mannitol without the risk of congestive heart failure (118).

Furosemide acts directly on the kidney by increasing free water loss, with a resulting increase in serum osmolarity that decreases brain water due to the increased osmotic gradient. Furosemide may also decrease ICP by decreasing CSF production in the choroid plexus (79). Mannitol combined with furosemide (0.7 mg/kg) causes a greater and longer fall in ICP than does mannitol alone. This fall of ICP correlates well with an increase in osmotic gradient (79). Furosemide alone is useful in decreasing the ICP in patients with head injury (18), but in the presence of large areas of brain injury furosemide may be insufficiently effective to normalize ICP (30).

Warner and Boehland (114) found that postischemic cerebral edema developed to a similar extent whether the blood lost was replaced by saline, hetastarch, or blood (all iso-osmolar). Zornow et al (121) found that a decrease in osmolality of 5% acted to increase cortical water content whereas a 65% reduction in oncotic pressure (from 20 mm Hg to 7 mm Hg) produced no change in cortical water content.

For many years, solutions containing glucose were used routinely in managing patients under anesthesia. However, recent evidence suggests that the hyperglycemia produced by glucose-containing solutions may be detrimental to the ischemic brain (117). Surgical stress can result in hyperglycemia, the degree of which is modulated by the type of anesthesia. Thus, the choice of anesthesia may modulate the degree of ischemic injury based on the resulting serum glucose level. For example, high-dose fentanyl anesthesia greatly blunts the hormonal response to surgical stress (36, 48). Warner et al (117) found that hyperglycemia contributes to the increase in water content and seizure activity following cerebral ischemia.

It is extremely difficult to compare the hyperglycemic response to surgery that occurs with various anesthetics. However, studies in animals have shown that halothane causes hyperglycemia and decreases serum insulin, pentobarbital decreases insulin and causes a slight increase in glucose, and ketamine has little effect on serum glucose (6). Lanier et al (51) found, in a model of global ischemia, that the degree of neurologic injury was correlated with the blood glucose levels, even when the blood glucose was less than 250 mg/dl. Thus, an anesthetic that minimizes the surgical stress response should be used. In addition, strict control of blood glucose levels if necessary with insulin administration should be considered.

PERSPECTIVE

The optimal anesthetic for patients at risk of ischemic neurologic injury should minimize the hemodynamic abnormalities

Table 23.1.   Optimal Anesthetic Technique

Premedication	None; or avoid long-acting agents
Anesthesia induction	Short-acting barbiturate, etomidate, fentanyl
Neuromuscular blockade	Avoid succinylcholine if denervation exists
Anesthetic maintenance	Barbiturates; synthetic narcotics; low-dose isoflurane; ± nitrous oxide
Vasoactive drugs	Avoid nitroglycerin; maintenance of cerebral perfusion pressure is more important than direct drug effects

that impair oxygen delivery to the brain. We feel that this is generally best accomplished by narcotic-based anesthesia supplemented with low-dose volatile anesthesia (isoflurane). We also carefully titrate osmotic diuretics and vasopressors to preserve a normal CPP (Table 23.1). Although experienced anesthesiologists can safely use other agents, we feel that the versatility of this anesthetic technique, particularly in hemodynamically compromised patients, makes it the preferable alternative.

References

1. Adams HP, Olinger CP, Barsan WG, et al: A dose-escalation study of large doses of naloxone for treatment of patients with acute cerebral ischemia. *Stroke* 17:404–409, 1986.
2. Albrecht RF, Miletich DJ, Madala LR: Normalization of cerebral blood flow during prolonged halothane anesthesia. *Anesthesiology* 58:26–31, 1983.
3. Apuzzo MLJ, Weiss MH, Kurze T, et al: Influence of histamine on intracranial dynamics in dogs. *Surg Forum* 25:447–449, 1974.
4. Astrup J, Skovsted P, Gjerris F, et al: Increase in extracellular potassium in the brain during circulatory arrest: Effects of hypothermia, lidocaine, and thiopental. *Anesthesiology* 55:256–262, 1981.
5. Astrup J, Srensen OM, Srensen HR: Inhibition of cerebral oxygen and glucose consumption in the dog by hypothermia, pentobarbital, and lidocaine. *Anesthesiology* 55:263–268, 1981.
6. Aynsley-Green A, Biebuyck JF, Alberti KG: Anaesthesia and insulin secretion: The effects of diethyl ether, halothane, pentobarbitone sodium and ketamine hydrochloride on intravenous glucose tolerance and insulin secretion in the rat. *Diabetologia* 9:274–281, 1973.
7. Barry DI, Strandgaard S, Graham DI, et al: Cerebral blood flow during dihydralazine-induced hypotension in hypertensive rats. *Stroke* 15:102–108, 1984.
8. Batjer HH, Frankfurt AI, Purdy PD, et al: Use of etomidate, temporary arterial occlusion and intraoperative angiography in surgical treatment of large and giant cerebral aneurysms. *J Neurosurg* 68:234–240, 1988.
9. Bedford RF, Persing JA, Pobereskin L, et al: Lidocaine or thiopental for rapid control of intracranial hypertension? *Anesth Analg* 59:435–437, 1980.
10. Bell BA, Miller JD, Neto NG, et al: Effect of naloxone on deficits after aneurysmal subarachnoid hemorrhage. *Neurosurgery* 16:498–501, 1985.
11. Boarini DJ, Kassell NF, Coester HC, et al: Comparison of systemic and cerebrovascular effects of isoflurane and halothane. *Neurosurgery* 15:400–409, 1984.
12. Brain Resuscitation Clinical Trial I Study Group: Randomized clinical study of thiopental loading in comatose survivors of cardiac arrest. *N Engl J Med* 314:397–403, 1986.
13. Burchiel KH, Stockard JJ, Calverley RK, et al: Relationship to pre- and postanesthetic EEG abnormalities to enflurane-induced seizure activity. *Anesth Analg* 56:509–514, 1977.
14. Carlsson C, Smith DS, Keykhah M, et al: The effects of high dose fentanyl on cerebral circulation and metabolism in rats. *Anesthesiology* 57:375–380, 1982.
15. Chen CT, Toung TJK, Donham RT, et al: Fentanyl dosage of suppression of circulatory response to laryngoscopy and endotracheal intubation. *Anesth Rev* 13:37–42, 1986.
16. Chikovani O, Corkill G, McLeish I, et al: Effect on canine cerebral blood flow of two common pressor agents during prolonged halothane anesthesia. *Surg Neurol* 9:211–213, 1978.
17. Cottrell JE, Hartung J, Griffin JP, et al: Intracranial and hemodynamic changes after succinylcholine administration in cats. *Anesth Analg* 62:1006–1009, 1983.
18. Cottrell JE, Marlin AE: Furosemide and human head injury. *J Trauma* 21:805–806, 1981.
19. Cummings MF, Russell WJ, Frewin DB, et al: The effects of suxamethonium and D-tubocurarine on the pressor and plasma catecholamine responses to tracheal intubation. *Anaesth Intensive Care* 11:103–106, 1983.
20. Curran J, Crowley M, O'Sullivan G: Droperidol and endotracheal intubation. Attenuation of pressor response to laryngoscopy and intubation. *Anaesthesia* 35:290–294, 1980.
21. Dempsey RJ, Roy MW, Meyer KL, et al: Indomethacin-mediated improvement following middle cerebral artery occlusion in cats. Effects of anesthesia. *J Neurosurg* 62:874–881, 1985.
22. Drummond JC, Todd MM, Toutant SM, et al: Brain surface protrusion during enflurane, halothane, and isoflurane anesthesia in cats. *Anesthesiology* 59:288–293, 1983.
23. Dworacek B, De Vlieger M: Absence of electroencephalographic excitation pattern under isoflurane anesthesia. *Acta Anaesthesiol Belg* 35:211–217, 1984.
24. Estanol B, Aguilar F, Corona T: Diagnosis of

reversible versus irreversible cerebral ischemia by the intravenous administration of naloxone. *Stroke* 16:1006–1009, 1985.

25. Evans DE, Kobrine AI: Reduction of experimental intracranial hypertension by lidocaine. *Neurosurgery* 20:542–547, 1987.

26. Fitch W, Pickard JD, Digraham DI: Effects of hypotension induced with sodium nitroprusside on the cerebral circulation before, and one week after, the subarachnoid injection of blood. *J Neurol Neurosurg Psychiatry* 51:88–93, 1988.

27. Fleischer JE, Milde JH, Moyer TP, et al: Cerebral effects of high-dose midazolam and subsequent reversal with Ro 15-1788 in dogs. *Anesthesiology* 68:234–242, 1988.

28. Forster A, Juge O, Morel D: Effects of midazolam on cerebral blood flow in human volunteers. *Anesthesiology* 56:453–455, 1982.

29. Fragen RJ, Shanks CA, Molteni A, et al: Effects of etomidate on hormonal responses to surgical stress. *Anesthesiology* 61:652–656, 1984.

30. Gaab M, Knoblich OE, Schupp J, et al: Effect of furosemide (lasix) on acute severe experimental cerebral edema. *J Neurol* 220:185–197, 1979.

31. Hallmayer J, Hossmann KA, Miles G: Low dose of barbiturates for prevention of hippocampal lesions after brief ischemic episodes. *Acta Neuropathol (Berl)* 68:27–31, 1985.

32. Hamilton AJ, Black PM, Carr DB: Contrasting actions of naloxone in experimental spinal cord trauma and cerebral ischemia: A review. *Neurosurgery* 17:845–849, 1985.

33. Hart R, Hindman B: Mechanisms of perioperative cerebral infarction. *Stroke* 13:766–773, 1982.

34. Hennis PJ, Fahey MR, Canfell PC, et al: Pharmacology of laudanosine in dogs. *Anesthesiology* 65:56–60, 1986.

35. Hermans C, Fransen JF, Wauquier A: Survival and neurological outcome of the mongolian gerbil with or without bilateral carotid ligation after treatment with ether, thiopental or etomidate. *Arch Int Pharmacodyn Ther* 263:314–316, 1983.

36. Hicks HC, Mowbray AG, Yhap EO: Cardiovascular effects of and catecholamine responses to high dose fentanyl-O2 for induction of anesthesia in patients with ischemic coronary artery disease. *Anesth Analg* 60:563–568, 1981.

37. Hillered L, Ernster L: Respiratory activity of isolated rat brain mitochondria following in vitro exposure to oxygen radicals *J Cereb Blood Flow Metab* 3:207–214, 1983.

38. Hindman BJ: Perioperative stroke: The noncardiac surgery patient. *Int Anesthesiol Clin* 24:101–134, 1986.

39. Hoffman WE, Miletich DJ, Albrecht RF: Maintenance of cerebral blood flow and metabolism during pharmacological hypotension in aged hypertensive rats. *Neurobiol Aging* 3:101–104, 1982.

40. Hoffman WE, Miletich DJ, Albrecht RF: The influence of antihypertensive therapy on cerebral autoregulation in aged hypertensive rats. *Stroke* 13:701–704, 1982.

41. Ivankovich AD, Miletich DJ, Albrecht RF, et al: Sodium nitroprusside and cerebral blood flow in the anesthetized and unanesthetized goat. *Anesthesiology* 44:21–26, 1976.

42. Jobes DR, Kennell E, Bitner R, et al: Effects of morphine-nitrous oxide anesthesia on cerebral autoregulation. *Anesthesiology* 42:30–34, 1975.

43. John DA, Tobey RE, Homer LD, et al: Onset of succinylcholine induced hyperkalemia following denervation. *Anesthesiology* 45:294–299, 1976.

44. Kanto J, Maenpaa M, Mantyla R, et al: Effect of age on the pharmacokinetics of diazepam given in conjunction with spinal anesthesia. *Anesthesiology* 51:154–159, 1979.

45. Kassell NF, Peerless SJ, Durward QJ, et al: Treatment of ischemic deficits from vasospasm with intravascular volume expansion and induced arterial hypertension. *Neurosurgery* 11:337–343, 1982.

46. Keykhah MM, Smith DS, Carlsson C, et al: Influence of sufentanil on cerebral metabolism and circulation in the rat. *Anesthesiology* 63:274–277, 1985.

47. Keykhah MM, Welsh FA, Harp JR: Cerebral energy levels during trimethaphan-induced hypotension in the rat: Effects of light versus deep halothane anesthesia. *Anesthesiology* 50:36–39, 1979.

48. Kono K, Philbin DM, Coggins CH, et al: Renal function and stress response during halothane or fentanyl anesthesia. *Anesth Analg* 60:552–556, 1981.

49. Kruczek M, Albin MS, Wolf S, et al: Postoperative seizure activity following enflurane anesthesia. *Anesthesiology* 53:175–176, 1980.

50. Lanier WL, Milde JH, Michenfelder JD: Cerebral stimulation following succinycholine in dogs. *Anesthesiology* 64:551–559, 1986.

51. Lanier WI, Stangland KJ, Scheithauer BW, et al: The effects of dextrose infusion and head position on neurologic outcome after complete cerebral ischemia in primates: Examination of a model. *Anesthesiology* 66:39–48, 1987.

52. Liu PL, Gatt S, Gugino LD, et al: Esmolal for control of increases in heart rate and blood pressure during tracheal intubation after thiopentone and succinylcholine. *Can Anaesth Soc J* 33:556–562, 1986.

53. Lundar T, Lindegaard KF, Refsum L, et al: Cerebrovascular effects of isoflurane in man. Intracranial pressure and middle cerebral artery flow velocity. *Br J Anaesth* 59:1208–1213, 1987.

54. McLeskey CH, Cullen BF, Kennedy RD, et al: Control of cerebral perfusion pressure during induction of anesthesia in high-risk neurological patients. *Anesth Analg* 53:985–992, 1974.

55. McPherson RW, Eimerl D, Traystman RJ: Interaction of hypoxia and hypercapnia on cerebral hemodynamics and brain electrical activity in dogs. *Am J Physiol* 253(Part 2):H890–H897, 1987.

56. McPherson RW, Krempasanka E, Eimerl D, et al: Effects of alfentanil on cerebral vascular reactivity in dogs. *Br J Anaesth* 57:1232–1238, 1985.

57. McPherson RW, Traystman RJ: Fentanyl and cerebral vascular responsivity in dogs. *Anesthesiology* 60:180–186, 1984.

58. McPherson RW, Traystman RJ: Effects of isoflurane on cerebral autoregulation in dogs. *Anesthesiology* 69:493–499, 1988.

59. Michenfelder JD: The interdependency of cerebral functional and metabolic effects following

massive doses of thiopental in the dog. *Anesthesiology* 41:231–236, 1974.

60. Michenfelder JD, Sundt TM, Fode N, et al: Isoflurane when compared to enflurane and halothane decreases the frequency of cerebral ischemia during carotid endarterectomy. *Anesthesiology* 67:336–340, 1987.

61. Michenfelder JD, Theye RA: Cerebral protection by thiopental during hypoxia. *Anesthesiology* 39:510–517, 1973.

62. Michenfelder JD, Theye RA: Canine systemic and cerebral effects of hypotension induced by hemorrhage, trimethaphan, halothane, or nitroprusside. *Anesthesiology* 45:188–195, 1977.

63. Milde LN, Milde JH: The detrimental effect of lidocaine on cerebral metabolism measured in dogs anesthetized with isoflurane. *Anesthesiology* 67:180–184, 1987.

64. Milde LN, Milde JH, Michenfelder JD: Cerebral functional metabolic and hemodynamic effects of etomidate in dogs. *Anesthesiology* 63:371–377, 1985.

65. Miletich DJ, Ivankovich AD, Albrecht RF, et al: Absence of autoregulation of cerebral blood flow during halothane and enflurane anesthesia. *Anesth Analg* 55:100–109, 1976.

66. Minton MD, Grosslight K, Stirt JA, et al: Increases in intracranial pressure from succinylcholine: Prevention by prior nondepolarizing blockade. *Anesthesiology* 65:165–169, 1986.

67. Minton MD, Stirt JA, Bedford RF: Serum potassium following succinylcholine in patients with brain tumors. *Can Anaesth Soc J* 33:328–331, 1986.

68. Monsalve F, Rucabado L, Ruano M, et al: The neurologic effects of thiopental therapy after cardiac arrest. *Intensive Care Med* 13:244–248, 1987.

69. Moss E, Dearden NM, McDowall DG: Effects of 2% enflurane on intracranial pressure and cerebral perfusion pressure. *Br J Anaesth* 55:1083–1088, 1983.

70. Muizelaar JP, Becker DP: Induced hypertension for the treatment of cerebral ischemia after subarachnoid hemorrhage. Direct effect on cerebral blood flow. *Surg Neurol* 25:317–325, 1986.

71. Nehls DG, Todd MM, Spetzler RF, et al: A comparison of the cerebral protective effects of isoflurane and barbiturates during temporary focal ischemia in primates. *Anesthesiology* 66:453–464, 1987.

72. Nemoto EM, Shiu GK, Nemmer J, et al: Attenuation of brain free fatty acid liberation during global ischemia: A model for screening potential therapies for efficacy? *J Cereb Blood Flow Metab* 2:475–480, 1982.

73. Newberg LA, Michenfelder JD: Cerebral protection by isoflurane during hypoxemia or ischemia. *Anesthesiology* 59:29–35, 1983.

74. Nussmeier NA, Arlund C, Slogoff S: Neuropsychiatric complications after cardiopulmonary bypass: Cerebral protection by a barbiturate. *Anesthesiology* 64:165–170, 1986.

75. Ohm WW, Cullen BF, Amory DW, et al: Delayed seizure activity following enflurane anesthesia. *Anesthesiology* 42:367–368, 1976.

76. Ozyurt E, Graham DI, Woodruff GN, et al: Protective effect of the glutamate antagonist, MK-801 in focal cerebral ischemia in the cat. *J Cereb Blood Flow Metab* 8:138–143, 1988.

77. Pelligrino DA, Miletich DJ, Hoffman WE, et al: Nitrous oxide markedly increases cerebral cortical metabolic rate and blood flow in the goat. *Anesthesiology* 60:405–412, 1984.

78. Pickard JD, Matheson M, Patterson J, et al: Prediction of late ischemic complications after cerebral aneurysm surgery: The intraoperative measurement of cerebral blood flow. *J Neurosurg* 53:305–308, 1980.

79. Pollay M, Fullenwider C, Roberts PA, et al: Effect of mannitol and furosemide on blood brain osmotic gradient and intracranial pressure. *J Neurosurg* 59:945–950, 1983.

80. Pyrs-Roberts C, Greene LT, Meloche R, et al: Studies of anaesthesia in relation to hypertension. II. Haemodynamic consequences of induction and endotracheal intubation. *Br J Anaesth* 43:531–547, 1971.

81. Ravussin P, Archer DP, Meyer E, et al: The effects of rapid infusions of saline and mannitol on cerebral blood volume and intracranial pressure in dogs. *Can Anaesth Soc J* 32:506–515, 1985.

82. Roald OK, Steen PA, Milde JH: Reversal of the cerebral effects of diazepam in the dog by benzodiazepine antagonist Ro15-1788. *Acta Anaesthesiol Scand* 30:341–345, 1986.

83. Roberts PA, Pollay M, Engles C, et al: Effect on intracranial pressure of furosemide combined with varying doses and administration rates of mannitol. *J Neurosurg* 66:440–446, 1987.

84. Roelofse JA, Shipton EA, Joubert JJ, et al: A comparison of labetalol, acebutolol, and lidocaine for controlling the cardiovascular responses to endotracheal intubation for oral surgical procedures. *J Oral Maxillofac Surg* 45:835–840, 1987.

85. Rogers MC, Hamburger C, Owen K, et al: Intracranial pressure in the cat during nitroglycerin-induced hypotension. *Anesthesiology* 51:227–229, 1979.

86. Roizen MF, Horrigan RW, Frazer BM: Anesthetic doses blocking adrenergic (stress) and cardiovascular responses to incision—MAC BAR. *Anesthesiology* 54:390–398, 1981.

87. Rosa G, Orfei P, Sanfilippo M, et al: The effects of atracurium besylate (Tracrium) on intracranial pressure and cerebral perfusion pressure. *Anesth Analg* 65:381–384, 1986.

88. Rosen I, Soderberg M: Electroencephalographic activity in children under enflurane anesthesia. *Acta Anesthesiol Scand* 19:361–369, 1975.

89. Rosenberg H, Clofine R, Bialik O: Neurologic changes during awakening from anesthesia. *Anesthesiology* 54:125–130, 1981.

90. Rothberg CS, Weir B, Overton TR: Treatment of subarachnoid hemorrhage with sodium nitroprusside and phenylephrine: An experimental study. *Neurosurgery* 5:588–595, 1979.

91. Sakabe T, Kuramoto T, Kumagae S, et al: Cerebral responses to the addition of nitrous oxide to halothane in man. *Br J Anaesth* 48:957–962, 1976.

92. Sandor P, Gotoh F, Tomita M, et al: Effects of stable enkephalin analogue, (D-Met2, Pro5)-enkephalinamide, and naloxone on cortical blood flow and cerebral blood volume in experimental

brain ischemia in anesthetized cats. *J Cereb Blood Flow Metab* 6:553–558, 1986.

93. Scheller MS, Todd MM, Drummond JC, et al: The intracranial pressure effects of isoflurane and halothane administered following cryogenic brain injury in rabbits. *Anesthesiology* 67:507–512, 1987.

94. Schroeder T, Sillesen H: Dihydralazine induces marked cerebral vasodilation in man. *Eur J Clin Invest* 17:214–217, 1987.

95. Schwedler M, Miletich DJ, Albrecht RF: Cerebral blood flow and metabolism following ketamine administration. *Can Anaesth Soc J* 29:222–226, 1982.

96. Shokunbi MT, Gelb AW, Peerless SJ: An evaluation of the effect of lidocaine in experimental focal cerebral ischemia. *Stroke* 17:962–966, 1986.

97. Siemkowicz E: Improvement of restitution from cerebral ischemia in hyperglycemic rats by pentobarbital or diazepam. *Acta Neurol Scand* 61:368–376, 1980.

98. Sivarajan M, Amory DW, McKenzie SM: Regional blood flows during induced hypotension produced by nitroprusside or trimethaphan in the rhesus monkey. *Anesth Analg* 64:759–766, 1985.

99. Smith AL, Hoff JT, Nielsen SI, et al: Barbiturate protection in acute focal cerebral ischemia. *Stroke* 5:1–7, 1974.

100. Steen PA, Newberg L, Milde JH, et al: Hypothermia and barbiturates: Individual and combined effects on canine cerebral oxygen consumption. *Anesthesiology* 58:527–532, 1983.

101. Stefansson T, Wickstrom I, Haljamae H: Hemodynamic and metabolic effects of ketamine anesthesia in the geriatric patient. *Acta Anesth Scand* 26:371–377, 1982.

102. Stullken EH Jr, Sokoll MD: Anesthesia and subarachnoid intracranial pressure. *Anesth Analg* 54:494–500, 1975.

103. Stullken EH Jr, Sokoll MD: Intracranial pressure during hypotension and subsequent vasopressor therapy in anesthetized cats. *Anesthesiology* 42:425–431, 1975.

104. Tang AH: Protection from cerebral ischemia by U-50,488E, a specific kappa opioid analgesic agent. *Life Sci* 37:1475–1482, 1985.

105. Todd MM: The effects of $PaCO_2$ on the cerebrovascular response to nitrous oxide in the halothane-anesthetized rabbit. *Anesth Analg* 66:1090–1095, 1987.

106. Todd MM, Drummond JC: A comparison of the cerebrovascular and metabolic effects of halothane and isoflurane in the cat. *Anesthesiology* 60:276–282, 1984.

107. Todd MM, Drummond JC, U HS: The hemodynamic consequences of high-dose metho-

hexital anesthesia in humans. *Anesthesiology* 61:495–501, 1984.

108. Todd MM, Drummond JC, U HS: The hemodynamic consequences of high-dose thiopental anesthesia. *Anesth Analg* 64:681–687, 1985.

109. Turner JM, Powell D, Gibson RM, et al: Intracranial pressure changes in neurosurgical patients during hypotension induced with sodium nitroprusside or trimethaphan. *Br J Anaesth* 49:419–425, 1977.

110. Unni VK, Johnston RA, Young HS, et al: Prevention of intracranial hypertension during laryngoscopy and endotracheal intubation. Use of a second dose of thiopentone. *Br J Anaesth* 56:1219–1223, 1984.

111. Venables GS, Strong AJ, Miller SA, et al: The effects of etomidate in the cat middle cerebral artery occlusion model of brain ischaemia. *Neurol Res* 8:209–213, 1986.

112. Walsh ES, Paterson JL, Oriordan JB, et al: Effect of high dose fentanyl anaesthesia on the metabolic and endocrine response to cardiac surgery. *Br J Anaesth* 53:1155–1165, 1981.

113. Warner DS, Boarini DJ, Kassell NF: Cerebrovascular adaptation to prolonged halothane anesthesia is not related to cerebrospinal fluid pH *Anesthesiology* 63:243–248, 1985.

114. Warner DS, Boehland LA: Effects of iso-osmolal intravenous fluid therapy on post-ischemic brain water content in the rat. *Anesthesiology* 68:86–91, 1988.

115. Warner DS, Deshpande JK, Wieloch T: The effect of isoflurane on neuronal necrosis following near-complete forebrain ischemia in the rat. *Anesthesiology* 64:19–23, 1986.

116. Warner DS, Godersky JC, Smith ML: Failure of pre-ischemic lidocaine administration to ameliorate global ischemic brain damage in the rat. *Anesthesiology* 68:73–78, 1988.

117. Warner DS, Smith ML, Siesjö BK: Ischemia in normo- and hyperglycemic rats: Effects on brain water and electrolytes. *Stroke* 18:464–471, 1987.

118. Wauquier A, Ashton D, Clincke G, et al: Antihypoxic effects of etomidate, thiopental and methohexital. *Arch Int Pharmacodyn Ther* 249:330–334, 1981.

119. Wieloch T: Neurochemical correlates to selective neuronal vulnerability. *Prog Brain Res* 63:69–85, 1985.

120. Yaster M, Simmons RS, Tolo VT, et al: A comparison of nitroglycerin and nitroprusside for inducing hypotension in children: A double-blind study. *Anesthesiology* 65:175–179, 1986.

121. Zornow MH, Todd MM, Moore SS: The acute cerebral effects of changes in plasma osmolality and oncotic pressure. *Anesthesiology* 67:936–941, 1987.

CHAPTER TWENTY-FOUR

Barbiturate Therapy for Brain Protection During Temporary Vascular Occlusion

Robert F. Spetzler, M.D.
Mark N. Hadley, M.D.
Peter A. Raudzens, M.D.

Cerebral ischemia during temporary vascular occlusion may cause irreversible postoperative neurologic sequelae. The temporary interruption of nutrient blood supply to the brain stem or hemispheres during neurosurgical vascular procedures may result in a profound reduction in cerebral blood flow (CBF). Clinical series and laboratory studies imply that focal reductions in CBF to 10 to 20 ml/100 g/minute cannot be tolerated for more than a few minutes and may result in significant cerebral tissue injury and infarction in a large number of cases (3, 10, 13, 14, 17, 21, 24, 30, 32, 33, 36).

Several management strategies have been suggested to combat focal cerebral ischemia during temporary vascular occlusion, including induced hypertension, vascular shunting, and the administration of barbiturates. Although each method has potential merits, all but the administration of barbiturates have significant liabilities (13, 14, 29). To date, the most commonly used and most extensively evaluated method for pharmacologic protection against temporary intraoperative ischemic brain injury is deep barbiturate anesthesia. To provide maximum cerebral protection with the least treatment risk, we advocate the administration of barbiturates before and during operative procedures that may require temporary occlusion of cerebral vascular channels.

A single pharmacologic agent that can be administered to protect the brain from ischemia during neurosurgical vascular procedures offers attractive benefits. It allows cross-clamping of vessels and permits precise, unhurried placement of an aneurysm clip or arterial anastomosis, reconstruction, or endarterectomy. It also obviates the need for induced hypertension with its attendant risks of intracerebral hemorrhage and perioperative myocardial infarction, which are particularly problematic in patients with severe atherosclerosis, prior cerebral infarction, or coronary artery disease. Vascular shunting, which is practical only during the reconstruction of large vessels or endarterectomy, and the attendant risks of intimal injury, air embolization during shunt insertion, and intraoperative embolization of atherosclerotic debris through the shunt are avoided as well.

Adjuvant procedures to improve CBF or to protect the brain from low-flow states appear to be necessary only when regional CBF drops into the range of 10 to 20 ml/100 g of tissue per minute (3, 10, 13, 14, 32, 33). (Fig. 24.1). The ability of central nervous system (CNS) tissues to tolerate this degree of ischemia is variable and time dependent (10, 13, 33; see also Chapter 1, this volume). Under such circumstances, barbiturates may be protective because of their ability to reduce the metabolic requirements of neural tissue and extend the tolerance of cerebral tissue for the reduced substrate supply that accompanies ischemia from temporary vascular occlusion (5, 7, 11, 14, 15, 20, 22, 24, 26).

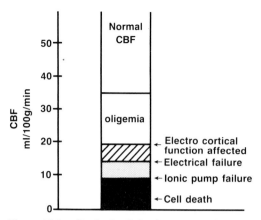

Figure 24.1. Cerebral cellular function is shown in relation to the level of cerebral blood flow (CBF). (From Spetzler RF, Nehls DG: Cerebral protection against ischemia. In Wood JH (ed): *Cerebral Blood Flow: Physiologic and Clinical Aspects*. New York, McGraw-Hill, 1988, pp 651–676. Adapted by permission of the American Heart Association, Inc., from Astrup J, Symon L, Branston NM, et al: Cortical evoked potential and extracellular K^+ and H^+ at critical levels of brain ischemia. *Stroke* 8:51–57, 1977.)

CEREBRAL AND CEREBRAL VASCULAR EFFECTS OF BARBITURATES

The best-known effect of barbiturates on the CNS is a dose-dependent, reversible depression of neurologic function (24). The precise mechanism of this effect is unknown but is thought to involve interference with synaptic transmission, inhibition of neurotransmission, and a direct local anesthetic effect on cellular membrane structures (11, 24–26). Associated with barbiturate depression of cerebral function is a parallel, dose-dependent reduction in cerebral metabolic rate (CMR) and CBF (11, 14, 24–26). These changes in CMR and CBF plateau when the electrical activity of the hemisphere drops to zero, the point at which the electroencephalographic (EEG) activity becomes isoelectric (14, 15, 17, 24, 35, 36). This reversible suppression of cerebral synaptic activity is associated with reductions in the CMR of oxygen and CBF of approximately 50% (15, 17, 24, 36).

The administration of barbiturates in high doses not only reduces CNS metabolic and electrical activity and thus cellular oxygen consumption and requirements, but also directly affects CBF. Shapiro (24) has shown that barbiturate-induced reductions in CBF are accompanied by increases in cerebral vascular resistance and reductions in cerebral blood volume which, in turn, reduce intracranial pressure (ICP). An additional benefit of barbiturates is that they appear to cause nonuniform alterations in local CBF (14, 24, 29). In cases of focal cerebral vascular disease, barbiturate-related increases in vascular resistance in nonischemic areas of the brain appear to cause shunting of CBF into regions of critically reduced CBF (14, 17, 24, 29). The same protective phenomenon is thought to occur during elective temporary vascular occlusion at surgery.

Several other neurochemical mechanisms have been proposed to play contributory roles in barbiturate-induced cerebral protection (8, 11, 14, 16, 21, 24–26), but irrespective of the mechanism(s), barbiturates, specifically thiopental and pentobarbital, clearly have the capacity to modify or prevent cerebral injury from focal ischemia (Table 24.1).

Barbiturate therapy is most effective if the agent is administered before the period of temporary ischemia (20–22, 30). Laboratory experience with a primate model of focal cerebral ischemia has established that preemptive administration of barbiturates provides dramatic cerebral protection even

Table 24.1. Beneficial Effects of Barbiturate Anesthesia

Reduction of cerebral metabolic rate and oxygen consumption
Parallel reduction of cerebral electrical activity (allows monitoring of dose and effects of barbiturate anesthesia)
Reduction of cerebral blood flow
Reduction of cerebral blood volume
Reduction of intracranial pressure
Increased cerebral vascular resistance
Favorable shunt from nonischemic regions to ischemic regions
Potential myocardial protection
Avoidance of induced hypertension, vascular shunting

during 6 hours of middle cerebral artery occlusion (11, 15, 20, 21, 23). These findings have been confirmed by our clinical experience (6, 9, 27–29). The protective effects of barbiturates in cases of temporary global cerebral ischemia due to cardiac arrest are less well established than for focal ischemia. However, recent evidence supports their efficacy when the agent is administered before cardiopulmonary bypass which most often results in focal postoperative ischemic deficits due to cerebral embolization (16, 28). Barbiturates provide less protection when administered after the onset of ischemia, whether focal or global, and they appear to offer no protection—or may be deleterious—if given in conjunction with permanent vascular occlusion (14, 19, 21,–23). The planned periods of temporary ischemia during carotid endarterectomy, arterial bypass, aneurysm clipping and/or aneurysmorrhaphy, and temporary complete cardiopulmonary circulatory arrest appear to be the ideal setting for the application of barbiturate therapy.

The degree of cerebral protection provided by barbiturates far exceeds that provided by other general anesthetic agents. Nehls et al (15) have shown the superiority of barbiturate administration over the use of isoflurane or nitrous-fentanyl anesthesia for cerebral protection in a primate model of temporary focal cerebral ischemia. Although isoflurane caused reductions in cortical electrical activity (EEG suppression) resembling barbiturate effects, isoflurane-treated animals had more strokes of greater magnitude and worse neurologic outcomes than did barbiturate-treated or control animals. Animals randomized to barbiturate therapy had significantly fewer strokes, smaller strokes, and better neurologic outcomes than animals in the other treatment groups.

Barbiturate therapy may also provide unexpected benefits, perhaps playing a role in the avoidance of cardiac complications. We have not encountered symptomatic myocardial ischemia as a perioperative complication in our surgical patients (9, 27, 29). The use of barbiturates obviates the need for induced hypertension during temporary vascular occlusion and may blunt the spontaneous hypertensive response that frequently accompanies vessel clamping and cerebral hypoperfusion, particularly in patients undergoing carotid endarterectomy (29, 32, 33). Barbiturates also reduce cardiac output and through these effects may reduce the myocardial stress associated with surgery. It is also tempting to speculate that barbiturates exert an as yet unidentified direct myocardial protective effect.

Clinical Application of Barbiturates

We advocate the use of cerebral protective doses of barbiturates in all neurosurgical cases that require temporary vascular occlusion of any vessel that provides nutrient flow to CNS structures. In these cases, a patient is given an initial dose of thiopental sodium (3 to 5 mg/kg) with the induction of anesthesia (17, 35, 36). Additional doses of thiopental sodium (50 to 100 mg) are administered intravenously throughout the period of temporary vessel occlusion, titrated to maintain barbiturate-induced EEG burst suppression. Cerebral electrical function is monitored by compressed spectral analysis of the raw EEG data using a two-channel, on-line Neurotrac spectral analyzer (Interspec, Philadelphia, PA) (1, 17, 18, 29, 35, 36).

Barbiturate administration may cause intraoperative hypotension. This has occurred in a few of our patients and can be reversed easily with the judicious use of vasopressors and intravascular volume expansion—the increase of blood volume by administration of intravenous crystalloid or colloid (plasma substitutes) solutions (9, 29). Deep barbiturate anesthesia prolongs the time it takes patients to wake up after surgery and requires that intubation be continued while they are in the recovery room. This effect rarely persists longer than 1 to 2 hours after surgery (9, 27, 29). Despite suppression of reflex activity, brain stem function can still be assessed in a neurologic examination. Most patients respond to the application of painful stimuli; therefore, gross motor movements may be observed.

We have used barbiturate therapy for cerebral protection in more than 400 consecutive carotid endarterectomies performed according to a standardized microsurgical protocol (29). The combined permanent perioperative morbidity and mortality in this series is 1.5%. Before the planned period of temporary vascular occlusion during surgery, all patients were given thiopental until the point of EEG burst suppression. This degree of cerebral protection has been adequate with respect to EEG response for most patients, but approximately 2% of patients will show a profound asymmetry in EEG activity, despite burst suppression, with depression of the ipsilateral hemisphere following occlusion of the carotid artery. These patients are treated with a temporary shunt in addition to barbiturate anesthesia.

We have also used barbiturate anesthesia in 200 patients treated with an extracranial-to-intracranial vascular anastomosis between 1978 and 1988 (6, 9). None of these patients had a perioperative infarction caused by temporary interruption of CBF during the bypass procedure, although such complications are rare (2% to 8%) even with standard anesthetic techniques (34). In the past 10 years, 50 additional patients have had extracranial vertebral artery revascularization procedures that required temporary interruption of the vertebral basilar blood supply (27). All were given barbiturate anesthesia before and during the vascular procedure. No patient had a perioperative stroke in the vertebral basilar distribution.

All intracranial aneurysms we have treated are operated on with the use of barbiturate cerebral protection. Few patients require temporary vessel occlusion to allow accurate placement of the aneurysm clip or thrombectomy and aneurysmorrhaphy; however, all patients benefit from the protective effects of barbiturates, which include a reduction and redistribution of CBF and reduction of ICP (6, 7). Although every effort is made to minimize retraction of cerebral structures during surgery, even the slightest retraction compresses the tissues and compromises local CBF. None of our patients treated for an aneurysm, including approximately 10% of aneurysm patients in whom temporary clipping was used, has had either immediate postoperative ischemic deficits or injury caused by retraction. We attribute this success, in large part, to the use of deep barbiturate anesthesia, although the incidence of ischemic deficits without deep barbiturate anesthesia is unknown.

Barbiturates are also an essential component of our surgical-anesthetic protocol for the treatment of intracranial aneurysms operated on with the patient in a temporary state of complete cardiopulmonary arrest (28). Between 1985 and 1988, nine patients with giant basilar artery aneurysms were treated with complete circulatory arrest, hypothermia, and barbiturate cerebral protection. Thus far, our results have been good. Of the nine patients treated in this fashion, six have had an excellent outcome (no neurologic deficit), one has had a good outcome (minimal deficit), one has had a fair outcome (ipsilateral third-nerve palsy with contralateral hemiparesis), and one died from brain stem stroke. These results are much better than others obtained using similar surgical adjuncts but without barbiturate cerebral protection (2, 4, 12, 31). It appears that the cerebral protective properties of barbiturate anesthesia and hypothermia are additive, increasing the tolerance of the cerebral tissues to temporary global ischemia.

The administration of barbiturates to patients with cerebral vascular disease who undergo neurovascular procedures has proved to be feasible and safe (6, 9, 27–29). We have not recognized any complication that we can attribute to barbiturate therapy. Intraoperative hypotension and a prolonged postoperative recovery time are potential drawbacks to the use of barbiturates that are easily managed. No randomized study has yet been performed to verify the protective effect of barbiturates in neurosurgery patients as compared with a control group receiving standard anesthesia. Nonetheless, on the basis of clinical experience and laboratory research, it appears that barbiturates may effectively protect the brain from transient ischemia during neurovascular surgery.

References

1. Archibald JE, Drazkowski JF, Wilkinson E, et al: Human variance to high dose thiopental therapy as determined by EEG/CSA monitoring. *Am J EEG Technol* 25:225–239, 1985.
2. Baumgartner WA, Silverberg GD, Ream AK, et al: Reappraisal of cardiopulmonary bypass with deep hypothermia and circulatory arrest for complex neurosurgical operations. *Surgery* 94:242–249, 1983.
3. Carter LP, Yamagata S, Erspamer R: Time limits of reversible cortical ischemia. *Neurosurgery* 12:620–623, 1983.
4. Drake CG, Barr HWK, Coles JC, et al: The use of extracorporeal circulation and profound hypothermia in the treatment of ruptured intracranial aneurysm. *J Neurosurg* 21:575–581, 1964.
5. Goldstein A Jr, Wells BA, Keats AS: Increased tolerance to cerebral anoxia by pentobarbital. *Arch Int Pharmacodyn Ther* 161:138–143, 1966.
6. Hadley MN, Spetzler RF: Contemporary application of the extracranial–intracranial bypass for cerebral revascularization. *Contemp Neurosurg* 9:1–6, 1987.
7. Hoff JT, Pitts LH, Spetzler RF, et al: Barbiturates for protection from cerebral ischemia in aneurysm surgery. *Acta Neurol Scand* 56 (Suppl 64):158–159, 1977.
8. Hoff JT, Smith AL, Hankinson HL, et al: Barbiturate protection from cerebral infarction in primates. *Stroke* 6:28–33, 1975.
9. Hopkins LN, Martin NA, Hadley MN, et al: Vertebrobasilar insufficiency. Part 2: Microsurgical treatment of intracranial vertebrobasilar disease. *J Neurosurg* 66:662–674, 1987.
10. Jones TH, Morawetz RB, Crowell RM, et al: Thresholds of focal cerebral ischemia in awake monkeys. *J Neurosurg* 54:773–782, 1981.
11. Michenfelder JD, Milde JH, Sundt TM Jr: Cerebral protection by barbiturate anesthesia: Use after middle cerebral artery occlusion in Java monkeys. *Arch Neurol* 33:345–350, 1976.
12. Morgan H, Norzinger JD, Robertson JT, et al: Hemorrhagic studies with severe hemodilution in profound hypothermia and cardiac arrest. *J Surg Res* 14:459–464, 1973.
13. Nehls DG, Spetzler RF: A review of cerebral protection against ischemia: Part I. *BNI Quarterly* 2(2):18–23, 1986.
14. Nehls DG, Spetzler RF: A review of cerebral protection against ischemia: Part III. *BNI Quarterly* 2(4):2–8, 1986.
15. Nehls DG, Todd MM, Spetzler RF, et al: A comparison of the cerebral protective effects of isoflurane and barbiturates during temporary focal ischemia in primates. *Anesthesiology* 66:453–464, 1987.
16. Nussmeier NA, Arlund C, Slogoff S: Neuropsychiatric complications after cardiopulmonary bypass: Cerebral protection by a barbiturate. *Anesthesiology* 64:165–170, 1986.
17. Raudzens PA, Spetzler RF, Carter LP, et al: Cerebral electrical activity during low flow states. In Spetzler RF, Carter LP, Selman WR, et al (eds): *Cerebral Revascularization for Stroke*. New York, Thieme-Stratton, 1985, pp 189–196.
18. Selman W, Spetzler R: Neurophysiological monitoring of barbiturate induced coma. *Acta Neurol Scand* 60 (Suppl 72):74–75, 1979.
19. Selman WR, Spetzler RF, Jackson D, et al: Regional cerebral blood flow following middle cerebral artery occlusion and barbiturate therapy in baboons. *J Cereb Blood Flow Metab* 1 (Suppl 1):S214–S215, 1981.
20. Selman WR, Spetzler RF, Roessmann UR, et al: Barbiturate-induced coma therapy for focal cerebral ischemia: Effect after temporary and permanent MCA occlusion. *J Neurosurg* 55:220–226, 1981.
21. Selman WR, Spetzler RF, Roski RA: Barbiturate resuscitation from focal cerebral ischemia—a review. *Resuscitation* 9:189–196, 1981.
22. Selman WR, Spetzler RF, Roski RA, et al: Barbiturate coma in focal cerebral ischemia: Relationship of protection to timing of therapy. *J Neurosurg* 56:685–690, 1982.
23. Selman WR, Zabramski JM, Spetzler RF: The therapeutic window of barbiturate protection in focal cerebral ischemia: Ineffectiveness of enhancement of protection with DMSO or naloxone. In Spetzler RF, Carter LP, Selman WR (eds): *Cerebral Revascularization for Stroke* New York, Theime-Stratton, 1985, pp 275–281.
24. Shapiro HM: Barbiturates in brain ischemia. *Br J Anaesth* 57:82–95, 1985.
25. Smith AL: Barbiturate protection in cerebral hypoxia. *Anesthesiology* 47:285–293, 1977.
26. Smith DS, Rehncrona S, Siesjö BK: Barbiturates as protective agents in brain ischemia and as free radical scavengers in vitro. *Acta Physiol Scand* Suppl 492:129–134, 1980.
27. Spetzler RF, Hadley MN, Martin NA, et al: Vertebrobasilar insufficiency. Part 1: Microsurgical treatment of extracranial vertebrobasilar disease. *J Neurosurg* 66:648–661, 1987.
28. Spetzler RF, Hadley MN, Rigamonti D, et al: Aneurysms of the basilar artery treated with circulatory arrest, hypothermia and barbiturate cerebral protection. *J Neurosurg* 68:868–879, 1988.
29. Spetzler RF, Martin NA, Hadley MN, et al: Microsurgical endarterectomy under barbiturate protection: A prospective study. *J Neurosurg* 65:63–73, 1986.
30. Spetzler RF, Selman WR, Roski RA, et al: Cerebral revascularization during barbiturate coma in primates and humans. *Surg Neurol* 17:111–115, 1982.
31. Sundt TM Jr, Pluth JR, Gronert GA: Excision of giant basilar aneurysm under profound hypothermia. Report of a case. *Mayo Clin Proc* 47:631–634, 1972.
32. Sundt TM Jr, Sharbrough FW, Anderson RE, et al: Cerebral blood flow measurements and electroencephalograms during carotid endarterectomy. *J Neurosurg* 41:310–320, 1974.
33. Trojaborg W, Boysen G: Relation between EEG, regional cerebral blood flow and internal carotid

artery pressure during carotid endarterectomy. *Electroencephalogr Clin Neurophysiol* 34:61–69, 1973.

34. Weinstein PR, Rodriguez y Baena R, Chater NL: Results of extracranial–intracranial arterial bypass for intracranial internal carotid artery stenosis: Review of 105 cases. *Neurosurgery* 15:787–794, 1984.

35. Wilkinson E, Spetzler RF, Archibald J: Barbiturate protection and EEG monitoring in neurovascular surgery. *BNI Quarterly* 2(2):5–10, 1986.

36. Wilkinson E, Spetzler RF, Carter LP, et al: Intraoperative barbiturate therapy during temporary vessel occlusion in man. In Spetzler RF, Carter LP, Selman WR, et al (eds): *Cerebral Revascularization for Stroke*. New York, Thieme-Stratton, 1985, pp 397–402.

CHAPTER TWENTY-FIVE

Calcium Channel Blockers

David A. Greenberg, M.D., Ph.D.

Cerebral ischemia frequently results in necrosis of brain tissue and permanent neurologic deficits. However, clinical experience with transient ischemic attacks and the excellent recovery of some patients following cardiac arrest indicate that cerebral dysfunction related to ischemia is initially reversible. Although the pathophysiology of brain ischemia has been examined in considerable detail, at least one question with important therapeutic implications has not been answered: What is the critical cellular event that seals the fate of the reversibly injured ischemic neuron?

CALCIUM AND NEURONAL INJURY

To answer this question, some investigators have looked to studies of ischemic, hypoxic, or chemical injury to nonneuronal cells, particularly hepatocytes and cardiac myocytes. Several such studies appear to implicate intracellular calcium overload as a final common pathway for irreversible cytotoxicity. For example, the ability of various chemical toxins to kill cultured hepatocytes is calcium dependent (18) and reperfusion of ischemic myocardium with calcium-containing, but not calcium-free, solutions leads to myocardial cell death—a phenomenon known as the *calcium paradox* (2). Calcium overload is also demonstrable in selectively vulnerable neurons of the hippocampus following experimental cerebral ischemia (20).

Although it is generally agreed that excessive accumulation of intracellular calcium is a common feature of irreversible cell injury from diverse causes, the contention that calcium overload and cell death

are causally and inevitably linked has been disputed. Whereas excitotoxic injury increases the calcium content of hippocampal nerve cell bodies approximately tenfold (23), it is not certain that free intracellular calcium levels in living hypoxic cells exceed levels achieved with nontoxic physiologic stimulation. Another objection to the theory that calcium overload is the critical event leading to cell death is that, at least in hepatocytes and cardiac cells, morphologic or physiologic evidence of severe cellular injury induced by chemical hypoxia precedes marked elevation of intracellular calcium levels (3, 10). In contrast, accumulation of calcium in ischemic CA1 pyramidal cells of the hippocampus may precede ischemic cell death (5). In summary, whether calcium overload is the cause of or simply a consequence of irreversible ischemic injury is still controversial.

CALCIUM INFLUX INTO NEURONS

Under physiologic conditions, unbound calcium is present at only very low concentrations in the cytoplasm, whereas extracellular calcium is approximately 10,000 times more concentrated. During ischemia, intracellular calcium rises and extracellular calcium falls, presumably reflecting calcium influx into neurons. If elevation of intracellular calcium is important in the pathogenesis of ischemic neuronal injury, then its prevention by inhibiting calcium influx could be therapeutically useful. Two principal pathways for the entry of calcium into neurons have been identified (9), but it is uncertain which pathway is most important in ischemia.

Receptor-Operated Calcium Channels

Receptor-operated calcium channels are pores in the cell membrane that open in response to the occupation of a receptor by a neurotransmitter or drug, permitting calcium entry from the extracellular space. Although many different types of receptors may be coupled to calcium entry in this fashion, the receptor best characterized in brain is the N-methyl-D-aspartate (NMDA)-preferring excitatory amino acid receptor. This receptor is associated with an ion channel that exhibits high permeability to calcium (11), is activated by compounds such as glutamate and NMDA, and is competitively blocked by 2-amino-7-phosphonoheptanoic acid (AP-7) and 3-3(2-carboxypiperazine-4-y1)propyl-1-phosphonic acid (CPP). NMDA-receptor-operated calcium channels are blocked by magnesium in a voltage-dependent manner (12, 16), but are relatively resistant to blockade by cadmium. Evidence favoring a role for NMDA-receptor-operated channels in ischemic neuronal injury and the therapeutic approaches that such a role suggests are discussed by Simon (*see* Chapter 20, this volume).

Voltage-Dependent Calcium Channels

In contrast to receptor-operated channels, voltage-dependent calcium channels open in response to depolarization of the cell membrane (9). They are unaffected by excitatory amino acids and are less sensitive to magnesium and more sensitive to cadmium than are NMDA channels. Several types of voltage-dependent calcium channels can be distinguished on physiologic and pharmacologic grounds (14).

T channels open only briefly and are relatively insensitive to drugs and toxins that block other calcium channel subtypes (Table 25.1). Their role in neuronal functioning is poorly understood.

L channels remain open for more prolonged periods, and their activity is modulated by drugs termed *calcium channel an-*

Table 25.1. Pharmacologic Classification of Voltage-Dependent Calcium Channels

Calcium channel subtype	Inhibited by calcium channel blockers	Inhibited by conotoxin
T	−	−
L (neuronal)	+	+
L (nonneuronal)	+	−
N	−	+

tagonists or *calcium channel blockers,* which are considered in detail shortly. L channels in neurons are also blocked by conotoxin, a peptide derived from the venom of the piscivorous marine snail, *Conus geographus,* whereas L channels in nonneuronal tissues are unaffected by the toxin (4). The functional significance of neuronal L channels has not been established, but they may be preferentially localized to nerve cell bodies and dendrites. One piece of evidence for such a localization is that L channels do not appear to have a major role in neurotransmitter release from nerve terminals (14). In addition, L channels are depleted from human striatum in Huntington's disease, which is associated with loss of striatal nerve cell bodies, whereas they are present in normal numbers in the same tissue from patients with Parkinson's disease, in which only nigrostriatal nerve terminals are destroyed (25).

Finally, N channels, channels that are neither T nor L, share properties of the other calcium channel subtypes: They conduct currents that are intermediate in size between those of T and L channels, are inhibited by conotoxin, and are resistant to inhibition by calcium channel blockers. N channels appear to be important for linking nerve terminal depolarization to neurotransmitter release in brain (14).

Several mechanisms can be envisioned whereby voltage-dependent calcium channels could be involved in neuronal calcium overload during ischemia. One possibility is that ischemia-induced neuronal depolarization activates voltage-dependent channels directly to promote calcium influx into cells that are targets for ischemic injury. Calcium influx through N channels on nerve terminals could also be important in stimulating the release of excitotoxic neurotransmitters onto preferentially vulnerable neurons. Finally, the depolarizing effects of such endogenous excitotoxins might elicit secondarily the influx of calcium through voltage-dependent channels. The relative importance of these putative mechanisms of ischemic neuronal injury has yet to be determined.

CALCIUM CHANNEL BLOCKERS

A variety of chemical compounds that are otherwise distinct share the ability to inhibit the influx of extracellular calcium through voltage-dependent channels, apparently by reducing the probability that channels will open in response to cell membrane depolarization. Because both vascular smooth muscle and neurons express calcium channels that can be inhibited by calcium channel blockers, these drugs could ameliorate ischemic brain injury either by inducing changes in cerebral blood flow (CBF) to reversibly damaged neurons or by directly preventing calcium influx into neurons.

The major classes of calcium channel blockers can be categorized according to their chemical structures as dihydropyridines (nifedipine, nimodipine, nitrendipine, nicardipine, niludipine, PN200-110, and PY108-068), phenylalkylamines (verapamil, D600, and D888), diphenylalkylamines (flunarizine, cinnarizine, prenylamine, and lidoflazine), and benzothiazepines (diltiazem). Of these drugs, nifedipine, nimodipine, verapamil, and diltiazem are currently available for nonexperimental clinical use in the United States, while flunarizine has been widely employed as an experimental neurotherapeutic agent. The various classes of calcium channel blocking drugs appear to act at different sites on the channel. In addition to the classic calcium channel blockers listed above, which selectively inhibit L channels, several drugs that may have neuroprotective effects in ischemia also possess calcium channel antagonist activity. These

include cyproheptadine (17), phenytoin (13), and dextromethorphan (1).

Nifedipine, verapamil, and diltiazem are all well absorbed when administered orally, but appear to penetrate only poorly into the central nervous system. This is an important drawback in attempts to use these agents to treat cerebral disorders, but the use of more penetrant drugs, such as nimodipine or flunarizine, may be a solution. It is also important to consider the cardiovascular side effects of calcium channel blockers when they are proposed for use in cerebral ischemia. Systemic hypotension, which could exacerbate cerebral ischemia, is most common with dihydropyridines such as nifedipine, whereas atrioventricular conduction disturbances may be associated with administration of verapamil (9).

CALCIUM CHANNEL BLOCKERS AND CEREBRAL ISCHEMIA

Animal Studies

Numerous studies have been conducted to evaluate the possible beneficial effects of calcium channel blockers in animal models of cerebral ischemia. In interpreting the results, it is important to consider the following issues:

1. Is the experimental model one of global cerebral ischemia, which is analogous to cardiac arrest in human patients, or focal ischemia, which more closely corresponds to stroke?
2. Is the drug effective only if administered before the onset of ischemia, or can it be given during or after the ischemic period, when patients typically come to medical attention?
3. If a favorable effect is found, does this reflect a change in long-term outcome or simply the speed of recovery?
4. Are the criteria for drug-related improvement clinically relevant?

Outcome measures that have been used include neurologic outcome, electroencephalography findings, regional CBF, cerebral metabolic rate of oxygen, and histologic change in selectively vulnerable brain regions. However, not all of these may predict long-term clinical recovery.

Results of animal studies of global cerebral ischemia support a beneficial effect on clinical outcome at 12 to 96 hours when nimodipine is administered before the ischemic insult (22) or when lidoflazine (26) or nimodipine (21) is given after ischemia. Drug-related improvement in regional CBF is sometimes (22, 26) but not always (22) associated with improved clinical outcome. Attenuation of histologic neuronal damage following global ischemia has also been reported with nimodipine (21) or flunarizine (6), but this has not always been found (24).

In studies of focal ischemia, pretreatment with nimodipine improved regional CBF and histopathology 3 hours after coagulation and division of the middle cerebral artery of the rat (15). Using a similar technique for producing focal ischemia, Germano et al (8) determined that nimodipine produced a better neurologic outcome and reduced infarct size when given 1 to 6 hours after the induction of ischemia, although these results have not been replicated in subsequent studies in the same laboratory. Another group found that administration of the dihydropyridine calcium channel blocker PY108-068, beginning 90 minutes after microsphere embolization of one hemisphere of the rat brain, improved recovery of neurologic function (27).

Clinical Studies

The promising results of animal studies have prompted investigation of the possible role of calcium channel blockers in the clinical treatment of global cerebral ischemia (cardiac arrest) and stroke.

A retrospective study examined the clinical outcome following cardiac arrest in 18 patients who received either the organic calcium channel blocker verapamil or the ionic calcium channel blocker magnesium and 11 patients who were given neither

drug (19). Among the treated patients, 39% regained consciousness and 33% were neurologically normal at 3 and 6 months, whereas only 27% of control patients emerged from coma and none had a full neurologic recovery.

In a prospective study, 186 patients enrolled within 24 hours of the onset of ischemic stroke received either standard therapy (in this case, a 5-day course of dextran for hemodilution) or standard therapy plus nimodipine, given at a dosage of 30 mg, orally or via nasogastric tube, four times per day for 28 days (7). At the end of this period, neurologic outcome was significantly better in the patients who received nimodipine; those with moderately severe deficits at the beginning of the study obtained the greatest benefit. Nimodipine also reduced mortality from 20% to 9% at 4 weeks and from 29% to 17% at 6 months, although this effect was significant only in men. Nimodipine did not appear to alter systemic blood pressure. Side effects of the drug included reversible azotemia, dizziness, and vomiting, each of which occurred in one patient. Thus, treatment with nimodipine appeared to be associated with improved neurologic outcome and with decreased mortality rates in men.

The initial clinical data concerning the use of nimodipine in the treatment of global cerebral ischemia and stroke are thus encouraging, and additional studies of nimodipine treatment in ischemic stroke are currently being conducted. The results of these investigations will be important in determining the role of calcium channel blockers in the pharmacologic management of cerebral ischemia.

Acknowledgments—The author's work is supported in part by USPHS Research grants no. NS14543 and NS24728 from the National Institute of Neurologic Diseases and Stroke and AA07032 from the National Institute on Alcohol Abuse and Alcoholism, an Alfred P. Sloan Research Fellowship in Neuroscience awarded by Alfred P. Sloan Foundation, New York, NY, the Alcoholic Beverage Medical Research Foundation, Baltimore, MD, and the Dr. Louis Sklarow Memorial Fund, Buffalo, NY.

References

1. Carpenter CL, Marks SM, Watson DL, et al: Dextromethorphan and dextrorphan as calcium channel antagonists. *Brain Res* 439:372–375, 1988.
2. Cheung JY, Bonventre JV, Malis CD, et al: Calcium and ischemic injury. *N Engl J Med* 314:1670–1676, 1986.
3. Cobbold PH, Bourne PK: Aequorin measurements of free calcium in single heart cells. *Nature* 312:444–446, 1984.
4. Cruz LJ, Johnson DS, Olivera BM: Characterization of the *w*-conotoxin target. Evidence for tissue-specific heterogeneity in calcium channel types. *Biochemistry* 26:820–824, 1987.
5. Deshpande JK, Siesjö BK, Wieloch T: Calcium accumulation and neuronal damage in the rat hippocampus following cerebral ischemia. *J Cereb Blood Flow Metab* 7:89–95, 1987.
6. Deshpande JK, Wieloch T: Flunarizine, a calcium entry blocker, ameliorates ischemic brain damage in the rat. *Anesthesiology* 64:215–224, 1986.
7. Gelmers HJ, Gorter K, De Weerdt CJ, et al: A controlled trial of nimodipine in acute ischemic stroke. *N Engl J Med* 318:203–207, 1988.
8. Germano IM, Bartkowski HM, Cassel ME, et al: The therapeutic value of nimodipine in experimental focal cerebral ischemia. *J Neurosurg* 67:81–87, 1987.
9. Greenberg DA: Calcium channels and calcium channel antagonists. *Ann Neurol* 21:317–330, 1987.
10. Lemasters JJ, DiGuiseppi J, Nieminen A-L, et al: Blebbing, free Ca^{2+}, and mitochondrial membrane potential preceding cell death in hepatocytes. *Nature* 325:78–81, 1987.
11. MacDermott AB, Mayer ML, Westbrook GL, et al: NMDA-receptor activation increases cytoplasmic calcium concentration in cultured spinal cord neurones. *Nature* 321:519–522, 1986.
12. Mayer ML, Westbrook GL, Guthrie PB: Voltage-dependent block by Mg^{2+} of NMDA responses in spinal cord neurones. *Nature* 309:261–263, 1984.
13. Messing RO, Carpenter CL, Greenberg DA: Mechanism of calcium channel inhibition by phenytoin: Comparison with classical calcium channel antagonists. *J Pharmacol Exp Ther* 235:407–411, 1985.
14. Miller RJ: Multiple calcium channels and neuronal function. *Science* 235:46–52, 1987.
15. Mohamed AA, Gotoh O, Graham DI, et al: Effect of pretreatment with the calcium antagonist nimodipine on local cerebral blood flow and histopathology after middle cerebral artery occlusion. *Ann Neurol* 18:705–711, 1985.
16. Nowak L, Bregestovoski P, Ascher P, et al: Magnesium gates glutamate-activated channels in mouse central neruones. *Nature* 307:462–465, 1984.
17. Peroutka SJ, Allen GS: The calcium antagonist properties of cyproheptadine: Implications for antimigraine action. *Neurology* 34:304–309, 1984.
18. Schanne FAX, Kane AB, Young EE, et al: Calcium dependence of toxic cell death: A final common pathway. *Science* 206:700–702, 1979.
19. Schwartz AC: Neurological recovery after cardiac arrest: Clinical feasibility trial of calcium blockers. *Am J Emerg Med* 3:1–10, 1985.
20. Simon RP, Griffiths T, Evans MC, et al: Calcium overload in selectively vulnerable neurons of the hippocampus during and after ischemia: An EM study in the rat. *J Cereb Blood Flow Metab* 4:350–361, 1984.
21. Steen PA, Gisvold SE, Milde JH, et al: Nimodipine improves outcome when given after complete cerebral ischemia in primates. *Anesthesiology* 62:406–414, 1985.
22. Steen PA, Newberg LA, Milde JH, et al: Cerebral blood flow and neurologic outcome when nimodipine is given after complete cerebral ischemia in the dog. *J Cereb Blood Flow Metab* 4:82–87, 1984.
23. Stodieck LS, Miller JJ: Direct evidence for an increase in intracellular free calcium in amino acid neurotoxicity of selectively vulnerable hippocampal neurons. *Soc Neurosci Abstr* 13:9, 1987.
24. Vibulsreth S, Dietrich WD, Busto R, et al: Failure of nimodipine to prevent ischemic neuronal damage in rats. *Stroke* 18:210–216, 1987.
25. Watson DL, Carpenter CL, Marks SM, et al: Striatal calcium channel antagonist receptors in Huntington's disease and Parkinson's disease. *Ann Neurol* 23:303–305, 1988.
26. White BC, Winegar CD, Wilson RF, et al: Calcium blockers in cerebral resuscitation. *J Trauma* 23:788–794, 1983.
27. Wiernsperger N, Gygax P, Hofmann A: Calcium antagonist PH 108-068: Demonstration of its efficacy in various types of experimental brain ischemia. *Stroke* 15:679–685, 1984.

CHAPTER TWENTY-SIX

Role of Opiate Antagonists in the Treatment of Stroke

Alan I. Faden, M.D.

Since 1981, a substantial body of experimental data has shown that opiate-receptor antagonists can improve physiologic variables, histopathology, and neurologic outcome following traumatic or ischemic injuries to the central nervous system (CNS) (15). Initial studies (23) examined the role of the relatively nonspecific opiate antagonist naloxone in experimental spinal cord trauma. Subsequently, many studies evaluated the potential therapeutic role of opiate-receptor antagonists, particularly naloxone, in the treatment of experimental global and focal ischemia. Although most studies have shown that opiate-receptor antagonists improve outcome following ischemic brain and spinal cord injury in a variety of animal models, a number of negative reports have raised questions about the effectiveness of such treatment. This review critically assesses the experimental and clinical literature with particular emphasis on methodologic issues and interpretation of experimental data.

OPIOIDS, OPIATE RECEPTORS, AND OPIATE-RECEPTOR ANTAGONISTS

Since the identification of the first endogenous opioids—the penta-peptide enkephalins—in 1975, a variety of endogenous opioids and opiate receptors have been found (9). Most of the opioids and opioid fragments that have been identified are derived from one of three major prohormone precursors: (a) pro-enkephalin; (b) pro-dynorphin; and (c) pro-opiomelanocortin (11). These major opioid systems have different and distinct distributions within the brain and spinal cord and may subserve different physiologic and pathophysiologic roles (14). A variety of other opioid substances have also been identified that are not clearly derived from these classes; the roles of these substances are even less well defined (9).

At least five classes of opiate receptors have been proposed, called μ, δ, κ, σ, and ϵ; in addition, other receptors have been proposed, such as λ, as well as isoreceptors for the μ receptor and κ receptor (11, 14). Although certain opioids and opioid fragments have some selectivity for specific opiate receptors, in many cases opioids may act at multiple receptors. Thus, whereas β-endorphin has high affinity for μ receptors, it also acts at other receptors including δ and κ. Enkephalins have activity at both μ sites and δ sites, and whereas the large fragment of dynorphin (dynorphin A-[1-17]) may be relatively selective at κ sites, shorter dynorphin fragments (e.g. dynorphin A-[1-8]) have considerable activity at μ sites. This diversity of opioids and opiate antagonists, as well as the lack of a one-to-one correspondence between agonist and receptor, complicates interpretation of data pertaining to the possible pathophysiologic role of specific opioids or specific receptors in CNS injury.

Over the past few years, many newer and partially receptor-selective opiate antagonists have been developed. These include: the μ-receptor antagonists β-funaltrexamine and naloxonazine; the δ-selective antagonists ICI-154,129 and ICI-174,864; and most recently the κ-selective antagonists binaltorphimine (BNI) and nor-binaltorphimine (nor-BNI). A variety of selective agonists have also been developed, including the μ-receptor agonist [D-Ala^2-Me-Phe^4-Gly-Ol]-enkephalin, the δ-receptor agonists [D-Ala^{2}D-Leu^5]-enkephalin and [D-Ser^2-Leu^5-Thr^6]-enkephalin, and the κ-agonists U-50,488H and U-69,593. Although the data now available regarding use of these specific agonists or antagonists in CNS ischemia are not extensive, they can be used to provide information regarding possible roles of specific opiate receptors in the injury process.

ENDOGENOUS OPIOIDS AND POSTISCHEMIC CENTRAL NERVOUS SYSTEM INJURY

From investigations of experimental shock, we proposed that endogenous opioids are released following spinal cord trauma or spinal cord ischemia and contribute to secondary or delayed tissue damage, in part, by reducing microcirculatory blood flow (22, 24). Two groups have demonstrated that the opiate antagonist naloxone, when administered at very high doses (in the mg/kg range), reverses or prevents delayed ischemia of the spinal cord that follows contusive injury (22, 52). Although subsequent studies suggested that the endogenous opioid dynorphin may be a critical factor in secondary injury following trauma (17, 20, 25, 41), few studies have examined changes of tissue opioids in cerebral ischemia. Andrews et al (2) found no significant changes in levels of β-endorphin, leucine-enkephalin, or dynorphin-like immunoreactive material within the region of injury following focal cerebral ischemia in rats. Fried et al (28) reported a decline in dynorphin-like immunoreactive material within the hippocampus following experimental focal ischemia. However, neither of these studies examined the effects of varying degrees of injury or fully evaluated changes in opioids over time.

USE OF NONSELECTIVE ANTAGONISTS IN EXPERIMENTAL CENTRAL NERVOUS SYSTEM ISCHEMIA

The possible therapeutic effects of opiate-receptor antagonists have been studied extensively in experimental models of ischemia and stroke. Hosobuchi et al (33) were the first to report that naloxone treatment enhanced neurologic recovery in experimental stroke, using a common carotid artery occlusion model in gerbils. Subsequently, other groups evaluated naloxone treatment in related models of carotid artery occlusion in gerbils, but obtained inconclusive results. Avery et al (4) showed that naloxone treatment improved blood flow and survival, and reduced seizure activity, in gerbils subjected to temporary bilateral common carotid artery occlusion. Turcani et al (49) found that naloxone treatment increased cerebral blood flow (CBF) in gerbils subjected to sectioning of one common carotid artery and of the contralateral external carotid artery. In contrast, four other groups found no beneficial effect of naloxone treatment following unilateral or bilateral common carotid artery ligation in gerbils (32, 36, 39, 48). Similar naloxone doses (1 to 10 mg/kg) were used in each of these studies.

Whereas inconsistent effects have been reported in the gerbil, naloxone in similar doses has been found to improve outcome in most studies of focal or global ischemia in rats. Wexler (50) showed that naloxone administered prophylactically prevented stroke in spontaneously hypertensive rats fed a low-protein fish diet; treatment following stroke was also associated with improved outcome. Capdeville et al (10) found that neurologic scores improved after naloxone treatment in rats with temporary forebrain ischemia; the beneficial effects were dose dependent. Phillis et al (44) noted that naloxone increased basal CBF and prolonged reactive hyperemia after anoxia. Skarphendinsson and Thoren (47) reported improved cortical somatosensory-evoked responses after naloxone treatment in rats subjected to hypotensive hemorrhage. Hariri et al (31) observed that naloxone treatment given during or after transient global cerebral ischemia (four-vessel occlusion) blocked the hyperemic–oligemic CBF patterns characteristic of stroke in this model. In contrast, two studies using rats have not been positive. Shigeno et al (46) noted that naloxone did not significantly alter local cerebral glucose utilization after middle cerebral artery

(MCA) occlusion, although such treatment did prevent the decrease in glycogen phosphorylase activity observed after ischemia. Young et al (51), evaluating the effects of naloxone in hypoxic–ischemic brain injury induced by the Levine method in neonatal rats, found that treatment worsened outcome in a dose-dependent manner.

In studies of rabbits, Koskinen (38) reported that naloxone treatment did not affect CBF following cerebral ischemia produced by raised intracranial pressure. However, we have shown that naloxone treatment in the mg/kg range improves neurologic recovery following global spinal cord ischemia in rabbits (24).

Most of the studies in cats have noted a beneficial effect for opiate-receptor antagonists. Levy et al (40) found that naloxone reversed neurologic deficits after MCA occlusion, although cortical CBF in the ischemic hemisphere was decreased. In the same model, Baskin et al (8) observed that naloxone and naltrexone improved survival and motor function. Sandor et al (45) showed that CBF was improved by naloxone in the ischemic hemisphere after MCA occlusion; administration of an enkephalin analogue exacerbated such ischemia. The same group also found that naloxone was able to dilate pial arteries in cats (37). Although Hubbard and Sundt (34) reported no beneficial effects for naloxone treatment after MCA occlusion in cats, evaluation of their reported data indicates that such treatment significantly improved electroencephalographic (EEG) activity, and may have enhanced CBF.

We have evaluated the effects of naloxone in dogs using a stroke model produced by repeated air embolization of the carotid artery. Naloxone treatment (2 mg/kg bolus followed by 2 mg/kg/hour intravenously) significantly improved cortical somatosensory-evoked responses and focal CBF (18). Namba et al (42) showed that naloxone treatment improved somatosensory-evoked responses but not local CBF after transient focal ischemia in dogs; both naloxone and the opiate-receptor antagonist levallorphan reversed motor deficits in chronically injured animals, although the effect was not marked.

Several groups have also reported improvement following naloxone treatment of stroke in primates. Using permanent MCA occlusion models in baboons, both Baskin et al (7) and Zabramski et al (53) observed improved outcome with high-dose naloxone therapy. In contrast, Gaines et al (29) found no beneficial effects with naloxone following temporary or permanent MCA occlusion in awake cynomulgus monkeys; however, there were trends favoring naloxone-treated animals with regard to behavioral and histopathologic changes.

It is unfortunate that none of the negative studies reported provides information regarding the statistical power of their evaluations or justification of the use of the specific models for pharmacologic testing. Only in the gerbil studies have there been attempts to replicate the conditions of the previously reported positive studies.

In most models of cerebral ischemia substantial variability of collateral flow can be found among individual animals; thus, it may be difficult to demonstrate significant differences using relatively small numbers of animals. It should also be noted that optimal doses of naloxone may not have been used in many of the reported studies; rarely have escalating doses been evaluated. In this regard, it has been well demonstrated both in shock (19) and CNS ischemia (2, 21) that the beneficial effects of opiate antagonists show an inverted U-shaped curve, with diminished actions at both the higher and lower doses. The optimal dose range for naloxone appears to be 2 to 5 mg/kg, administered as a bolus intravenous injection followed by a continuous infusion of approximately 70% of the bolus dose each hour for a period of at least 4 hours.

ROLE OF SPECIFIC OPIOIDS AND OPIATE RECEPTORS IN CENTRAL NERVOUS SYSTEM ISCHEMIA

WIN44,441-3 (WIN) is a benzomorphan that appears to have increased activity at κ opiate receptors, although it is not highly selective. This compound significantly improves neurologic outcome following ischemic spinal cord injury in rabbits (21). This compound is approximately 50 times more potent than naloxone in treating ischemic spinal injury; moreover, the beneficial actions are stereospecific, strongly suggesting that effects are mediated by opiate receptors (21). More recently we have found that WIN significantly improved EEG change (using fast-Fourier transform analysis) following permanent MCA occlusion in rats (2). This beneficial effect is dose related, showing an inverted U-shaped pattern. In addition, the drug has beneficial effects on survival but does not appear to significantly affect histopathologic change. These observations suggest that κ opiate receptors might play a role in ischemic spinal cord and cerebral injury, just as they have been shown to play a role in traumatic CNS injury (16).

However, the role of dynorphin and κ opiate receptors in cerebral ischemia has recently been questioned. Baskin et al (6) reported that dynorphin(1-13), administered at relatively high doses systematically, improved survival following MCA occlusion in cats, although there was no reported effect on neurologic recovery. Tang (48) has reported that the compound U-50,448H, which has selective opiate agonist properties at κ receptors—but *not* dynorphin—improves neurologic outcome following MCA occlusion in rats. These apparent inconsistencies may have several explanations. First, U-50,488H, although selective for κ opiate receptors, may have other physiologic actions including possibly calcium antagonist effects and an ability to antagonize certain actions of excitatory amino acids; these actions of U-50,488H, independent of effects on κ opiate receptors, might serve to protect the brain against injury. In addition, there is some evidence to support the existence of κ isoreceptors (3), different populations of κ receptors which may have different physiologic actions. It is possible that various κ isoreceptors could mediate actions that are in opposite directions.

More recently, we have evaluated another opiate-receptor antagonist, nalmefene, in ischemic cerebral injury. Nalmefene is an exomethylene derivative of naltrexone, with enhanced activity and increased selectivity for κ receptors. Nalmefene treatment, at approximately 1% of the optimal naloxone dose, significantly improves cellular bioenergetic state and tissue acidosis, and reduces lactate accumulation following global cerebral ischemia and reperfusion in rats. Most recently, another opiate-receptor antagonist has been developed—nor-BNI—which is very highly selective for κ opiate receptors. We have recently found that this compound significantly improves neurologic recovery following traumatic spinal cord injury in rats (26), and we will soon begin to evaluate the effects of this selective agent in the treatment of cerebral ischemia.

OPIATE ANTAGONISTS IN CENTRAL NERVOUS SYSTEM ISCHEMIA AND STROKE: CLINICAL STUDIES

Several clinical anecdotes and papers have been published regarding the use of opiate antagonists in human stroke and they show conflicting results. Baskin and Hosobuchi (5) reported improved neurologic function in two patients who had motor dysfunction postoperatively following intracranial procedures. Jabaily and Davis (35) found transitory improvement of neurologic function in three of 13 patients with acute neurologic deficits: Diagnoses included cerebral ischemia, infarction, and intracranial hemorrhage. Handa et al (30) gave the nonselective opiate-receptor antagonist levellorphan to 19 patients with acute ischemic stroke and reported temporary improvement of motor deficits in 13. Namba et al (42) also reported that levellorphan improved neurologic deficits following stroke or angiospasm. In contrast, at least three studies have found little or no beneficial effects with opiate antagonists in stroke patients (12, 27, 43).

There are many methodologic problems

---

*R Shirane, personal communication, 1980.

with these earlier studies. The majority were neither randomized nor controlled. No attempt was made to control for type of stroke or time of treatment. In many cases, patients were treated as long as days after injury. In addition, the doses of opiate-receptor antagonists administered were approximately 1/1,000 of the doses shown to be required for therapeutic effect in experimental animals.

Recently, an attempt has been made to evaluate some of these important issues, including stroke etiology and time of treatment. Estanol et al (13) compared the effects of naloxone in four groups of patients: *(a)* computerized tomography (CT)-proven cerebral infarction of greater than 7 days' duration; *(b)* acute cerebral ischemia of less than 24 hours; *(c)* CT-proven intracerebral hemorrhage of less than 24 hours' duration; and *(d)* hyperacute cerebral ischemia observed during angiography. Naloxone treatment, at a dose of 0.8 mg, improved outcome in seven of 20 patients with acute ischemia and was markedly effective in each of three patients with hyperacute ischemia. In contrast, naloxone had no effect in chronic cerebral infarction or in intracerebral hemorrhage. The investigators concluded that naloxone treatment might be used in the evaluation of acute cerebral ischemia to determine the potential reversibility of such injury.

A phase 1 study of naloxone treatment of human cerebral ischemia has been reported (1). Naloxone treatment appeared to be safe at the very high doses (in the mg/kg range) required for beneficial effects in experimental animals. Patients received a bolus injection followed by an hourly infusion of 50% of the bolus dose for 24 hours. Total doses ranged from 52 to 4,978 mg. No major dose-related side effects occurred and 13 of 27 patients showed transient or sustained improvement. Subsequently, the same group completed a phase 2 study of naloxone treatment in human stroke. These results, which have not yet been reported, have been mixed. Although high doses of naloxone were used, few patients were treated following cerebral ischemia of relatively acute onset.

At the present time, there appear to be no plans for the institution of phase 3 trials of naloxone or other opiate-receptor antagonists in the treatment of human stroke. This is unfortunate, in view of the demonstrated safety of these compounds as well as the large number of positive experimental studies reported to date. However, it is possible that some of the more newly developed opiate-receptor antagonists, which have greater potency or activity than naloxone, may ultimately be evaluated in clinical trials.

INTERPRETATION OF EXPERIMENTAL AND CLINICAL STUDIES: METHODOLOGIC ISSUES

Interpretation of apparently conflicting findings related to the role of opiate antagonists in CNS ischemia has been confounded by the lack of uniformity with regard to injury models, choice of species, choice of anesthetic, drug dosage, and outcome measures employed. Furthermore, there has been little discussion regarding possible differences in pathophysiologic mechanisms, including the role of endogenous opioids, in various types of ischemia (focal versus global) or with differing severity of ischemic injury.

In the reporting of negative studies to date, there has been a uniform failure to address the issue of type II or β error, yet it is particularly important to recognize the possibility of a false-negative finding. There are many reasons a possible beneficial effect of a drug therapy might be missed. First, the injury model might be either so severe that no drug therapy could be expected to be effective, or so mild that injured animals show differences that are not significantly different from uninjured controls. The choice of number of animals in each study group is usually arbitrarily defined and generally represents a relatively small number, usually 10 or less. The choice of number of animals per treatment group should reflect expectations of possible differences between treatment and control animals, as well as the consistency of the particular model. For example, whereas we have found significant treatment effects in cats subjected to spinal cord injury using 6 to 10 cats per group, pharmacologic evaluations in rabbits or rats often require much larger numbers per group, 15 to 20 animals. The outcome measure chosen is also of considerable importance. Generally, the greater the number of independent outcome measures that are evaluated, the higher is the probability of distinguishing a drug effect if one exists. Finally, there has been relatively little appreciation of the importance of titrating drug dosage; few studies have examined wide-range, dose–response effects for any of the opiate antagonists in ischemia. This is particularly important in evaluating the effects of opiate-receptor antagonists considering the inverted U-shaped dose–response pattern, with diminished effects at both the lower and the higher doses (2, 21). For these reasons, negative studies may be of limited value, unless there has been an attempt to completely replicate the work of others.

In the interpretation of clinical studies, other methodologic issues should be noted. The majority of clinical investigators have used doses of opiate antagonists more than two orders of magnitude lower than those shown to be effective in experimental animals. In many of the studies, patients have been treated days after the onset of stroke, after cerebral infarction has occurred; at this time no drug might be expected to show therapeutic efficacy. Moreover, patient populations often have not been well defined and have included ischemia, infarction, and intracerebral hemorrhage.

References

1. Adams HP, Olinger CP, Barsan WG, et al: A dose-escalation study of large doses of naloxone for treatment of patients with acute cerebral ischemia. *Stroke* 17:404–409, 1986.
2. Andrews BT, McIntosh TK, Gonzalez MF, et al: Levels of endogenous opioids and effects of an opiate antagonist during regional cerebral ischemia in rats. *J Pharmacol Exp Thera* 247:1248–1254, 1988.
3. Attali B, Gouarderes C, Mazarquil H, et al: Evidence for multiple "kappa" binding sites by use of opioid peptides in the guinea-pig lumbo-sacral spinal cord. *Neuropeptides* 3:53–64, 1982.
4. Avery SF, Crockard H, Russel RW: Improved survival following severe cerebral ischemia using naloxone. *J Cereb Blood Flow Metab* 3(Suppl 1):S331–S332, 1983.
5. Baskin DS, Hosobuchi Y: Naloxone and reversal of ischemic neurological deficits in man. *Lancet* 2:272–275, 1981.
6. Baskin DS, Hosobuchi Y, Loh HH, et al: Dynorphin(1–13) improves survival in cats with focal cerebral ischaemia (letter). *Nature* 312:51–52, 1984.
7. Baskin DS, Kieck CF, Hosobuchi Y: Naloxone reversal of ischemic neurologic deficits in baboons is not mediated by systemic effects. *Life Sci* 31:220–224, 1982.
8. Baskin DS, Kuroda H, Hosobuchi Y, et al: Treatment of stroke with opiate antagonists—Effects of exogenous antagonists and dynorphin 1-13. *Neuropeptides* 5:307–310, 1985.
9. Bloom FE: The endorphins. A growing family of pharmacologically pertinent peptides. *Annu Rev Pharmacol Toxicol* 23:151–170, 1983.
10. Capdeville C, Pruneau D, Allix M, et al: Naloxone effect on the neurological deficit induced by forebrain ischemia in rats. *Life Sci* 38:437–442, 1986.
11. Cox BM: Endogenous opioid peptides: A guide to structures and terminology. *Life Sci* 31:1645–1658, 1982.
12. Cutler JR, Bredesen DE, Edwards R, et al: Failure of naloxone to reverse vascular neurologic deficits. *Neurology* 33:1517–1518, 1983.
13. Estanol B, Aguilar F, Corona T: Diagnosis of reversible versus irreversible cerebral ischemia by the intravenous administration of naloxone. *Stroke* 16:1006–1009, 1985.
14. Faden AI: Endogenous opioids: Physiologic and pathophysiologic actions. *J Am Osteopath Assoc* 84 (Suppl):129–134, 1984.
15. Faden AI: Opiate antagonists and thyrotropin-releasing hormone: II. Potential role in the treatment of central nervous system injury. *JAMA* 252:1452–1454, 1984.
16. Faden AI: Opiate receptor antagonist, thyrotropin-releasing hormone (TRH) and TRH-analogs in the treatment of spinal cord injury. *CNS Trauma* 4:217–226, 1987.
17. Faden AI: Opioid and non-opioid mechanisms may contribute to dynorphin's pathophysiologic actions in spinal cord injury. *Ann Neurol*, in press.
18. Faden AI, Hallenbeck JM, Brown CQ: Treatment of experimental stroke: Comparison of naloxone and thyrotropin releasing hormone. *Neurology* 32:1083–1087, 1982.
19. Faden AI, Holaday JW: Naloxone treatment of endotoxin shock: Stereospecificity of physiologic and pharmacologic effects in the rat. *J Pharmacol Exp Ther* 212:441–447, 1980.
20. Faden AI, Jacobs TP: Dynorphin induces partially reversible paraplegia in the rat. *Eur J Pharmacol* 20:321–324, 1983.
21. Faden AI, Jacobs TP: Opiate antagonist WIN44,441-3 stereospecificity improves neurologic recovery after ischemic spinal injury. *Neurology* 35:1311–1315, 1985.
22. Faden AI, Jacobs TP, Holaday JW: Endorphins in experimental spinal injury: Therapeutic effect of naloxone. *Ann Neurol* 10:326–332, 1981.

23. Faden AI, Jacobs TP, Holaday JW: Opiate antagonist improves neurologic recovery after spinal injury. *Science* 211:493–494, 1981.

24. Faden AI, Jacobs TP, Smith MT, et al: Naloxone in experimental spinal cord ischemia: Dose–response studies. *Eur J Pharmacol* 103:115–120, 1984.

25. Faden AI, Molineaux CJ, Rosenberg JG, et al: Increased dynorphin immunoreactivity in spinal cord after traumatic injury. *Reg Peptides* 11:35–41, 1985.

26. Faden AI, Takemori AI, Portoghese PS: κ-Selective opiate antagonist norbinaltorphimine improves outcome after traumatic spinal cord injury in rats. *CNS Trauma* 4:227–237, 1987.

27. Fallis RJ, Fisher M, Lobo R: A double-blind trial of naloxone in the treatment of acute stroke. *Stroke* 15:627–629, 1984.

28. Fried RL, Nowak TS Jr: Opioid peptide levels in gerbil brain after transient ischemia: Lasting depletion of hippocampal dynorphin. *Stroke* 18:765–770, 1987.

29. Gaines C, Nehls DG, Suess DM, et al: Effect of naloxone on experimental stroke in awake monkeys. *Neurosurgery* 14:308–314, 1984.

30. Handa N, Matsumoto M, Nakamura M, et al: Reversal of neurological deficits by levallorphan in patients with acute ischemic stroke. *J Cereb Blood Flow Metab* 5:469–472, 1985.

31. Hariri RJ, Supra EL, Roberts JP, et al: Effect of naloxone on cerebral perfusion and cardiac performance during experimental cerebral ischemia. *J Neurosurg* 64:780–786, 1986.

32. Holaday JW, D'Amato RJ: Naloxone or TRH fails to improve neurological deficits in gerbil models of 'stroke.' *Life Sci* 31:385–392, 1982.

33. Hosobuchi Y, Baskin WS, Woo SK: Reversal of induced ischemic neurologic deficit in gerbils by the opiate antagonist naloxone. *Science* 215:69–71, 1982.

34. Hubbard JL, Sundt TM: Failure of naloxone to affect focal incomplete cerebral ischemia and collateral blood flow in cats. *J Neurosurg* 59:237–244, 1983.

35. Jabaily J, Davis JN: Naloxone administration to patients with acute stroke. *Stroke* 15:36–39, 1984.

36. Kastin AJ, Nissen C, Olson RD: Failure of MIF or naloxone to reverse ischemic-induced neurologic deficits in gerbils. *Pharmacol Biochem Behav* 17:1083–1085, 1982.

37. Kobari M, Gotoh F, Fukuuchi Y, et al: Effects of (D-Met^2,Pro^5)-enkephalinamide and naloxone on pial vessels in cats. *J Cereb Blood Flow Metab* 5:34–39, 1985.

38. Koskinen LOD: Effects of raised intracranial pressure on regional cerebral blood flow: A comparison of effects of naloxone and TRH on the microcirculation in partial cerebral ischaemia. *Br J Pharmacol* 85:489–497, 1985.

39. Levy DE, Pike CL, Rawlinson DG: Failure of naloxone to limit clinical or morphological brain damage in gerbils with unilateral carotid artery occlusion (abstract). *Soc Neurosci Abstr* 8:248, 1982.

40. Levy R, Feustel P, Severinghaus J, et al: Effect of naloxone on neurologic deficit and cortical blood flow during focal cerebral ischemia in cats. *Life Sci* 31:2206–2208, 1982.

41. Long JB, Martinez-Arizala A, Petras JM, et al: Endogenous opioids in spinal cord injury: A critical evaluation. *CNS Trauma* 3:295–315, 1986.

42. Namba S, Nishigaki S, Fujiwara N, et al: Opiate-antagonist reversal of neurological deficits—Experimental and clinical studies. *Japan J Psych Neurol* 40:61–79, 1986.

43. Perraro F, Tosolini G, Pertoldi F, et al: Double-blind placebo-controlled trial of naloxone on motor deficits in acute cerebrovascular disease (letter). *Lancet* 1:915, 1984.

44. Phillis JW, DeLong RE, Towner JK: Naloxone enhances cerebral reactive hyperemia in the rat. *Neurosurgery* 17:596–599, 1985.

45. Sandor P, Gotoh F, Tomita M, et al: Effects of a stable enkephalin analogue, (D-Met^2,Pro^5)-enkephalinamide, and naloxone on cortical blood flow and cerebral blood volume in experimental brain ischemia in anesthetized cats. *J Cereb Blood Flow Metab* 6:553–558, 1986.

46. Shigeno T, Teasdale GM, Kirkham D, et al: Effect of naloxone on cerebral glucose metabolism in normal rats with focal cerebral ischemia. *J Cereb Blood Flow Metab* 3(Suppl 1):S528–S529, 1983.

47. Skarphedinsson JO, Thoren P: The effects of naloxone on cerebral function in spontaneously hypertensive rats during hypotensive haemorrhage. *Acta Physiol Scand* 128:597–604, 1986.

48. Tang AH: Protection from cerebral ischemia by U-50,488E, a specific kappa opioid analgesic agent. *Life Sci* 37:1475–1482, 1985.

49. Turcani P, Gotoh F, Ishihara N, et al: Dual effect of naloxone on blood platelet aggregation and cerebral blood flow in gerbils. *Thromb Res* 44:817–828, 1986.

50. Wexler BC: Naloxone ameliorates the pathophysiologic changes which lead to and attend an acute stroke in stroke-prone/SHR. *Stroke* 15:630–634, 1984.

51. Young RSK, Hessert TR, Pritchard GA, et al: Naloxone exacerbates hypoxic–ischemic brain injury in the neonatal rat. *Am J Obstet Gynecol* 150:52–56, 1984.

52. Young W, Flamm ES, Demopoulos HB, et al: Naloxone ameliorates post-traumatic ischemia in experimental spinal contusion. *J Neurosurg* 55:209–219, 1981.

53. Zabramski JM, Spetzler RF, Selman WR, et al: Naloxone improves neurologic function during and outcome after temporary focal cerebral ischemia. *Stroke* 15:621–627, 1984.

CHAPTER TWENTY-SEVEN

Arachidonic Acid Metabolism in Ischemia

Keith L. Black, M.D.
Julian T. Hoff, M.D.

Arachidonic acid (AA) is one of the brain's most abundant lipids. Free AA is oxidized to a variety of biologically active compounds that have effects ranging from vasoconstriction to vasogenic edema. Several studies have demonstrated the importance of AA metabolites in cerebral ischemia (14, 18, 19). Our present knowledge about ischemic brain suggests that a goal of protective brain therapy during ischemia should be to increase levels of beneficial AA metabolites such as prostacyclin (PGI_2), a potent vasodilator and antiplatelet aggregator, and to inhibit compounds such as thromboxane and leukotrienes that cause vasoconstriction, platelet aggregation, and edema. In this chapter, we outline the rationale for approaches designed to achieve these objectives and review results from experiments in which these concepts have in part been implemented.

Because prostaglandins, thromboxanes, and leukotrienes are not stored in mammalian tissues, it is generally thought that the rate of their synthesis is limited by the release of AA from membrane phospholipids through the activation of phospholipase A_2 or phospholipase C (3, 23, 35). After severe ischemia, the tissue content of free AA is increased to 20 to 40 times greater than normal (28, 30, 37). Only small changes occur in the level of prostaglandins or leukotrienes in brain, however, because depletion of tissue oxygen in severely ischemic brain restricts the conversion of AA to prostaglandin or leukotriene intermediates by the respective cyclooxygenase or 5-lipoxygenase pathways because both pathways require molecular oxygen (21). In contrast, during reperfusion of the brain after episodes of brief ischemia, there is a large accumulation of AA metabolites in the brain (14, 15). Reestablishment of blood flow restores tissue oxygen and permits the conversion of AA to prostaglandins and leukotrienes (Fig. 27.1). Conversion of AA also occurs in border zones of ischemia or in the ischemic penumbra where molecular oxygen, although limited, is available.

The concept that the conversion of AA is modified during ischemia is not new. Indomethacin and aspirin have been shown to be effective in inhibiting cyclooxygenase and preventing the conversion of AA to its vasoactive and prothrombotic metabolites, prostaglandins, and thromboxane. Clinically, cooperative studies have demonstrated beneficial effects of aspirin in patients with transient ischemic attacks (TIAs) (*see* Chapter 21, this volume). It is now accepted that many TIAs result from platelet emboli forming on ulcerative plaques in the carotid artery and that aspirin prevents platelet conversion of prostaglandin endoperoxides to thromboxane A_2 (TXA_2), a potent platelet aggregator.

The ischemic penumbra is the zone bordering a focus of ischemia where flow is decreased and without further intervention will become infarcted tissue. Restoration of flow or pharmacologic intervention, if given before irreversible injury occurs, can preserve function within the penumbra. Experimental data from studies of reperfused brain have suggested that the low levels of oxygen available in the penumbra might allow the conversion of AA to deleterious metabolites (14, 15). These AA metabolites could contribute to cell death within the penumbra by causing

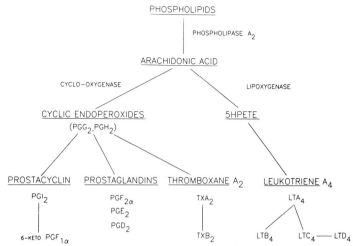

Figure 27.1. Oxidation of free arachidonic acid to prostaglandins and leukotrienes. Molecular oxygen is required.

platelet aggregation, edema, and vasoconstriction, leading to further impairment of the collateral microcirculation in ischemic areas. Increased levels of free AA within the penumbra may be converted by platelets to TXA_2 (32), which could result in platelet aggregates and vasoconstriction and could further occlude the microcirculation. Free AA and/or its metabolites, particularly leukotrienes, may also cause edema which could further compromise the microcirculation (5). Recent work to preserve tissue in the ischemic penumbra has therefore been directed in part toward attenuation of free AA accumulation and inhibition of its conversion to deleterious metabolites.

Published reports vary in their conclusions about the effectiveness of indomethacin in improving blood flow and preventing edema in ischemic animals (1, 18, 19). Hallenbeck and Furlow (18) concluded that impaired postischemic reperfusion could be prevented by pretreatment with indomethacin. Cyclooxygenase inhibition by indomethacin or aspirin before the onset of ischemia will attenuate the accumulation of TXA_2 but it will also block the conversion of AA to PGI_2 (Fig. 27.1), a potent vasodilator and antiplatelet aggregator. Thus, the beneficial effects of attenuated levels of TXA_2 by treatment with cyclooxygenase inhibitors is blunted by a concurrent inhibition of PGI_2.

Selective treatment with thromboxane synthetase inhibitors can avoid the problem of concurrent inhibition of PGI_2. Several compounds that have a selective effect on thromboxane synthetase have been synthesized and their effect in models of ischemia has been investigated (8, 16, 36). However, when administered alone, these compounds appear to have little benefit in ischemia.

PGI_2 has been administered intraarterially or intravenously, with or without indomethacin or selective thromboxane synthetase inhibitors, by several investigators (1, 18). One drawback to this approach has been the development of hypotension associated with PGI_2 infusions, which apparently is caused by vasodilation in systemic vascular beds. Hypotension in already ischemic brain that has lost its autoregulation could potentially have a greater negative impact on cerebral blood flow (CBF) and ultimate brain injury than the positive impact caused by the local vasodilation theoretically produced by the PGI_2 infusion.

Eicosapentaenoic acid (EPA) is structurally similar to AA (Fig. 27.2). It competitively inhibits the oxidation of AA by both cyclooxygenase and lipoxygenase (9, 27). As does aspirin or indomethacin, EPA prevents prostaglandin formation and thromboxane formation in platelets (17). Unlike indomethacin, however, EPA is itself oxi-

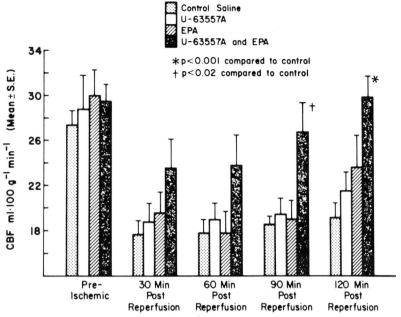

Figure 27.2. Cerebral blood flow (CBF) in gerbils before carotid artery occlusion and during 2 hours of reperfusion after ischemia in four treatment groups. U-63557A is a selective thromboxane synthetase inhibitor. EPA = eicosapentaenoic acid; SE = standard error of the mean.

dized by cyclooxygenase to a Δ^{17} prostacyclin (PGI_3).

A therapeutic potential for EPA was first suggested by the findings of Dyerberg et al (12), who noted the high content of EPA in the maritime diet of Eskimos in Greenland. EPA was implicated as an important factor in the low incidence of myocardial infarction in Eskimos (2, 10, 12). In a control group of Danes, platelet fatty acids contained 22% arachidonate, but only 0.5% EPA. In contrast, platelet fatty acids in the Eskimo group contained 8.5% arachidonate and 8% EPA. This accounted for an eicosapentaenoate/arachidonate ratio of 0.02 in Danes and 0.94 in Eskimos (11). Coagulation factors II, VII, and X, prothrombin time, and activated partial thromboplastin time were the same in Eskimos and Danes. However, platelets in 10 of 21 Eskimos tested did not aggregate in the presence of adenosine diphosphate or collagen.

Dyerberg and colleagues (10, 12) indicated that EPA could have an antiaggregatory action as a result of competitive inhibition of TXA_2 synthesis. This notion is in accord with the observation that EPA

is bound to the enzyme cyclooxygenase from the sheep vesicular gland with affinities (1.7 to 15 μM) equal to or greater than the Michaelis constant (Km) value for arachidonate. EPA is thus an effective competitive inhibitor (9, 22). On that basis, Moncada and Vane (24), citing evidence observed by Raz et al (29), have concluded that the use of EPA could afford a "dietary protection against thrombosis" (24). Nevertheless, they regard the protective effect to be due to the possibility that EPA could be used by the vessel wall to make "an antiaggregating substance, probably a . . . Δ^{17} PGI_3" and an accompanying TXA_3 that is not a "proaggregatory agent." Morita et al (25), challenging this concept, could find neither conversion of EPA to Δ^{17} 6-keto $PGF_{1\alpha}$ by cultured murine smooth muscle cells from rat aortas nor to thromboxane B_3 by rat platelets. Dyerberg et al (13) subsequently reported that human umbilical blood vessel wall transforms EPA to PGI_3 and suggested that rat cyclooxygenase may have a greater specificity in its requirements of AA than human cyclooxygenase does, and that this difference could explain why experiments using rats have failed to show a conversion of EPA to PGI₃.

Dietary supplements of EPA were shown to have a protective effect on ischemia in gerbils after bilateral carotid occlusions and reperfusion (7). In animals fed a menhaden fish-oil-enriched diet, their levels of EPA in brain—both the free and total fatty acids—significantly increased after 2 months. After severe ischemia in control animals, there was a significant decrease in CBF during reperfusion. No decrease in CBF occurred in animals receiving EPA supplements. Moreover, EPA supplements appeared also to protect animals from postischemic edema.

EPA was also shown to be beneficial in ischemia after acute administration (8). Gerbils were infused intravenously with 0.835 mg of EPA over 5 minutes before the occlusion of both carotid arteries; the infusion was continued during occlusion. With reperfusion and EPA infusion at 1 mg/hour, the gerbils showed a return of CBF to preischemic values 120 minutes after reperfusion. In contrast, the CBF in control gerbils remained depressed. The protective effect of EPA on postischemic CBF was potentiated, moreover, by concurrent administration of a selective thromboxane synthetase inhibitor, sodium 5-(3′-pyridinylmethyl)benzofuran-2-carboxylate (U-63557A) (8). In these experiments, immediately after ischemia, gerbils were given either an intravenous bolus of EPA (0.167 mg) followed by a continuous infusion of EPA (1 mg/hour), U-63557A (10 mg/kg intraperitoneally), a combination of U-63557A and EPA, or a saline solution. Regional CBF was again measured by the hydrogen clearance method. Preischemic CBFs ranged from 27.4 ml/100 g/minute to 29.5 ml/100 g/minute for all four groups. After ischemia and 2 hours of reperfusion, CBF in the saline-infused gerbils was significantly decreased to 19.2 ml/100 g/minute. Gerbils treated with only EPA had a CBF of 23.7 ml/100 g/minute, and those with only U-63557A had a CBF of 21.6 ml/100 g/minute. However, postischemic CBF in gerbils treated with a combination of U-63557A and EPA was 30.0 ml/100 g/min-

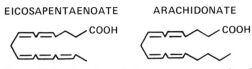

Figure 27.3. Structure of eicosapentaenoic acid and arachidonic acid.

ute, a level significantly higher than that in the saline-infused gerbils (Fig. 27.3).

EPA offers a unique potential for the treatment of ischemic injury. It is the precursor of the triene prostaglandins. It will compete with arachidonate for cyclooxygenase and 5-lipoxygenase and thus acts as an effective competitive inhibitor of AA oxidation to diene prostaglandins, TXA₂, and leukotrienes. EPA is itself, however, oxidized to PGI₃, which is a potent vasodilator and antiplatelet aggregator. It is converted to an inactive TXA₃ and also to less active leukotrienes which could act as competitive receptor blockers for the active TXA₂ and AA leukotrienes.

The potentiation of EPA's protective effects by a selective thromboxane synthetase inhibitor further denotes the importance of the prostacyclin–thromboxane balance in ischemia. In experiments where EPA and U-63557A were administered together, the prostacyclin metabolite 6-keto PGF₁α was significantly increased in ischemic brain tissue (8). This finding suggests that blockade of the thromboxane pathway may also result in shunting of EPA metabolites toward prostacyclin formation.

An advantage of EPA and thromboxane synthetase inhibition therapy over infusions of pure prostacyclin is that it avoids the systemic hypotension which occurs with pure prostacyclin infusions (1, 34). Culp et al (9) reported that EPA is a poor substrate for cyclooxygenase at peroxide levels which occur in nonischemic tissue. Increasing peroxide tone in an incubate containing cyclooxygenase increased the conversion of EPA considerably. Accordingly, in areas of ischemia where peroxide tone is higher, the formation in platelets of cyclic endoperoxides from EPA may be increased. This increase, in turn, could produce an increased transfer of these endoperoxides to the vessel wall and, subsequently, increased formation of PGI_3. In nonischemic areas, without platelet adhesion to the vessel wall and with lower peroxide levels, the formation of PGI_3 may be reduced. Prostacyclin has a very short half-life. Although levels of PGI_3 may be high in ischemic areas, the levels of circulating PGI_3—which can affect systemic resistance vessels and produce hypotension—may be low.

Leukotrienes have only recently been recognized as potentially important compounds in the chemistry of brain ischemia (20, 26, 33). Leukotrienes are hydroxylipids (LTB_4, the *LT* denoting leukotriene) and peptidolipids (LTC_4, D_4, E_4, and F_4), formally known as the slow-reacting substances of anaphylaxis which are formed from AA through the epoxide intermediate LT_{A4} (31). Peptidoleukotrienes are vasoconstrictors of the cerebral circulation (33) and increase vascular permeability in a variety of tissues, including brain (5). Leukotrienes injected directly into the brain parenchyma at doses as low as 100 ng have resulted in vasogenic edema in rats (5). Topical application of leukotrienes on the brain surface, however, does not result in large increases in vascular permeability, probably as a consequence of differences between the blood–brain barrier and the blood–pial barrier. Leukotrienes are significantly increased after a variety of brain injuries, including ischemia. There is also a significant correlation between leukotriene levels measured in brain tumors in humans and the amount of edema surrounding these tumors (6). High affinity binding sites for LTC_4 also exist on isolated brain capillaries (4). The hydroxy leukotriene LTB_4 is a potent chemotactic factor for leukocytes and generates superoxide radicals in neutrophils. During ischemia, leukotrienes may therefore contribute to edema, vasoconstriction, and free-radical-induced injury.

Several drugs inhibit AA conversion to leukotrienes by 5-lipoxygenase. Some compounds, such as BW755C, have dual actions on both cyclooxygenase and 5-lipoxygenase (5), whereas others, such as nordihydroguaiaretic acid, are more specific for 5-lipoxygenase. Inhibition of 5-lipoxygenase alone, however, may be deleterious in ischemia because AA metabolism may be shunted toward prostaglandins and thromboxane.

From a theoretical point of view, AA modification might be most beneficial if drugs were given to inhibit both 5-lipoxygenase and thromboxane synthetase concurrently. This regimen would block production of multiple deleterious products (TXA_2, leukotrienes) and might also shunt AA oxidation toward increased prostacyclin formation. Concurrent administration of the PGI_3 precursor EPA could have an additive effect.

Ischemia is a multifactorial event that is influenced by mechanisms extending beyond the AA cascade. AA metabolites can produce either beneficial or deleterious effects. Future therapies increasingly will be designed specifically to block formation of thromboxane and leukotrienes while concurrently maximizing the local production of prostacyclin in ischemic tissue.

References

1. Awad I, Little JR, Lucas F, et al: Modification of focal cerebral ischemia by prostacyclin and indomethacin. *J Neurosurg* 58:714–719, 1983.
2. Bang HO, Dyerberg J, et al: Composition of food consumed by Greenland Eskimos. *Acta Med Scand* 200:69–73, 1976.
3. Bazan NG: Free arachidonic acid and other lipids in the nervous system during early ischemia and after electroshock. In Porcellati G, Amaducci L, Galli C (eds): *Advances in Experimental Medicine and Biology. Vol 72: Function and Metabolism of Phospholipids in the Central and Peripheral Nervous System.* New York, Plenum Press, 1976, pp 317–335.
4. Black KL, Betz AL, Ar B: Leukotriene C4 receptors in isolated brain capillaries. *Adv Prostaglandin Thromboxane Leukotriene Res* 17:508–511, 1987.
5. Black KL, Hoff JT: Leukotrienes increase blood–brain barrier permeability in rats. *Ann Neurol* 18:349–351, 1985.
6. Black KL, Hoff JT, McGillicuddy JE, et al: Increased leukotriene C4 and vasogenic edema surrounding brain tumors in humans. *Ann Neurol* 19:592–595, 1986.
7. Black KL, Hoff JT, Radin NS, et al: Eicosapentaenoic acid: Effect on brain prostaglandins, cerebral blood flow and edema in ischemic gerbils. *Stroke* 15:65–69, 1984.
8. Black KL, Hsu S, Radin NS, et al: Sodium 5-(3'-pyridinylmethyl)benzofuran-2-carboxylate (U-63557A) potentiates protective effect of intravenous eicosapentaenoic acid on impaired CBF

in ischemic gerbils. *J Neurosurg* 61:453–457, 1984.

9. Culp BR, Titus BG, Lands WEM: Inhibition of prostaglandin biosynthesis by eicosapentaenoic acid. *Prostaglandins and Medicine* 3:269–278, 1979.

10. Dyerberg J, Bang HO: Dietary fat and thrombosis. *Lancet* 1:152, 1978.

11. Dyerberg J, Bang HO: Hemostatic function and platelet polyunsaturated fatty acids in Eskimos. *Lancet* 2:433–435, 1979.

12. Dyerberg J, Bang HO, Stoffersen E, et al: Eicosapentaenoic acid and prevention of thrombosis and atherosclerosis. *Lancet* 2:117–119, 1978.

13. Dyerberg J, Joregensen KA, Arnfred T: Human umbilical blood vessel converts all cis-5,8,11,14,17 eicosapentaenoic acid to prostaglandin I3. *Prostaglandins* 22:857–862, 1981.

14. Gaudet RJ, Alam I, Levine L: Accumulation of cyclooxygenase products of arachidonic acid metabolism in gerbil brain during reperfusion after bilateral common carotid artery occlusion. *J Neurochem* 35:653–658, 1980.

15. Gaudet RJ, Levine L: Transient cerebral ischemia and brain prostaglandins. *Biochem Biophys Res Commun* 86:893–901, 1979.

16. Gorman RR, Johnson RA, Spilman CH, et al: Inhibition of platelet thromboxane A2 synthase activity by sodium 5-(3′-pyridinylmethyl) benzofuran-2-carboxylate. *Prostaglandins* 26:325–342, 1983.

17. Haddeman EA: Fish oil feeding and prostaglandin synthesis. In Foerster W (ed): *Proceedings of the Third International Symposium on Prostaglandins, Thromboxane, and the Cardiovascular System.* Oxford, England, Pergamon, 1981, pp. 191–195.

18. Hallenbeck JM, Furlow TW: Prostaglandin I2 and indomethacin prevent impairment of post-ischemic brain reperfusion in the dog. *Stroke* 10:629–637, 1979.

19. Iannotti F, Crockard A, Ladds G, et al: Are prostaglandins involved in experimental ischemic edema in gerbils? *Stroke* 12:301–306, 1981.

20. Kiwak KJ, Moskowitz MA, Levine L: Leukotriene production in gerbil brain after ischemic insult, subarachnoid hemorrhage, and concussive injury. *J Neurosurg* 62:865–869, 1985.

21. Lands WEM: The biosynthesis and metabolism of prostaglandins. *Annu Rev Physiol* 41:633–652, 1979.

22. Lands WEM, LeTellier PR, Rome LH, et al: Inhibition of prostaglandin biosynthesis (abstract). *Advances in Biosciences* 9:15, 1973.

23. Lands WEM, Samuelsson B: Phospholipid precursor of prostaglandins. *Biochim Biophys Acta* 164:426–429, 1968.

24. Moncada S, Vane JR: The role of prostacyclin in vascular tissue. *Fed Proc* 38:66–71, 1979.

25. Morita I, Saito Y, Chang WC, et al: Effects of purified eicosapentaenoic acid on arachidonic acid metabolism in cultured murine aortic smooth muscle cells, vessel walls and platelets. *Lipids* 18:42–49, 1983.

26. Moskowitz MA, Kiwak KJ, Hekimian K, et al: Synthesis of compounds with properties of leukotrienes C4 and D4 in gerbil brains after ischemia and reperfusion. *Science* 224:886–888, 1984.

27. Needleman P, Raz A, Minkes MS, et al: Triene prostaglandins: Prostacyclin and thromboxane biosynthesis and unique biological properties. *Proc Natl Acad Sci USA* 76:944–948, 1979.

28. Porcellati G, DeMedio GE, Fini C, et al: Phospholipid and its metabolism in ischemia. In Neuhoff V (ed): *European Society for Neurochemistry.* Weinheim, Verlag Chemie, 1978, pp 285–303.

29. Raz A, Minkes MS, Needleman P: Endoperoxides and thromboxanes. Structural determinants for platelet aggregation and vasoconstriction. *Biochim Biophys Acta* 488:305–311, 1977.

30. Rehncrona S, Westerberg E, Akesson B, et al: Brain cortical fatty acids and phospholipids during and following complete and severe incomplete ischemia. *J Neurochem* 38:84–93, 1982.

31. Samuelsson B: Leukotrienes: Mediators of immediate hypersensitivity reactions and inflammation. *Science* 220:568–575, 1983.

32. Smith JB, Araki H, Lefer AM: Thromboxane A2, prostacyclin and aspirin: Effects on vascular tone and platelet aggregation. *Circulation (Suppl V):* 62:V19—V25, 1980.

33. Tagari P, Du Boulay GH, Aitken V, et al: Leukotriene D4 and the cerebral vasculature in vivo and in vitro. *Prostaglandins Leukotrienes Med* 11:281–297, 1983.

34. van den Kerckhoff W, Hossmann KA, Hossmann V: No effect of prostacyclin on blood flow, regulation of blood flow and blood coagulation following global cerebral ischemia. *Stroke* 14:724–730, 1983.

35. Wolfe LS: Eicosanoids, prostaglandins, thromboxanes, leukotrienes, and other derivatives of carbon-20 unsaturated fatty acids. Short review. *J Neurochem* 38:1–14, 1982.

36. Wynalda MA, Liggett WF, Fitzpatrick FA: Sodium 5-(3′-pyridinylmethyl) benzofuran-2-carboxylate (U-63557A), a new, selective thromboxane synthase inhibitor: Intravenous and oral pharmacokinetics in dogs and correlations with ex situ thromboxane B2 production. *Prostaglandins* 26:311–324, 1983.

37. Yoshida S, Inoh S, Asano T, et al: Brain free fatty acids and their peroxidation in ischemic and post ischemic brain injury (abstract). *Stroke* 11:128–1980.

CHAPTER TWENTY-EIGHT

Intravascular Techniques for Angioplasty and Thrombolysis

Randall T. Higashida, M.D.
Grant B. Hieshima, M.D.
Van V. Halbach, M.D.

Interventional neurovascular techniques for increasing perfusion to the cerebral circulation are gaining acceptance as favorable results are reported from a growing number of centers. This chapter describes two of those techniques: angioplasty and thrombolysis. Percutaneous transluminal angioplasty (PTA) may be used to treat hemodynamically significant stenosis of the innominate, subclavian, internal and external carotid, and vertebral arteries (3, 7, 16, 22, 26, 28, 30). It is most effective for atherosclerotic disease, but has also been used to treat fibromuscular dysplasia (2, 11), vasculitis (17), postoperative stenosis (29), and intracranial arterial vasospasm after subarachnoid hemorrhage (SAH) (36). Thrombolytic therapy for acute thromboembolic disease is performed by superselective catheterization of intracranial arteries to deliver streptokinase or urokinase directly to the site of occlusion (34).

PERCUTANEOUS TRANSLUMINAL ANGIOPLASTY

Preliminary Considerations

PTA techniques should be used only after careful consideration of the clinical and radiologic findings and consultation with the vascular surgeon, neurosurgeon, and interventional neuroradiologist. Only patients who have recurrent symptoms of cerebral vascular insufficiency that localize to the territory of the involved artery and do not respond to medical therapy should be considered for angioplasty.

The basic preliminary examination should include Doppler studies of blood flow; angiography to determine the extent of stenosis, seek evidence of ulceration, and evaluate collateral blood flow; and computerized tomographic (CT) brain scanning to rule out infarction. More sophisticated imaging techniques may supply additional information. These include magnetic resonance imaging of blood flow; cerebral blood flow (CBF) and cerebral blood volume studies with acetazolamide or carbon dioxide; positron emission tomography to determine CBF, cerebral blood volume, and cerebral oxygen use; fast scanning, contrast-enhanced CT of the supraaortic vessels; and echotomography of the carotid bifurcation (4, 10, 12, 19, 26, 31).

Initially, PTA was used to treat patients with symptomatic lesions in vessels that are difficult or impossible to access surgically, such as the innominate, proximal carotid, and prevertebral subclavian arteries. The favorable results from early studies and the low morbidity and mortality rates, particularly in patients with thromboembolic complications, shown by follow-up studies led to application of PTA for high cervical and intracranial carotid lesions and lesions of the cervical carotid bifurcation (11, 16, 30).

Technique

Balloon angioplasty for atherosclerotic disease involves mechanical disruption of the calcified plaque surrounding the intima and media. Histologically, it can be seen that the plaque is disrupted and split, leading to actual dehiscence of the intimal layer of the vessel wall. In areas where this has occurred, platelets are deposited and a layer of fibrin forms over the site of injury. As healing occurs over time, the intimal flaps retract, and scar tissue and neointima form (5, 35).

Patients undergoing PTA of the supraaortic vessels are given oral or parenteral anticoagulants for at least 5 days before the procedure. Under local anesthesia (5 ml of 1% lidocaine), a 5.0 to 7.5 French sheath is placed in the femoral or axillary artery by the Seldinger technique. Five thousand units of heparin are given intravenously for systemic anticoagulation. Under fluoroscopic guidance, a 5.5 French catheter is advanced to the site of stenosis, and a 260-cm exchange guide wire 0.035 inch in diameter is advanced beyond the area to be treated. Over this guide wire, a smoothly tapered 5.0 to 7.0 French polyethylene catheter is guided across the atherosclerotic plaque to mechanically dilate the lesion to 7.0 French diameter (2.34 mm). The catheter is immediately removed, and a balloon angioplasty catheter is passed over the guide wire. The balloon is inflated once or twice across the atheromatous plaque for 8 to 10 seconds until the stenosis is seen to dilate fluoroscopically.

The balloon catheter and guide wire are removed, and the patient is rechecked neurologically. An arteriogram is obtained to assess the patency of the vessel and the extent of intimal and medial injury and to evaluate the intracranial circulation for evidence of distal embolization. The patient is closely monitored for 24 hours and, if stable, is discharged on a regimen of aspirin (325 to 650 mg/day) and/or dipyridamole (75 to 150 mg/day). This therapy is continued for at least 6 months after the procedure. Patients are followed clinically at 1-, 3-, and 12-month intervals, and angiography is repeated at 3 to 12 months to assess the angioplasty site.

Vertebral Basilar Insufficiency

The vast majority of patients with symptoms of vertebral basilar insufficiency, transient ischemic attacks, or strokes involving the posterior circulation can be managed conservatively with antiplatelet agents and anticoagulants (8, 18, 33). Clinically, these patients present with symptoms of subclavian "steal" syndrome, vertigo, drop attacks, vascular headaches, ataxia, weakness, and diplopia. Other, less common symptoms include transient cortical blindness, memory disturbance, nystagmus, visual agnosia, and poor eye–hand coordination. Most patients with stenosis or occlusion of one vertebral artery are asymptomatic. In patients with high-grade stenoses of both subclavian and/or vertebral arteries who do not respond to medical therapy, PTA may be beneficial (Fig. 28.1).

Innominate and Carotid Arteries

Transluminal angioplasty of the innominate and carotid arteries arising from the aortic arch has been reported from several centers (27, 32). Patients with stenosis of these vessels present with transient ischemic events involving the anterior circulation, ophthalmic symptoms, repetitive strokes, and/or subclavian steal syndrome.

Whether to treat atherosclerotic disease of the carotid bifurcation medically or surgically has been controversial. The operative morbidity and mortality rates have been reported to be 1% to 8%. Similar risks have been reported for PTA in this territory (3, 26, 30), although long-term follow-up data are still not available. In most cases, carotid endarterectomy remains the procedure of choice unless medical risks are a contraindication to surgical treatment (Fig. 28.2).

Results of Percutaneous Transluminal Angioplasty

PTA of brachiocephalic vessels for hemodynamically significant atherosclerotic lesions has been successfully performed in the following territories as documented in two large studies (15, 26): innominate artery (12 cases), proximal subclavian artery (106 cases), vertebral artery (36 cases), common carotid artery (29 cases), external carotid artery (5 cases), and internal ca-

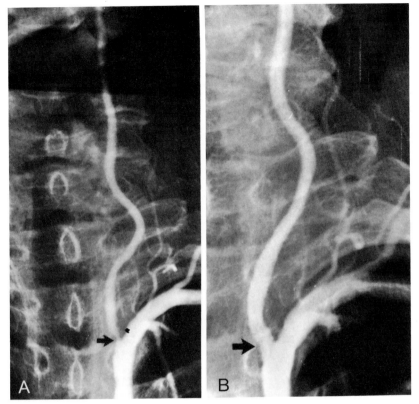

Figure 28.1.   Vertebral artery angioplasty. *A,* angiogram showing high-grade stenosis of the proximal left vertebral artery *(arrow)* in a patient with symptoms of vertebral basilar insufficiency. *B,* after successful dilatation with a 4.0-mm balloon catheter, luminal diameter of the vertebral artery returned to normal *(arrow),* and the symptoms resolved.

rotid artery (37 cases). There were no deaths related to the procedure, and only two of the 225 angioplasty procedures caused significant morbidity. One patient had transient cerebral ischemia that resolved after 5 minutes, and one patient suffered permanent unilateral blindness after carotid angioplasty. Angiograms obtained 3 to 12 months after the procedure showed that the angioplasty sites were widely patent in all cases; no patient required a second angioplasty. Clinical follow-up of these patients ranged from 6 months to 4 years (mean, 27 months).

INTRACRANIAL ARTERIAL VASOSPASM

Many pharmacologic agents have been used in an attempt to prevent or reverse the effects of cerebral vasospasm after SAH, including sympathomimetic amines, adrenergic blocking agents, parasympathomimetic drugs, prostaglandins, local anesthetics, and calcium antagonists, but no regimen consistently decreases the serious morbidity associated with vasospasm resulting in ischemia and infarction (6, 24, 25).

Transluminal angioplasty for arterial vasospasm after SAH was first reported by Zubkov et al (36) in 1984; they performed 105 dilatations of vasospastic arteries in 33 patients. Focal as well as diffuse areas of vasospasm were effectively dilated under local anesthesia, and there was radiographic and clinical evidence of improved cerebral perfusion after the procedure. The effect of angioplasty, they concluded, was stable and long lasting; the functional state of the brain improved, and focal neurologic signs regressed.

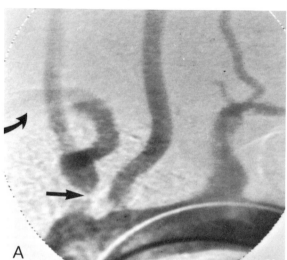
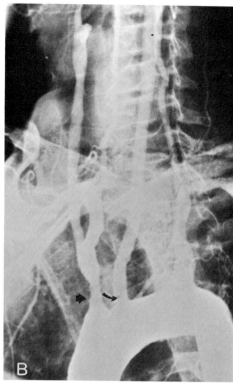

Figure 28.2. *A,* angiogram showing a high-grade (>90%) stenosis of innominate artery *(straight arrow)* due to severe atherosclerotic disease. Note very poor filling of the right subclavian artery *(curved arrow)*. *B,* after transluminal angioplasty, angiogram shows that the innominate artery is widely patent *(straight arrow)* and perfusion to subclavian artery is improved. Angioplasty of the common carotid artery was also performed *(curved arrow)*.

We have performed angioplasty of vasospastic vessels with a nondetachable, custom-designed, silicone microballoon (Interventional Therapeutics Corporation, San Francisco, CA). In our series of 13 patients (14), we have dilated focal and diffuse areas of spasm in the basilar, posterior cerebral, internal carotid, anterior cerebral, and middle cerebral arteries in 36 vascular territories. After angioplasty, particularly when performed within 24 hours after the onset of neurologic deficit, we have seen immediate improvement in neurologic function and angiographic demonstration of increased cerebral blood flow. Despite angioplasty, four patients continued to deteriorate and eventually died.

Thus, PTA for vasospasm of intracranial vessels after SAH appears to be feasible, although more research in animal models and clinical trials in patients who do not respond to medical therapy are needed. In

some instances (e.g. when medical therapy including hypertension and hypervolemia fails), PTA may reverse the state of hypoperfusion in the larger vessels at the base of the brain (Fig. 28.3) (13).

Thrombolytic Techniques

Fibrinolysis is the continuous physiologic process by which insoluble fibrin is broken down into soluble degradation products in order to maintain vascular patency (23). The agent mediating fibrinolysis is plasmin, a proteolytic enzyme derived from plasminogen. It is the activation of plasminogen to plasmin that stimulates fibrinolysis. Streptokinase and urokinase are the pharmacologic agents most commonly used to activate this system (20).

The idea of using thrombolytic agents to increase blood supply to the ischemic area

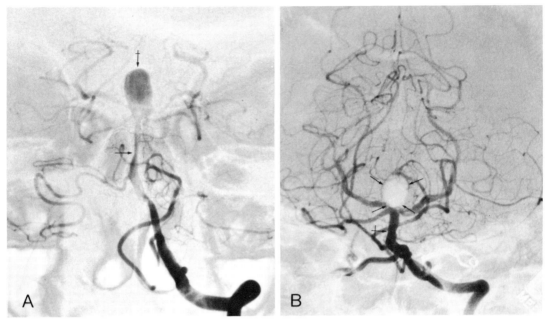

Figure 28.3. Angioplasty for vasospasm of the basilar artery. *A,* angiogram showing vasospasm of the midbasilar artery *(arrow)* caused by hemorrhage of a large distal basilar artery aneurysm *(crossed arrow). B,* angiogram obtained after transluminal angioplasty of the basilar artery and placement of a detachable balloon into the aneurysm shows normal luminal diameter of the basilar artery *(crossed arrow),* and complete obliteration of the aneurysm by the balloon *(arrows).* (From Hieshima GB, Higashida RT, Wapenski J, et al: Balloon embolization of a large distal basilar artery aneurysm. *J Neurosurg* 65:413–416, 1986.)

and surrounding viable tissue in acute cerebral infarction is controversial, but theoretically attractive. In early studies, thrombolytic agents were administered systemically by the intravenous route, but the results were disappointing owing to hemorrhagic complications (1, 9, 21). More recently, local intraarterial thrombolysis has been used, particularly for thromboembolic disease in the vertebral basilar territory. In 1983, Zeumer et al (34) reported five cases in which a transfemoral catheter was guided into the vertebral and basilar arteries, and streptokinase, 200,000 IU over 4 hours, was delivered directly to the site of occlusion to lyse the thrombus. The procedure was successful in three cases. In 1986, Bruckmann et al* reported 67 patients with acute basilar thrombosis; 14

were treated with local intraarterial streptokinase. Seven of the patients died, and seven survived with moderate to mild neurologic complications.

Although the risk of intracranial bleeding limits the use of thrombolytic agents for cerebral vascular occlusion, this approach may be justified for patients with impending brain stem infarction.

References

1. Abe T, Kazama M: Thrombolytic therapy of cerebrovascular occlusive disease. In Yamori Y, Lovenberg W, Freis ED (eds): *Prophylactic Approach to Hypertensive Diseases.* New York, Raven Press, 1977, pp 441–447.
2. Belan A, Vesela M, Vanek I, et al: Percutaneous transluminal angioplasty of fibromuscular dysplasia of the internal carotid artery. *Cardiovasc Intervent Radiol* 5:79–81, 1982.
3. Bockenheimer S, Mathias K: Percutaneous transluminal angioplasty in arteriosclerotic internal carotid artery stenosis. *AJNR* 4:791–792, 1983.
4. Bullock R, Mendelow AD, Bone I, et al: Cerebral blood flow and CO_2 responsiveness as an indicator of collateral reserve capacity in patients with carotid arterial disease. *Br J Surg* 14:882–886, 1982.

*H Bruckmann, A Ferbert, H Zeumer: The acute basilar thrombosis. Angiological, clinical comparison and therapeutic implications. Presented at the 13th Symposium Neuroradiologicum, Stockholm, Sweden, 1986.

5. Castaneda-Zuniga WR, Sibley R, Amplatz K: The pathologic basis of angioplasty. *Angiology* 35:195–205, 1984.

6. Chyatte D, Rusch N, Sundt TM Jr: Prevention of chronic experimental cerebral vasospasm with ibuprofen and high-dose methylprednisolone. *J Neurosurg* 59:925–932, 1983.

7. Damuth HD Jr, Diamond AB, Rappoport AS, et al: Angioplasty of subclavian artery stenosis proximal to the vertebral origin. *AJNR* 4:1239–1242, 1983.

8. Dyken ML: Anticoagulant and platelet antiaggregating therapy in stroke and threatened stroke. *Neurol Clin* 1:223–242, 1983.

9. Fletcher AP, Alkjaersig N, Lewis M, et al: A pilot study of urokinase therapy in cerebral infarction. *Stroke* 7:135–142, 1976.

10. Gibbs JM, Wise RJS, Leenders KL, et al: Evaluation of cerebral perfusion reserve in patients with carotid artery occlusion. *Lancet* 1:182–186, 1984.

11. Hasso AN, Bird CR, Zinke DE, et al: Fibromuscular dysplasia of the internal carotid artery. Percutaneous transluminal angioplasty. *AJNR* 2:175–180, 1981.

12. Hauge A, Nicolaysen G, Thoresen M: Acute effects of acetazolamide on cerebral blood flow in man. *Acta Physiol Scand* 177:233–239, 1983.

13. Hieshima GB, Higashida RT, Wapenski J, et al: Balloon embolization of a large distal basilar artery aneurysm. *J Neurosurg* 65:413–416, 1986.

14. Higashida RT, Halbach VV, Cahan LC, et al: Transluminal angioplasty of intracerebral vessels for treatment of intracranial arterial vasospasm. *J Neurosurg*, in press.

15. Higashida RT, Halbach VV, Tsai FY, et al: Percutaneous transluminal angioplasty of brachiocephalic vessels. In Margulis AR, Gooding CA (eds): *Diagnostic Radiology*. San Francisco, University of California, 1987, pp 303–308.

16. Higashida RT, Hieshima GB, Tsai FY, et al: Transluminal angioplasty of the vertebral and basilar artery. *AJNR* 8:745–749, 1987.

17. Hodgins EW, Dutton JW: Subclavian and carotid angioplasties for Takayasa's arteritis. *J Can Assoc Radiol* 33:305–307, 1982.

18. Kistler JP, Roppo AH, Heros RC: Therapy of ischemic cerebral vascular disease due to atherothrombosis. *N Engl J Med* 311:100–105, 1984.

19. Lesson MD, Cacayorin ED, Iliya AR, et al: Atheromatous extracranial carotid arteries: CT evaluation correlated with arteriography and pathologic examination. *Radiology* 156:397–402, 1985.

20. Marder V: The use of thrombolytic agents: Choice of patient, drug administration and laboratory monitoring. *Ann Intern Med* 90:802–808, 1979.

21. Meyer JS, Gilroy S, Bonnhart MI, et al: Anticoagulant plus streptokinase therapy in progressive stroke. *JAMA* 189:373, 1964.

22. Motarjeme A, Keifer JW, Zuaka AJ: Percutaneous transluminal angioplasty of the brachiocephalic arteries. *AJNR* 3:169–174, 1982.

23. Sharma G, Cella G, Parisi A, et al: Thrombolytic therapy. *N Engl J Med* 306:1268–1276, 1982.

24. Sundt TM Jr: Chemical management of cerebral vasospasm. In Whisnant JP, Sandok BA (eds): *Cerebral Vascular Disease* (Transactions of the 9th Princeton Conference). New York, Grune & Stratton, 1974, pp 77–81.

25. Tani E, Maeda Y, Fukumori T: Effect of selective inhibitor of thromboxane A_2 synthetase on cerebral vasospasm after early surgery. *J Neurosurg* 61:24–29, 1984.

26. Theron JG: Angioplasty of supraaortic arteries. *Semin Intervent Radiol* 4:331–342, 1987.

27. Theron J, Courtheoux P, Henriet JP, et al: Angioplasty of supraaortic arteries. *J Neuroradiol* 11:187–200, 1984.

28. Theron J, Melancon D, Ethier R: "Pre" subclavian steal syndromes and their treatment by angioplasty. *Neuroradiology* 27:265–270, 1985.

29. Tievsky AL, Dray EM, Mardiat JG: Transluminal angioplasty in postsurgical stenosis of the extracranial artery. *AJNR* 4:800–802, 1983.

30. Tsai FY, Matovich V, Hieshima GB, et al: Percutaneous transluminal angioplasty of the carotid artery. *AJNR* 7:349–358, 1986.

31. Tsuruda J, Halbach V, Higashida RT, et al: MR evaluation of large and giant aneurysms using cine low flip angle gradient-refocused imaging. *AJNR* 9:415–424, 1988.

32. Vitek JJ, Raymond BC, Oh SJ: Innominate artery angioplasty. *AJNR* 5:113–114, 1984.

33. Waksler BB, Lewin MC: Anticoagulation in cerebral ischemia. *Stroke* 14:658–663, 1983.

34. Zeumer H, Hacke W, Ringelstein EB: Local intraarterial thrombolysis in vertebrobasilar thromboembolic disease. *AJNR* 4:401–404, 1983.

35. Zollikofer CL, Salomonowitz E, Sibley R, et al: Transluminal angioplasty evaluated by electron microscopy. *Radiology* 153:369–374, 1984.

36. Zubkov YN, Nikiforov BM, Shustin VA: Balloon catheter technique for dilatation of constricted cerebral arteries after aneurysmal SAH. *Acta Neurochir (Wien)* 70:665–679, 1984.

CHAPTER TWENTY-NINE

Surgical Revascularization for Acute Occlusion: Theoretical and Practical Considerations

Robert M. Crowell, M.D.
Jafar J. Jafar, M.D.

EMERGENCY CEREBRAL REVASCULARIZATION

Emergency cerebral revascularization is a controversial approach to the treatment of acute ischemia. On the one hand, there is a rationale for the approach. Some experimental data indicate that, during a period of some 4 to 6 hours after arterial occlusion, focal cerebral ischemia may be fully reversible (13, 15, 27). Medical measures that have been proposed for future evaluation could prolong this "golden period" (29, 47, 49). Clinical and experimental observations suggest that, at least theoretically, rapid revascularization could restore circulation to resuscitate paralyzed but still viable neurons (19, 23, 34, 41). On the other hand, some other experimental and clinical data suggest the inadequacy or even deleterious effects of emergency revascularization (20, 43). In this chapter, we review the rationale and techniques for several forms of emergency brain revascularization, as well as their results and complications. We offer an opinion about current indications for this approach and possible future applications.

THRESHOLDS OF ISCHEMIA AND INFARCTION

Adequate perfusion is required to maintain the normal function and structure of the brain. Specific thresholds for minimal levels of adequate cerebral blood flow (CBF) have been identified for a variety of reversible dysfunctions (2).

CBF determinations and the electroencephalogram (EEG) during carotid endarterectomy show EEG slowing when hemispheric blood flow falls to 16 to 20 ml/100 g/minute (39). Baboons lose somatosensory evoked potentials when regional CBF (rCBF) falls below 15 ml/100 g/minute (8). Neuronal firing in anesthesized cats ceases when rCBF falls below 18 ml/100 g/minute (24). In monkeys, average hemispheral CBF below 23 ml/100 g/minute causes a mild neurologic deficit (Fig. 29.1) and CBF below 8 ml/100 g/minute causes flaccid hemiplegia (27).

The threshold of energy failure to a level producing loss of membrane function is a lethal insult that causes cellular damage (3). Infarction corresponds to the zones with CBF of less than 10 ml/100 g/minute in baboons. According to Morawetz et al (33), infarction is a function of intensity and duration of ischemia. Monkeys with very brief middle cerebral artery (MCA) occlusions tolerate marked ischemia without evidence of infarction. For permanent MCA occlusion, local CBF of 17 to 18 ml/100 g/minute causes infarction (*see also* Chapter 1, this volume). Data from these studies suggests an infarction threshold, rising over 6 to 8 hours to a plateau.

The concept of a threshold for infarction in a core region, with a surrounding penumbra of moderate ischemia in which there is loss of synaptic transmission without cell necrosis, is useful in the management of acute ischemic stroke. It implies that some cases of fresh hemiplegia with CBF

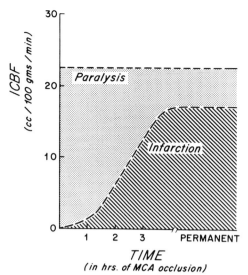

Figure 29.1. Thresholds of ischemia and infarction. Correlation of reduction in cerebral blood flow (CBF) with infarction in awake monkeys with temporary middle cerebral artery (MCA) occlusion. CBF below 23 ml/100 g/minute results in reversible paralysis. Long-lasting ischemia below 17 to 18 ml/100 g/minute results in permanent infarction. Note that CBF recovery to levels above 23 ml/100 g/minute may result in full recovery unless CBF previously has fallen below the infarction threshold. lCBF = local cerebral blood flow. (From Jones TH, Morawetz RB, Crowell RM, et al: Thresholds of focal cerebral ischemia in awake monkeys. *J Neurosurg* 54:773–782, 1981.)

in the range in which neurons become inactivated might improve with surgical revascularization. Recovery of animals and patients observed after the restoration of MCA blood flow following a few hours of occlusion supports this theory. However, in cases of acute hemiplegia with a core region of CBF in the range of infarction for a sufficiently long interval, restoration of CBF will be of no benefit. Moreover, ischemic edema may be exacerbated by reperfusion because it may extend infarction by further reducing flow in the penumbra.

DIAGNOSIS OF ACUTE ISCHEMIA AND INFARCTION

There are no clinically applicable methods that unequivocally distinguish infarction from reversible ischemia (3, 16, 48). Magnetic resonance (MR) imaging may be a promising diagnostic method, however, because it can detect experimentally induced cerebral infarction within 3 hours after its onset (17). Emergency computerized tomographic (CT) determination of regional CBF (rCBF) using the xenon-133 inhalation technique or single photon emission CT might be useful to select patients for surgical revascularization or to document transgression of the infarction threshold that has been defined in experimental studies of primates (27); *see also* Chapter 8, this volume).

Angiographic studies are helpful in determining the mechanism of vascular insult. The angiographic pathology may include distal emboli or occlusion of conducting and perforating arterial branches. Collateral circulation and vessels suitable for anastomosis may also be visualized. Carotid endarterectomy or distal bypass is unlikely to remedy ischemia resulting from multiple embolic occlusions or obstruction of deep perforating branches.

PROTECTIVE THERAPY

Many medical therapies have been evaluated experimentally to assess their effectiveness in improving the outcome after revascularization for ischemia, but none has been established as clinically effective (*see* Chapter 18, this volume). Osmotic agents such as mannitol reduce cerebral edema and improve CBF (26, 47). Barbiturate coma may, under certain experimental conditions, diminish the size of the infarct (40, 41), but its clinical use is controversial (*see* Chapter 24, this volume). Hypervolemic hemodilution has been shown to increase CBF and decrease infarct size in experimental animals (49). Induced hypertension has been shown to be of some benefit (28), and perfluorochemicals may improve oxygenation of the brain (47).

EMERGENCY CAROTID ENDARTERECTOMY

Observations that focal cerebral ischemia may be reversible in its early stages provide a rationale for attempting emergency carotid endarterectomy to restore flow through occluded or stenotic internal carotid arteries in patients with incomplete or unstable stroke (31). During the 1960s, discouraging results appeared in several reports which indicated that emergency endarterectomy led to cerebral hemorrhage and neurologic deterioration (9). Careful scrutiny of these reports indicates, however, that hemorrhage sometimes occurred on the opposite side from surgery and almost always occurred in conjunction with postoperative hypertension (11). Later experience has suggested that, in selected cases, good results can be obtained with emergency endarterectomy if meticulous efforts to control blood pressure are applied during the postoperative period (35). For patients who have unstable ischemic neurologic syndromes with mild to moderate disability which may progress to severe disability without treatment, we believe a diagnosis should be established as quickly as possible and then a rational program of treatment instituted, which in appropriate candidates could include emergency endarterectomy. This approach has been taken in several centers with encouraging results in the surgical treatment of selected acute stroke patients. (22, 44).

Evaluation for Emergency Endarterectomy

A thorough medical history and careful neurologic examination will lead to a correct diagnosis in a high percentage of patients with acute ischemia. Almost every patient admitted to the hospital for an acute stroke should have an electrocardiogram (ECG) and an immediate CT scan to differentiate between infarction and hemorrhage (10). Laboratory tests should include a complete blood count, blood chemistry determinations, and coagulation studies.

If the medical history, the findings of the examination, or both suggest carotid arterial disease, then angiography should be done immediately (Fig. 29.2A). Angiograms are particularly important if the patient has had an increasing frequency severity of transient ischemic attacks (TIAs)

during the days preceding evaluation or has the sudden onset of a mild to moderate progressive or fluctuating neurologic deficit. TIAs that last more than 1 hour and those involving face, arm, and leg are particularly worrisome and should be investigated promptly. If there is a severe stenosis with delayed perfusion, thrombus in the lumen distal to stenosis, or carotid occlusion with reflux to the intrapetrous segment of the carotid artery, then emergency endarterectomy should be performed in order to allow maximum blood flow to ischemic brain tissue, to prevent extension of a thrombus, and to remove a potential source of embolization. Intraluminal thrombi within the internal carotid artery may be treated medically with heparin, thus obviating the need for emergency endarterectomy, according to recent reports (7, 36). A stenosis with residual lumen diameter greater than 2.0 mm (not hemodynamically significant) or ulceration in the plaque at the carotid bifurcation suggests that an embolus is the cause of the problem; the patient should be considered for anticoagulation therapy rather than surgical therapy. If an acute neurologic deficit occurs with loss of a previously documented carotid bruit, emergency endarterectomy should be undertaken without CT scan or angiography. In such a case, the family should be involved in the decision-making and should see the patient to appreciate the devastating deficit before surgical intervention (32). When the patient has a reduced level of consciousness, restoration of blood flow, whether by emergency carotid endarterectomy or extracranial-to-intracranial (EC–IC) arterial bypass graft, has not been beneficial.

Surgical Technique

The technique of carotid endarterectomy is modified for emergency use (34). Every effort is made to expedite the procedure in order to minimize the progressive damage of acute ischemia. If there is a complete occlusion, then EEG monitoring may be omitted. While efforts to prepare for endarterectomy are underway, the blood pressure is elevated with intravenous blood

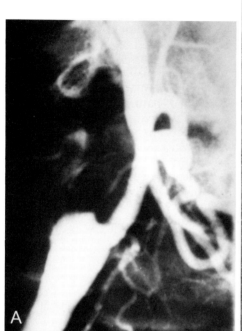
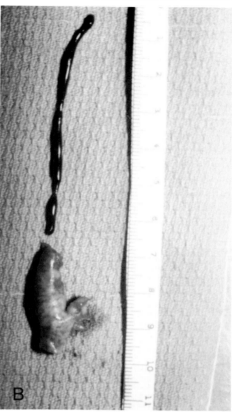

Figure 29.2.   Emergency carotid endarterectomy. *A*, angiogram shows complete occlusion of the left internal carotid artery 8 hours after the onset of moderate dysphasia and right hemiparesis. *B*, plaque and fresh thrombus were removed at endarterectomy, resulting in excellent backflow. The patient gradually achieved complete recovery within a few hours.

volume expansion, a dopamine infusion, or both to increase mean arterial blood pressure (MABP) by 30%. The carotid bifurcation is rapidly exposed. In the case of complete or nearly complete occlusion, a shunt is usually not required; occasionally, when a patient has a large common-to-external carotid collateral circulation to the brain, we have used a common-to-external carotid intraluminal shunt during surgery.

When the angiogram indicates that the internal carotid artery is completely occluded, in most cases a thrombus will be disclosed at surgery. In many of these patients there will be good backflow, but some will have a further obstruction distally. If there is a long-standing occlusion, the thrombosed artery may be a firm, fibrous cord. Hugenholtz and Elgie (25) noted that the angiographic pattern correlates with

the ability to obtain backflow. They were able to reopen the vessel in 19 (53%) of their 35 patients with an occluded carotid artery. There was good correlation between observations of internal carotid backflow and the collateral circulation to the distal internal carotid artery: The artery could be reopened in six (33%) of 18 patients who had modest retrograde filling of the intracranial carotid, and in 13 (87%) of 15 patients with good retrograde filling of the intracranial internal carotid arteries.

Certain techniques may help in opening the completely occluded artery. If a thrombus is encountered in the internal carotid artery, an effort is made to withdraw it gradually using a hand-over-hand technique (Fig. 29.2*B*). Thrombi as long as 20 cm have been removed in this way. If this technique fails, a smooth-ended suction catheter is introduced into the internal carotid lumen and suction is applied to withdraw the thrombus. If this method also fails, a Fogarty No. 3 catheter is passed gently into the occluded artery as far as the base of the skull, then is inflated and withdrawn; care is required to avoid injuring the distal internal carotid artery and causing development of a carotid–cavernous fistula. Measurements made on the angiogram from the internal carotid bifurcation to the base of the skull may be helpful in determining the length of catheter which may be inserted safely. A single lateral intraoperative angiogram made after injection of 10 ml of contrast agent is recommended to document restoration of blood flow while confirming that no initial flap or distal thrombus is present.

If good backflow and a satisfactory angiographic confirmation cannot be achieved, then the internal carotid artery is doubly ligated with 0 silk suture and its origin is plicated with 3–0 continuous suture to avoid formation of a stump that might release emboli to the external carotid circulation. In such cases, anticoagulation therapy may be considered to avert propagation of clot or embolization. When flow can be reestablished, anticoagulation should be continued throughout the postoperative period in order to avoid recurrent thrombosis at the operative site. Heparin at 500 U/hour for 12 hours is recommended, followed by full heparinization to maintain a partial thromboplastin time of about 60 seconds. Heparinization may be continued for several days, after which a decision is made regarding therapy with warfarin sodium. For patients who have had carotid occlusion or in whom recurrent thrombosis is particularly feared, we have favored warfarin sodium therapy for a period of approximately 3 months.

Results of Emergency Endarterectomy

Because the reported results obtained with emergency carotid endarterectomy cannot be compared with angiographically controlled natural history data and because a randomized prospective study has not yet been accomplished, support for advocating the use of emergency endarterectomy relies on cumulative empirical evidence. We base indications for surgical treatment on our previous experience with emergency carotid endarterectomy in 55 consecutive patients (34). Table 29.1 correlates the outcome of surgery with the patient's preoperative status. Patients with crescendo TIAs had severe stenosis with either an intraluminal thrombus or marked reduction of flow in the distal internal carotid artery. Patients with mild to moderate neurologic deficits may have been stable or have had progressing or fluctuating deficits. In the series of 36 patients with recurrent or crescendo TIAs, acute mild to moderate deficit, or progressive or fluctuating deficit, 29 patients had an excellent or good outcome. There was one death in this group; the patient had complete neurologic recovery but then died of a cardiopulmonary complication. There were two patients whose neurologic deficit was worse after the operation. Several patients had substantial neurologic recoveries in the immediate postoperative period. In the series reported by Goldstone and Moore (22), 27

Table 29.1. Results of Emergency Carotid Endarterectomy

Preoperative neurologic status	Outcome								Total
	Excellent		Good		Poor		Death		
	n	Percent	n	Percent	n	Percent	n	Percent	n
Transient ischemic attacks	4	100							4
Mild deficit	2	50	2	50					4
Moderate deficit	7	25	14	50	6	21.4	1	3.6	28
Sudden severe deficit	1	5.3	5	26.3	6	31.6	7	36.8	19
Total	14	25.5	21	38.2	12	21.9	8	14.5	55

of 28 patients presenting with crescendo TIAs or stroke-in-evolution made a prompt recovery after emergency carotid endarterectomy; one patient died from a brain stem stroke.

Patients who have sudden severe onset of neurologic deficit rarely benefit from endarterectomy (34). In 19 such cases, we noted seven deaths, six poor outcomes, and only one recovery to an excellent condition—a development that may be related to operating on this patient within 1 hour of the onset of neurologic deficit. Five of the seven deaths were related to extensive cerebral infarction and edema and two were from myocardial infarction. These cases were early in our experience, and we now rarely operate on such patients.

The correlation between the surgical finding and outcome is positive: 18 of 21 patients with total occlusion and restoration of internal carotid flow improved (Table 29.2) (34). Only one of eight patients in whom occlusion could not be reopened showed improvement. These findings strongly suggest that restoration of blood flow is the major factor determining neurologic improvement in these cases. The time elapsed from the onset of symptoms to revascularization in our study was usually less than 24 hours, but an excellent result was observed as late as 36 hours after the onset of symptoms. In other reports, it was possible to restore and maintain patency in patients who underwent surgery within 48 hours (44) or within 1 week after occlusion (25). However, better methods of patient selection are needed to predict viability of ischemic brain and presence of surgically removable intraluminal thrombus.

EMERGENCY BYPASS

Emergency arterial bypass procedures are technically feasible, but indications are difficult to define. Laboratory results obtained using these procedures vary: Crowell and Olsson (14), in an experimental model of MCA occlusion in dogs, found a favorable effect of the superficial temporal-to-middle cerebral artery (STA–MCA) bypass, provided that revascularization was completed within 6 hours. Levinthal et al (30) reported similar results. If the blood–brain barrier is damaged, however, revascularization may produce hemorrhage. Moreover, the STA may supply too little blood to overcome clinical ischemia. Experimental results in dogs reported by Diaz et al (19) indicate that STA–MCA bypass performed at 4 hours or 24 hours after MCA occlusion resulted in greater neurologic deficit, infarct size, and incidence of hemorrhagic infarction as compared with the results obtained when the procedure was performed after only 2 hours.

The cooperative EC/IC bypass study (21) has shown that bypass surgery is no more effective than medical treatment in reducing stroke. There has been considerable controversy regarding interpretation of the results of this study (1, 4, 5, 37, 42). Moreover, it should be noted that the investigators did not evaluate results of surgical revascularization for acute occlusions.

Reports of findings from clinical applications of STA–MCA bypass grafting for acute stroke have varied, but in general beneficial results have been rare. In the series of Gratzl et al (23), five of seven patients undergoing STA–MCA bypass for stroke-in-evolution died; they concluded

Table 29.2. Surgical Findings and Outcome of Emergency Carotid Endarterectomy

Preoperative neurologic status	Outcome								Total *n*
	Excellent		Good		Poor		Death		
	n	Percent	*n*	Percent	*n*	Percent	*n*	Percent	*n*
Stenosis	8	30.7	11	42.3	4	15.4	3	11.5	26
Occluded									
Flow restored	5	23.8	11	52.4	2	9.5	3	14.3	21
Flow not restored			1	12.5	5	62.5	2	25	8
Total	13	23.6	23	41.8	11	20	8	14.5	55

that emergency bypass surgery was contraindicated. Crowell (12) reported that 11 of 12 patients undergoing emergency STA–MCA bypass procedures had poor results. Various factors, including occlusion of perforating vessels and delay in surgery, may have influenced outcomes. Samson et al (38) warned that an STA–MCA bypass might not sustain a hemisphere afflicted with acute MCA occlusion. However, Sundt (45) reported four good results in five cases with STA–MCA bypass for progressive stroke. Diaz et al (18) used STA–MCA bypass in treating 15 patients with crescendo TIAs, stroke-in-evolution, and completed stroke (Fig. 29.3). Two of their patients with fixed preoperative deficit showed no improvement; there were no deaths in this series. A review of 63 cases of emergency bypass grafting from the literature (18) showed 27 instances of therapy-related improvement (if delayed improvement unrelated to surgery is included), 26 cases without improvement, and 10 deaths (Table 29.3). This review contained a mixture of cases, some procedures performed concomitantly with intracranial occlusion and others several days after the onset of symptoms. Most of the patients who improved were operated on after a short interval, usually within 6 hours.

Suzuki et al (47) performed STA–MCA bypass procedures in 10 patients with acute occlusion of the internal carotid artery or MCA. For cerebral protection, the patients received mannitol and oxygen-delivery enhancement with perfluorochemicals. Six patients did well, one had a small hematoma, and three had cerebral edema. These preliminary observations suggest that perioperative protective medical therapy combined with EC–IC bypass is an approach that could provide a better outcome than the natural history of acute cerebrovascular occlusion. Batjer et al (6) have also reported performing emergency STA–MCA bypass surgery for patients suffering from vasospasm secondary to subarachnoid hemorrhage, but this indication for surgical treatment awaits further verification and should be considered as under evaluation at present.

Table 29.3. Results of Emergency Superficial Temporal-to-Middle Cerebral Artery Bypass

Source	Outcome		
	Better	Same	Dead
Diaz et al[a]	13	2	0
Literature	27	26	10
Total	40	28	10
Percent	51	36	13

[a]Data from Diaz FG, Ausman JI, Mehta B, et al: Acute cerebral revascularization. *J Neurosurg* 63:200–209, 1985.

INTRAOPERATIVE OCCLUSION AND REVASCULARIZATION

Theoretically, the best opportunity for emergency bypass surgery should be immediately after surgical occlusion of an internal carotid artery or MCA in aneurysm or tumor cases. This situation could afford the opportunity for immediate, or even prophylactic, medical therapy with mannitol (47) and hypertension (49) before vascular occlusion, which could be preceded or followed immediately by revascularization. Although Samson et al (38) found that immediate STA–MCA bypass under such circumstances may be inadequate to prevent infarction, in the case reported by Lawner and Simeone (29) STA–MCA bypass was adequate to sustain an entire hemisphere after forced occlusion of the MCA. Samson et al (38) suggested that, in some cases, the grafting procedure should be a saphenous vein EC–IC graft to provide higher flow immediately. Successful experiences of Spetzler et al (41) support this concept. Consideration of collateral circulation that is available in each case might be helpful in selecting the most appropriate grafting procedure.

MIDDLE CEREBRAL EMBOLECTOMY

The results of embolectomy as compared with the natural history of embolic MCA occlusion remain inconclusive on the basis of case reports (Fig. 29.4) published

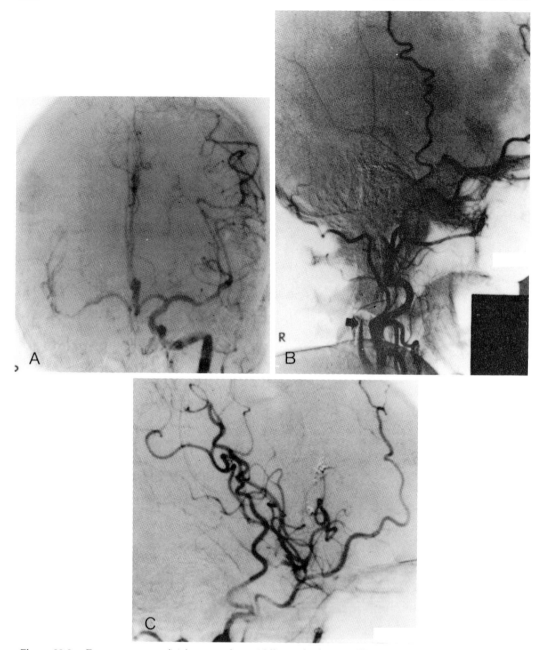

Figure 29.3. Emergency superficial temporal-to-middle cerebral artery (STA–MCA) bypass. *A* and *B*, angiogram shows occlusion of the right internal carotid artery and fair collateral circulation in a 42-year-old woman 6 hours after onset of left hemiparesis. *C*, angiogram shows excellent MCA filling via an STA–MCA bypass. The patient achieved a complete recovery. (From Diaz FG, Ausman JI, Mehta B, et al: Acute cerebral revascularization (*see* Case 13). *J Neurosurg* 63:200–209, 1985.)

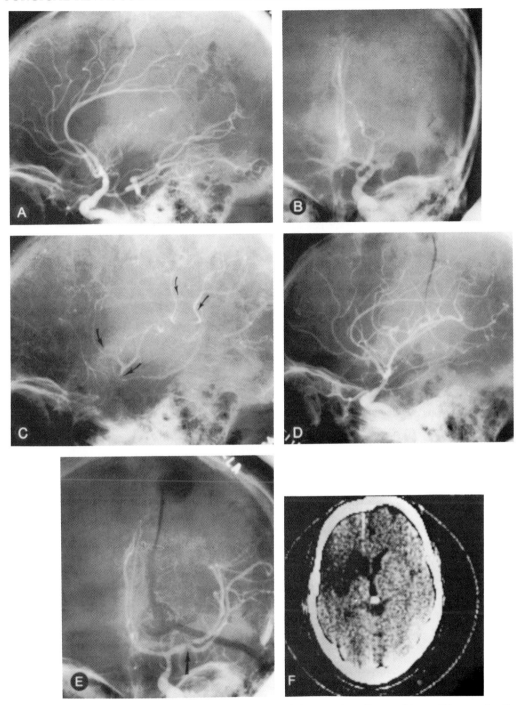

Figure 29.4.   Emergency middle cerebral artery (MCA) embolectomy in a 42-year-old man 2 hours after the onset of aphasia and hemiplegia. *A* and *B*, immediate angiogram shows complete left MCA occlusion with good collateral circulation. *C*, good retrograde filling of the distal MCA branches is observed back to the bifurcation *(arrows)*. *D* and *E*, postoperative angiography documents patency; note the site of embolectomy *(arrow)*. *F*, the postoperative CT scan shows a region of hypodensity in the left frontal temporal area but the patient had gradual partial improvement with residual right brachial monoparesis and dysphasia. (From Ojemann RG, Heros RC, Crowell RM: *Surgical Management of Cerebrovascular Disease*. Baltimore, Williams & Wilkins, 1988, p 141.)

to date. The natural history of MCA acute occlusion is not well defined. Dr. C. Miller Fisher* believes that 90% of patients who have MCA occlusion will sustain a disabling deficit. Experimental results of embolectomy are encouraging, provided that the operation is done within 4 hours (20).

Rapid evaluation of patients considered for MCA embolectomy is imperative if revascularization is to be of benefit. In most cases the diagnosis can be inferred from the clinical history and examination. The sudden onset of a substantial hemispheric deficit, particularly when there is a known cardiac source or embolus, strongly suggests MCA occlusion. The diagnosis must be confirmed by cerebral angiography to pinpoint the site of occlusion, to investigate possible multiple distal emboli, and to evaluate the collateral circulation. Administration of mannitol therapy (26) together with hypervolemic hemodilution (49) may offer benefit during the evaluation phase.

Operative technique is aimed at rapid exposure of the MCA–internal carotid artery complex (50). Ordinarily, this involves opening the Sylvian fissure. Occasionally we have found it advantageous to enter the fissure through a superior temporal gyrus corticectomy if the fissure is difficult to open (34). Temporary aneurysm clips are placed on the M1 segment and main divisions of the MCA distal to the embolus. The location of the embolus is identified by bluish discoloration of the nonpulsatile artery. Preferably a short axial arterotomy is made in one of the divisions of the artery, although in some cases the main trunk of the MCA may be incised. The embolus is milked out by means of suction and forceps, with sequential use of anterograde and retrograde flow to the MCA complex. After the embolus is removed, the arterotomy is closed with 9–0 monofilament sutures. Patients may be given mannitol (100 g intravenously) at the beginning of the operation and MABP is elevated to 30% to enhance collateral flow (46).

Results of the largest single series of

patients treated with emergency embolectomy are reported from the Mayo Clinic by Meyer et al (32) (Table 29.4). The 20 patients reported had preoperative neurologic deficits of varied severity. Flow was restored in 16 patients (80%). It was technically most difficult to achieve patency with arteriosclerotic emboli from the aorta. Two patients (10%) had an excellent result with no neurologic deficit, five (25%) were left with a minimal deficit but were able to return to work, seven (35%) had a fair result but were still independent and employable, four (20%) did poorly, and two (10%) died. Patients with an associated ipsilateral carotid artery occlusion did poorly. Collateral flow, as judged from preoperative angiograms, was the best predictor of outcome. A review of the literature (32) disclosed 64 cases of MCA embolectomy (Table 29.4), but only 24 of the procedures were performed within 24 hours of the onset of symptoms. In these 24 cases, time for reestablishment of flow ranged from 40 minutes to 18 hours after occlusion. Fourteen (58%) of the patients were improved, one was unchanged, and nine (37.5%) died. Three of these deaths were indirectly related to surgery or the actual ischemic event. There were two hemorrhagic infarctions, one resulting from use of anticoagulation therapy. Eighteen of 24 arteries were demonstrated to be patent. Seven of eight patients in whom good preoperative collateral flow was observed angiographically demonstrated improvement after surgery.

In the Mayo Clinic series (32), seven of 20 patients (35%) improved after MCA embolectomy. Outcome in seven patients with delayed improvement cannot be distin-

Table 29.4. Results of Middle Cerebral Arterial Embolectomy

Source	Outcome		
	Better	Same	Dead
Meyer et al[a]	7	11	2
Literature	14	1	9
Total	21	12	11
Percent	48	27	25

[a]Data from Meyer FD, Piepgras TG, Sundt TM Jr, et al: Emergency embolectomy for acute occlusion of the middle cerebral artery. *J Neurosurg* 62:639–647, 1985.

*Massachusetts General Hospital, Boston, MA; personal communication, 1980.

guished from the natural history of the disease; that is, they might have improved to that stage without surgery. Analysis of the preoperative cerebral angiograms in these cases suggests that collateral flow was sufficient to prevent irreversible cell damage in the majority of the ischemic regions, maintaining them within the penumbra.

Although additional data are needed to establish whether indications can be defined for emergency embolectomy, tentative guidelines for the procedure can be proposed on the basis of the results of preliminary observations: *(a)* The embolic source should be thrombotic rather than atheromatous because only rarely can large atheroma from the aorta be removed resulting in restoration of flow. *(b)* Embolectomy should probably not be performed later than 6 hours after the onset of neurologic deficit. *(c)* If there is an ipsilateral carotid occlusion, the prognosis is poor and embolectomy is unwarranted. *(d)* Substantial collateral flow to the MCA complex shown on the preoperative angiogram favors a good operative result. As an alternative, thrombolysis therapy with tissue-type plasminogen activator could be considered in these patients.

PERSPECTIVE

There is a theoretical rationale for emergency surgical revascularization to restore flow to the ischemic brain. However, results indicate that, in many cases, the required reperfusion will come too late. Therefore, at present, emergency revascularization is warranted only under certain specific circumstances.

On the basis of experience obtained to date, we recommend the following guidelines:

1. *Carotid endarterectomy* may be offered to patients with crescendo TIAs, with mild to moderate deficit without drowsiness, and without CT evidence of hemorrhage or extensive edema. Angiography performed within 24 hours of onset of neurologic deficit should show occlu-

sion or hemodynamically significant stenosis. This will be the most commonly indicated emergency revascularization procedure.

2. *STA–MCA bypass* might be considered for patients with crescendo TIAs or mild to moderate deficit in whom CT or MR imaging studies are negative for infarction. Angiography should show ICA or MCA occlusion with patent perforating branches. Patients should be ready for operation within 6 hours after onset of deficit. These cases will be extremely rare. It will remain difficult to distinguish the results of surgical therapy from the varied outcomes of the natural history of acute stroke.

3. *MCA embolectomy* may be considered for patients with moderate to severe deficit who are evaluated within 6 hours of the onset of neurologic deficit and in whom angiography discloses an MCA trunk occlusion, patent branches, and good collateral circulation. These cases will be rare. In such situations, thrombolytic therapy may also be attempted.

4. *Immediate bypass* surgery may be indicated for intraoperative ICA or MCA occlusion. Intraoperative institution of cerebral protection therapy is warranted. Saphenous vein bypass may be advisable to achieve adequate bypass flow.

Intensive medical therapy must be initiated in all cases considered for emergency revascularization. Certainly hypotension is to be avoided, and for cases in which hemorrhage is not present hypertension (MABP increased by 30%) may be induced with volume expansion and/or hypertensive agents. Hemodilution or transfusion to achieve an optimum hematocrit (about 33%) for improved microcirculation flow has been recommended (49), but its benefit is unproven (*see* Chapter 18, this volume). Mannitol therapy can be safely administered and may be beneficial during evaluation and surgery (26, 47). Deep barbiturate anesthesia can be considered but, because of its complexity, potentially deleterious systemic hemodynamic effects, and the resulting coma, it is more difficult to institute preceding surgery; this issue is, however, a subject of debate (see Chapter 24, this volume).

Another critical variable is the experience of the surgical team. Emergency cerebral revascularization requires speed and accuracy to be effective and it carries a high risk. Therefore, the approach can be recommended only for an organized and experienced surgical team.

Prevention of stroke is the goal of acute cerebral revascularization surgery. Successful reversal of ischemia by emergency revascularization, despite the tempting rationale for it, is likely to remain elusive. Emergency surgical revascularization might become more practical with the development of education for both the public and the medical community, to encourage prompt referral and rapid evaluation. More effective protective therapy to extend the period of time during which ischemia is reversible is also needed. A diagnostic method to distinguish ischemia from infarction needs to be developed as well. More effective thrombolytic medical therapy to restore patency of occluded branch vessels may also be of value.

References

1. The American Association of Neurological Surgeons Committee: The EC–IC bypass study. N Engl J Med 316:817–820, 1987.
2. Astrup J, Siesjö BK, Symon L: Thresholds in cerebral ischemia—the ischemic penumbra. Stroke 12:723–725, 1981.
3. Astrup J, Symon L, Branston NM, et al: Cortical evoked potential and extracellular K$^+$ and H$^+$ at critical levels of brain ischemia. Stroke 8:51–57, 1977.
4. Ausman JI, Diaz FG: Critique of the EC–IC bypass study. Surg Neurol 26:218–221, 1986.
5. Barnett HJ, Sachett D, Taylor DW, et al: Are the results of the EC–IC bypass trial generalizable? N Engl J Med 316:820–824, 1987.
6. Batjer H, Samson D: Use of EC–IC bypass in the management of symptomatic vasospasm. Neurosurgery 19:235–246, 1986.
7. Biller J, Adams HP, Boarini D, et al: Intraluminal clot of the carotid artery. A clinical–angiographic correlation of nine patients and literature review. Surg Neurol 25:467–477, 1986.
8. Branston NM, Symon L, Crockard HA, et al: Relationship between the cortical evoked potential and local cortical blood flow following acute middle cerebral artery occlusion in the baboon. Exp Neurol 45:195–208, 1974.
9. Bruetman ME, Fields WS, Crawford ES, et al: Cerebral hemorrhage in carotid artery surgery. Arch Neurol 9:458, 1963.
10. Buonanno F, Toole JF: Management of patients with established cerebral infarction. Stroke 12:7–16, 1978.
11. Caplan LR, Skillman J, Ojemann RG, et al: Intracerebral hemorrhage following carotid endarterectomy: A hypertensive complication. Stroke 9:457–460, 1978.
12. Crowell RM: STA–MCA bypass for acute focal cerebral ischemia. In Schmiedek P, Gratzl O, Spetzler RF (eds): Microsurgery for Stroke. Berlin, Springer-Verlag, 1977, pp 244–250.
13. Crowell RM, Marcoux FW, DeGirolami U: Variability and reversibility of focal cerebral ischemia in unanesthetized monkeys. Neurology 31:1295–1302, 1981.
14. Crowell RM, Olsson Y: Effect of extracranial–intracranial vascular bypass graft on experimental acute stroke in dogs. J Neurosurg 38:26–31, 1973.
15. Crowell RM, Olsson Y, Klatzo I, et al: Temporary occlusion of the middle cerebral artery in the monkey. Clinical and pathological observations. Stroke 1:439–448, 1970.
16. Davis KR, Ackerman RH, Kistler JP, et al: Computed tomography of cerebral infarction: Hemorrhage, contrast enhancement, and time of appearance. Comput Tomogr 1:71–86, 1977.
17. DeWitt LD, Buonanno FS, Kistler JP, et al: Nuclear magnetic resonance imaging in evaluation of clinical stroke syndromes. Neurology 16:535–545, 1984.
18. Diaz FG, Ausman JI, Mehta B, et al: Acute cerebral revascularization. J Neurosurg 63:200–209, 1985.
19. Diaz FG, Mastri AR, Ausman JI, et al: Acute cerebral revascularization after regional cerebral ischemia in the dog. Part II: Clinical pathological correlation. J Neurosurg 51:644–653, 1979.
20. Dujovny M, Osgood CP, Barrionuevo PJ, et al: Middle cerebral artery microneurosurgical embolectomy. Surgery 80:336–339, 1976.
21. EC/IC Bypass Study Group: Failure of EC–IC arterial bypass to reduce the risk of ischemic stroke: Results of an international randomized trial. N Engl J Med 313:1191–1200, 1985.
22. Goldstone J, Moore WS: Emergency carotid artery surgery in neurologically unstable patients. Arch Surg 111:1284–1291, 1976.
23. Gratzl O, Schmiedek P, Spetzler R, et al: Clinical experience with extra–intracranial arterial anastomosis in 65 cases. J Neurosurg 44:313–324, 1976.
24. Heiss WD, Hayakawa T, Waltz EG: Cortical neuronal function during ischemia. Effects of occlusion of one MCA on single unit activity in cats. Arch Neurol 33:813–820, 1976.
25. Hugenholtz H, Elgie RG: Carotid thromboendarterectomy: A reappraisal. J Neurosurg 53:776–783, 1980.
26. Jafar JJ, Johns LM, Mullan SF: The effect of mannitol on cerebral blood flow. J Neurosurg 64:754–759, 1986.
27. Jones TH, Morawetz RB, Crowell RM, et al: Thresholds of focal cerebral ischemia in awake monkeys. J Neurosurg 54:773–782, 1981.
28. Kassel NF, Peerless SJ, Drake CG: Reversal of

ischemic deficits by induced arterial hypertension. *Stroke* 9:104–105, 1978.

29. Lawner PM, Simeone FA: Treatment of intraoperative middle cerebral occlusion with phenobarbital and extracranial–intracranial bypass. Case report. *J Neurosurg* 51:710–712, 1979.

30. Levinthal R, Mosley JI, Brown WG, et al: Effect of STA–MCA anastomosis on the course of experimental acute MCA embolic occlusion. *Stroke* 10:371–375, 1979.

31. Meyer FB, Piepgras DG, Sandok BA, et al: Emergency carotid endarterectomy for patients with acute carotid occlusion and profound neurologic deficits. *Ann Surg* 203:82–89, 1986.

32. Meyer FB, Piepgras TG, Sundt TM Jr, et al: Emergency embolectomy for acute occlusion of the middle cerebral artery. *J Neurosurg* 62:639–647, 1985.

33. Morawetz RB, DeGirolami U, Ojemann RG, et al: Cerebral blood flow determined by hydrogen clearance during middle cerebral artery occlusion in unanesthetized monkeys. *Stroke* 9:143–149, 1978.

34. Ojemann RG, Crowell RM: *Surgical Management of Cerebrovascular Disease.* Baltimore, Williams & Wilkins, 1983.

35. Ojemann RG, Crowell RM, Fisher CM, et al: Surgical treatment of extracranial carotid occlusive disease. *Clin Neurosurg* 22:214–263, 1975.

36. Pelz DM, Buchanan A, Fox A, et al: Intraluminal thrombus of the internal carotid arteries: Angiographic demonstration of resolution with anticoagulation therapy alone. *Radiology* 160:369–373, 1986.

37. Relman A: The EC–IC arterial bypass study. What have we learned (editorial): *N Engl J Med* 316:809–810, 1987.

38. Samson DS, Neuwelt EA, Beyer CW, et al: Failure of extracranial–intracranial arterial bypass in acute middle cerebral artery occlusion: Case report. *Neurosurgery* 6:185–188, 1980.

39. Sharbrough FW, Messick JM, Sundt TM Jr: Correlation of continuous electroencephalograms with CBF measurements during carotid endarterectomy. *Stroke* 4:674–683, 1973.

40. Smith AL, Hoff JT, Nielsen SL, et al: Barbiturate protection in acute focal cerebral ischemia. *Stroke* 5:1–7, 1974.

41. Spetzler RF, Selman WR, Roski RA, et al: Cerebral revascularization during barbiturate coma in primates and humans. *Surg Neurol* 17:111–115, 1982.

42. Sundt TM Jr: Was the international randomized trial of EC–IC arterial bypass representative of the population at risk? *N Engl J Med* 316:814–816, 1987.

43. Sundt TM Jr, Grant WC, Garcia JH: Restoration of middle cerebral artery flow in experimental infarction. *J Neurosurg* 31:311–322, 1969.

44. Sundt TM Jr, Sandok DA, Whisnant JP: Carotid endarterectomy: Complications and preoperative assessment of risk. *Mayo Clin Proc* 50:301–306, 1975.

45. Sundt TM Jr, Siekert RG, Piepgras DG, et al: Bypass surgery for vascular disease of the carotid system. *Mayo Clin Proc* 51:667–692, 1976.

46. Suzuki J, Yoshimoto T, Kayama T: Surgical treatment of middle cerebral artery aneurysms. *J Neurosurg* 61:17–22, 1984.

47. Suzuki J, Yoshimoto T, Kodama N, et al: A new therapeutic method for acute brain infarction: Revascularization following the administration of mannitol and perfluorochemicals—a preliminary report. *Surg Neurol* 17:325–332, 1982.

48. Wall SD, Brant-Zawadzki M, Jeffrey RB, et al: High frequency CT findings within 24 hours after cerebral infarction. *AJR* 138:307–311, 1982.

49. Wood JH: Hypervolemic hemodilution: Rheologic therapy for acute cerebral ischemia. *Contemp Neurosurg* 4:1–6, 1982.

50. Yasargil MG, Krayenbuhl HA, Jacobson JH II: Microneurosurgical arterial reconstruction. *Surgery* 67:221–233, 1970.

Index

Page numbers in *italics* denote figures; those followed by "t" denote tables.